ADVANCES IN PROSTAGLANDIN, THROMBOXANE, AND LEUKOTRIENE RESEARCH
VOLUME 13

Platelets, Prostaglandins, and the Cardiovascular System

Advances in Prostaglandin, Thromboxane, and Leukotriene Research

Series Editors: Bengt Samuelsson and Rodolfo Paoletti

(Formerly *Advances in Prostaglandin and Thromboxane Research* Series)

Vol. 15: Advances in Prostaglandin, Thromboxane, and Leukotriene Research, *edited by O. Hayaishi and S. Yamamoto,* 1985.

Vol. 14: Chemistry of Prostaglandins and Leukotrienes, *edited by J. E. Pike and D. R. Morton, Jr.,* 1985.

Vol. 13: Platelets, Prostaglandins, and the Cardiovascular System, *edited by G. G. Neri Serneri, J. C. McGiff, R. Paoletti, and G. V. R. Born,* 424 pages, 1985.

Vol. 12: Advances in Prostaglandin, Thromboxane, and Leukotriene Research, *edited by B. Samuelsson, R. Paoletti, and P. W. Ramwell,* 544 pp., 1983.

Vol. 11: Advances in Prostaglandin, Thromboxane, and Leukotriene Research, *edited by B. Samuelsson, R. Paoletti, and P. W. Ramwell,* 576 pp., 1983.

Vol. 10: Prostaglandins and the Cardiovascular System, *edited by John A. Oates,* 400 pp., 1982.

Vol. 9: Leukotrienes and Other Lipoxygenase Products, *edited by B. Samuelsson and R. Paoletti,* 382 pp., 1982.

Vol. 8: Advances in Prostaglandin and Thromboxane Research, *edited by B. Samuelsson, P. W. Ramwell, and R. Paoletti,* 609 pp., 1980.

Vol. 7: Advances in Prostaglandin and Thromboxane Research, *edited by B. Samuelsson, P. W. Ramwell, and R. Paoletti,* 606 pp., 1980.

Vol. 6: Advances in Prostaglandin and Thromboxane Research, *edited by B. Samuelsson, P. W. Ramwell, and R. Paoletti,* 600 pp., 1980.

Vol. 5: Methods in Prostaglandin Research, *edited by J. C. Frölich,* 256 pp., 1978.

Vol. 4: Prostaglandins and Perinatal Medicine, *edited by F. Coceani and P. M. Olley,* 432 pp., 1978.

Vol. 3: Prostaglandins and Phospholipases, *edited by C. Galli, G. Galli, and G. Porcellati,* 224 pp., 1978.

Vol. 2: Advances in Prostaglandin and Thromboxane Research, *edited by B. Samuelsson and R. Paoletti,* 1028 pp., 1976.

Vol. 1: Advances in Prostaglandin and Thromboxane Research, *edited by B. Samuelsson and R. Paoletti,* 506 pp., 1976.

Advances in Prostaglandin, Thromboxane,
and Leukotriene Research
Volume 13

Platelets, Prostaglandins, and the Cardiovascular System

Editors

Gian G. Neri Serneri, M.D.
Professor and Chairman
Clinica Medica I
University of Florence
Florence, Italy

John C. McGiff, M.D.
Professor and Chairman
Department of Pharmacology
New York Medical College
Valhalla, New York

Rodolfo Paoletti, M.D.
Professor and Chairman
Institute of Pharmacology and
Pharmacognosy
University of Milan
Milan, Italy

Gustav V. R. Born, F.R.C.P.,F.R.S.
Professor and Chairman
Department of Pharmacology
King's College
London, England

Raven Press ■ New York

EB

Raven Press, 1140 Avenue of the Americas, New York, New York 10036

Library of Congress Cataloging in Publication Data
Main entry under title:

Platelets, prostaglandins, and the cardiovascular system.

(Advances in prostaglandin, thromboxane, and leukotriene research ; v. 13)
Proceedings of a meeting held Feb. 1984 in Florence, Italy.
Includes bibliographies and index.
1. Blood platelets—Congresses. 2. Prostaglandins— Congresses. 3. Hypertension—Congresses. 4. Cardio- vascular system—Diseases—Congresses. I. Born, Gustav V. R. II. Series. [DNLM: 1. Blood Platelets— drug effects - congresses. 2. Blood Platelets—physiology - congresses. 3. Cardiovascular Diseases—physiopatho- logy - congresses. 4. Prostaglandins—physiology - con- gresses. W1 AD788 v.13 QU 90 P716 1984]
QP801.P68A36 vol. 13   599'.01927 s   84-29840
[QP97]   [599'.011]
ISBN 0-88167-062-6

Made in the United States of America

rev. 10/8/87
8-15-85

Preface

In this volume of **Advances in Prostaglandin, Thromboxane, and Leukotriene Research,** international authorities and researchers in the field of platelets, prostaglandins, and leukotrienes present the results of their recent work. In the past few years, in addition to pharmacological-type investigations many studies were carried out on the role of prostaglandins in the control of physiological systems.

Prostaglandins are crucial in modulating vascular tone and vascular response to sympathetic stimulation, in regulating tubular function and extracellular fluid volume, and in modulating platelet functions. Prostaglandins are very much involved in such processes as pre- and postjunctional modulation of adrenergic nerve function, renin release, and thrombus formation. Prostaglandins have been shown to mediate the activity of many cardiovascular drugs. However, many of these basic discoveries have remained limited to the restricted circles of biochemists and pharmacologists; they have not yet entered the broader world of the clinicians.

The enormous development of scientific knowledge has necessarily fragmented the field of medicine, creating specializations and superspecializations. However, clinicians must have a global view of the patient. The aim of this volume is to offer the clinician a view of the importance of prostaglandins in the physiology of the cardiovascular diseases. In arranging the volume, we selected those topics that not only are relevant to platelets and prostaglandins, but also are of interest to clinicians.

This volume will be of interest to cardiologists, nephrologists, and hematologists, as well as to pharmacologists and scientists involved in the field of prostaglandins and inflammatory processes.

The Editors

Acknowledgments

This volume presents the proceedings of a meeting held February 1984 in Florence, Italy.

As a president of the meeting, I would like to thank the members of the Scientific Committee, Professors G. V. R. Born, J. C. McGiff, R. Paoletti, and B. Samuelsson, and all those who have contributed to this book.

I would like also to thank all my co-workers of the Clinica Medica of the University of Florence and specially Professors G. Masotti and G. F. Gensini, who carried most of the load of organization. Sincere gratitude is extended to the Boehringer Ingelheim, who generously supported the meeting.

Professor Gian Gastone Neri Serneri

Contents

Platelet Pathophysiology

Prostaglandin Pathophysiology

Leukotrienes: Physiology and Pathophysiology

Platelets, Prostaglandins, and Myocardial Ischemia

Cerebral Circulation

Prostaglandins and the Kidney

Prostaglandins, Kinins, and Hypertension

Prostaglandins in Transplant Rejection

Platelet Functions in Diabetes and Hyperlipoproteinemia

Antiplatelet Drugs: Therapy and Clinical Pharmacology

Contributors

B. Abdel-Haq
Clinica Medica I
University of Pisa
Pisa, Italy

U. Aehringhaus
Department of Pharmacology
Ruhr-University Bochum
Im-Lottental
D-4630 Bochum, Federal Republic of
  Germany

G. C. Agnoli
Cattedra di Fisiopatologia Medica
University of Bologna
Policlinico S. Orsola
40138 Bologna, Italy

M. R. Alijani
Department of Surgery
Division of Transplantation
Georgetown University Medical Center
Washington, D.C. 20007

Luigi Amaducci
Department of Neurology
Medical School
University of Florence
Viale Morgagni, 85
50134 Florence, Italy

P. Andreone
Cattedra di Fisiopatologia Medica
University of Bologna
Policlinico S. Orsola
40138 Bologna, Italy

Corrado Argentino
Department of Neurological Sciences
University of Rome, "La Sapienza"
Viale dell'Universitá, 30
00185 Rome, Italy

Philip G. Baer
Department of Pharmacology
University of Tennessee Center for the
  Health Sciences
874 Union Avenue—100 Crowe
Memphis, Tennessee 38163

H. J. M. Barnett
Department of Clinical Neurological
  Sciences
University of Western Ontario
P.O. Box 5339, Stn. A
Room 1-3
London, Ontario N6A 5A5, Canada

L. Bastagli
Istituto di Clinica Medica II
University of Bologna
40138 Bologna, Italy

Mohamed A. Bayorh
Morehouse School of Medicine
Department of Pharmacology
720 West View Drive
S.W. Atlanta, Georgia 30310

J. J. F. Belch
University Department of Medicine
Royal Infirmary
10 Alexandra Parade
Glasgow G31 2ER, Scotland

Jacques Benveniste
INSERM U 200
Université Paris-Sud
32 rue des Carnets
92140 Clamart, France

Bo Berglund
Department of Clinical Physiology
Karolinska Hospital
S-104 01 Stockholm, Sweden

U. Berglund
Department of Internal Medicine
University Hospital
S-581 85 Linköping, Sweden

P. Bernardi
Istituto di Clinica Medica II
University of Bologna
40138 Bologna, Italy

W. Bernini
C.N.R. Institute of Clinical Physiology
Istituto di Patologia Medica I
University of Pisa
Pisa, Italy

A. Bertoldi
Istituto di Clinica Medica II
University of Bologna
40138 Bologna, Italy

M. Boddi
Clinica Medica I
University of Florence
Viale Morgagni, 85
50134 Florence, Italy

A. Boem
C.N.R. Institute of Clinical Physiology
Istituto di Patologia Medica I
University of Pisa
Pisa, Italy

Lawrence E. Boerboom
Department of Cardiothoracic Surgery
Medical College of Wisconsin
8700 W. Wisconsin Avenue
Milwaukee, Wisconsin 53226

Lawrence I. Bonchek
Department of Medicine
Medical College of Wisconsin
8700 W. Wisconsin Avenue
Milwaukee, Wisconsin 53226

G. V. R. Born
Department of Pharmacology
King's College
London WC2R 2LS, England

A. Bosia
Cattedra di Chimica e Propedeutica
  Biochimica
Istituto di Igiene
Università of Turin
Turin, Italy

Thomas Brecht
Medical Department
University Hospital
Bonn, Federal Republic of Germany

H. Bricaud
Unité 8 de Cardiologie
INSERM
33600 Pessac, France

H. Bull
Department of Haematology
Middlesex Hospital and University
  College Hospital
London, England

F. Bussolino
Cattedra di Chimica e Propedeutica
  Biochimica
Istituto di Igiene
University of Turin
Turin, Italy

M. Cacciari
Cattedra di Fisiopatologia Medica
University of Bologna
Policlinico S. Orsola
40138 Bologna, Italy

L. Caparrotta
Department of Pharmacology
University of Padua
35100 Padua, Italy

Antonio Carolei
Department of Neurological Sciences
University of Rome, "La Sapienza"
Viale dell'Universitá, 30
00185 Rome, Italy

A. Carpi
Department of Pathophysiology
Istituto Superiore di Sanità
Rome, Italy

Gian Carlo Casolo
Clinica Medica I
University of Florence
Viale Morgagni, 85
50134 Florence, Italy

A. Casonato
Istituto di Semeiotica Medica
University of Padua Medical School
Padua, Italy

S. Castellani
Clinica Medica I
University of Florence
Viale Morgagni, 85
50134 Florence, Italy

F. Catella
Department of Pharmacology
Catholic University School of Medicine
Via Pineta Sacchetti 644
00168 Rome, Italy

M. Cavazza
Istituto di Clinica Medica II
University of Bologna
40138 Bologna, Italy

A. M. Cerbone
Istituto di Medicina Interna e Malattie
   Dismetaboliche
II Facoltà di Medicina e Chirurgia
University of Naples
80131 Naples, Italy

L. S. Chen
Second Department of Internal Medicine
Nagoya University School of Medicine
Nagoya, Japan

J. H. Chesebro
Division of Cardiology
Mayo Clinic and Mayo Foundation
Rochester, Minnesota 55905

M. Chiavarelli
Department of Cardiac Surgery
University of Rome
Rome, Italy

R. Chiavarelli
Department of Cardiac Surgery
University of Rome
Rome, Italy

G. Ciabattoni
Department of Pharmacology
Catholic University School of Medicine
Via Pineta Sacchetti 644
00168 Rome, Italy

F. Cirillo
Istituto di Medicina Interna e Malattie
   Dismetaboliche
II Facoltà di Medicina e Chirurgia
University of Naples
80131 Naples, Italy

C. Clo
Istituto di Chimica Biologica
University of Bologna
40138 Bologna, Italy

S. Colli
Institute of Pharmacology and
   Pharmacognosy
University of Milan
Milan, Italy

Mario Condorelli
Istituto di Clinica Medica I
II Facoltà di Medicina e Chirurgia
Via S. Pansini
University of Naples
80131 Naples, Italy

G. Covi
Clinica Medica
University of Verona
Verona, Italy

Alberto Cuocolo
Istituto di Clinica Medica I
II Facoltà di Medicina e Chirurgia
Via S. Pansini
University of Naples
80131 Naples, Italy

C. Curradi
*Istituto di Patologia Medica e
    Farmacologia Clinica*
University of Florence
Viale Morgagni, 85
50134 Florence, Italy

R. Dal Bo Zanon
Istituto di Semeiotica Medica
University of Padua Medical School
Padua, Italy

A. Danieli
*Servizio di Fisiopatologia della
    Riproduzione*
Policlinico S. Orsola
40138 Bologna, Italy

D. Daret
Unité 8 de Cardiologie
INSERM
33600 Pessac, France

G. Davì
*Istituto di Clinica Medica Generale e
    Terapia Medica I*
University of Palermo
Palermo, Italy

R. De Caterina
C.N.R. Institute of Clinical Physiology
Istituto di Patologia Medica I
University of Pisa
56100 Pisa, Italy

G. de Gaetano
*Mario Negri Institute for
    Pharmacological Research*
Milan, Italy

M. Degan
Clinica Medica
University of Verona
Verona, Italy

E. Dejana
*Mario Negri Institute for
    Pharmacological Research*
Milan, Italy

A. Del Maschio
*Mario Negri Institute for
    Pharmacological Research*
Milan, Italy

M. De Nes
C.N.R. Institute of Clinical Physiology
Istituto di Patologia Medica I
University of Pisa
56100 Pisa, Italy

Antonio De Simone
Istituto di Clinica Medica I
II Facoltà di Medicina e Chirurgia
Via S. Pansini
University of Naples
80131 Naples, Italy

L. De Zanche
Clinica Neurologica
University of Padua Medical School
Padua, Italy

G. Di Minno
*Istituto di Medicina Interna e Malattie
    Dismetaboliche*
II Facoltà di Medicina e Chirurgia
University of Naples
80131 Naples, Italy

Michael J. Dunn
Department of Medicine
*Case Western Reserve University and
    Division of Nephrology*
University Hospitals of Cleveland
Cleveland, Ohio 44106

Meltem Elyilmaz-Ayaz
Medical Department
University Hospital
Bonn, Federal Republic of Germany

David Ezra
Neurobiology Research Unit
*Uniformed Services University of the
    Health Sciences*
Bethesda, Maryland 20814

G. Fabbri
Istituto di Clinica Medica IV
(Cattedra di Patologia Speciale Medica
II)
University of Florence
Viale Morgagni, 85
50134 Florence, Italy

F. Fabi
Department of Pathophysiology
Istituto Superiore di Sanità
Rome, Italy

F. Fabris
Istituto di Semeiotica Medica
University of Padua Medical School
Padua, Italy

F. Fanara
Clinica Tisiologica e delle Malattie
dell'Apparato Respiratorio
II Facoltà
University of Naples
Naples, Italy

G. Fassina
Department of Pharmacology
University of Padua
35100 Padua, Italy

Nicholas R. Ferreri
Department of Molecular Immunology
Scripps Clinic & Research Foundation
10666 North Torrey Pines Road
La Jolla, California 92037

Giora Feuerstein
Neurobiology Research Unit
Uniformed Services University of the
Health Sciences
Bethesda, Maryland 20814

Cesare Fieschi
Department of Neurological Sciences
University of Rome, "La Sapienza"
Viale dell'Universitá, 30
00185 Rome, Italy

P. Filabozzi
Department of Pharmacology
Catholic University School of Medicine
Via Pineta Sacchetti, 644
00168 Rome, Italy

M. Finesso
Department of Cytopharmacology
Fidia Research Laboratories
Via Ponte della Fabbrica 3/A
Abano Terme, Italy

M. Floreani
Department of Pharmacology
University of Padua
35100 Padua, Italy

M. L. Foegh
Department of Medicine
Division of Nephrology
Georgetown University Medical Center
Washington, D.C. 20007

C. D. Forbes
University Department of Medicine
Royal Infirmary
10 Alexandra Parade
Glasgow G31 2 ER, Scotland

L. Forni
Department of Pharmacology
Catholic University School of Medicine
Via Pineta Sacchetti 644
00168 Rome, Italy

F. Franchi
Istituto di Clinica Medica IV
(Cattedra di Patologia Speciale Medica
II)
University of Florence
Viale Morgagni, 85
50134 Florence, Italy

Laura Fratiglioni
Department of Neurology
Medical School
University of Florence
Viale Morgagni, 85
50134 Florence, Italy

Valentin Fuster
Division of Cardiology
Mount Sinai Medical Center
New York, New York 10029

V. Gallo
Istituto di Clinica Medica Generale e
Terapia Medica I
University of Palermo
Palermo, Italy

C. Garutti
Cattedra di Fisiopatologia Medica
University of Bologna
Policlinico S. Orsola
40138 Bologna, Italy

G. F. Gensini
Clinica Medica I
University of Florence
Viale Morgagni, 85
50134 Florence, Italy

F. Ghezzi
Istituto di Clinica Medica II
University of Bologna
40138 Bologna, Italy

D. Ghigo
Cattedra di Chimica e Propedeutica
Biochimica
Istituto di Igiene
University of Turin
Turin, Italy

D. Giannessi
C.N.R. Institute of Clinical Physiology
Istituto di Patologia Medica I
University of Pisa
Pisa, Italy

A. Girolami
Istituto di Semeiotica Medica
University of Padua Medical School
Padua, Italy

Matthias Goerig
University of Heidelberg Medical School
Bergheimer Strasse 58
6900 Heidelberg, Federal Republic of
Germany

M. Goldman
Department of Surgery
Charing Cross Hospital
London, England

M. H. Goldman
Division of Cardiac Surgery
Medical College of Virginia
Richmond, Virginia 23298

Robert E. Goldstein
Departments of Pharmacology and
Medicine
Uniformed Services University of the
Health Sciences
Bethesda, Maryland 20814

R. Golin
Istituto di Clinica Medica IV
University of Milan; and
Centro di Fisiologia Clinica e
Ipertensione
Ospedale Maggiore
Milan, Italy

A. Gorio
Department of Cytopharmacology
Fidia Research Laboratories
Via Ponte della Fabbrica 3/A
Abano Terme, Italy

R. A. Greatorex
Department of Surgery
Wittington Hospital
London N19 5NF, England

R. Grimaldi
Istituto di Clinica Medica II
University of Bologna
40138 Bologna, Italy

Hermann-Josef Gröne
Medizinische Klinik
Universität Göttingen
Robert-Koch-Strasse 40
3400 Göttingen, Federal Republic of
Germany

Rainer Gronwald
University of Heidelberg Medical School
Bergheimer Strasse 58
6900 Heidelberg, Federal Republic of
  Germany

Jürgen Grulich
University of Heidelberg Medical School
Bergheimer Strasse 58
6900 Heidelberg, Federal Republic of
  Germany

Ryszard J. Gryglewski
Department of Pharmacology
Copernicus Academy of Medicine
Grzegórzecka 16
31-531 Cracow, Poland

Andreas J. R. Habenicht
University of Heidelberg Medical School
Bergheimer Strasse 58
6900 Heidelberg, Federal Republic of
  Germany

Edward Hayes
Merck, Sharp, & Dohme
126 East Lincoln Avenue
Rahway, New Jersey 07065

G. B. Helfrich
Department of Surgery
Division of Transplantation
Georgetown University Medical Center
Washington, D.C. 20007

J. Henri
Unité 8 de Cardiologie
INSERM
33600 Pessac, France

Thomas H. Hintze
Department of Physiology
New York Medical College
Valhalla, New York 10595

E. Ikonomu
Cattedra di Fisiopatologia Medica
University of Bologna
Policlinico S. Orsola
40138 Bologna, Italy

M. Imaizumi
Second Department of Internal Medicine
Nagoya University School of Medicine
Nagoya, Japan

Domenico Inzitari
Department of Neurology
Medical School
University of Florence
Viale Morgagni, 85
50134 Florence, Italy

T. Ito
Second Department of Internal Medicine
Nagoya University School of Medicine
Nagoya, Japan

Y. Ito
Second Department of Internal Medicine
Nagoya University School of Medicine
Nagoya, Japan

Lennart Kaijser
Department of Clinical Physiology
Karolinska Hospital
S-104 01 Stockholm, Sweden

Gabor Kaley
Department of Physiology
New York Medical College
Valhalla, New York, 10595

B. S. Khirabadi
Department of Physiology and Biophysics
Georgetown University Medical Center
Washington, D.C. 20007

M. R. Kichuk
Department of Physiology
New York Medical College
Valhalla, New York 10595

R. L. Kinlough-Rathbone
Department of Biochemistry
University of Toronto
Toronto, Ontario M5S 1A8, Canada

Ahmed H. Kissebah
Department of Medicine
Medical College of Wisconsin
8700 W. Wisconsin Avenue
Milwaukee, Wisconsin 53226

Burkhard Kommerell
University of Heidelberg Medical School
Bergheimer Strasse 58
6900 Heidelberg, Federal Republic of
Germany

Irwin J. Kopin
Laboratory of Clinical Science
National Institute of Mental Health
Bethesda, Maryland 20205

A. L'Abbate
C. N. R. Institute of Clinical Physiology
Istituto di Patologia Medica I
University of Pisa
56100 Pisa, Italy

L. R. Languino
Mario Negri Institute for
Pharmacological Research
Milan, Italy

J. Larrue
Unité 8 de Cardiologie
INSERM
33600 Pessac, France

A. Lechi
Istituto di Farmacologia
University of Verona
Verona, Italy

C. Lechi
Cattedra di Chimica e Microscopia
Clinica
University of Verona
Verona, Italy

James B. Lefkowith
Department of Pharmacology
Washington University Medical School
660 South Euclid Avenue
St. Louis, Missouri 63110

Gian Luigi Lenzi
Department of Neurological Science
University of Rome, "La Sapienza"
Viale dell'Universitá, 30
00185 Rome, Italy

P. Lo Sapio
Istituto di Clinica Medica IV
(Cattedra di Patologia Speciale Medica
II)
University of Florence
Viale Morgagni, 85
50134 Florence, Italy

R. R. Lower
Division of Cardiac Surgery
Medical College of Virginia
Richmond, Virginia 23298

S. J. Machin
Department of Haematology
Middlesex Hospital and University Collge
Hospital
London, England

I. J. Mackie
Department of Haematology
Middlesex Hospital and University
College Hospital
London, England

P. Maderna
Institute of Pharmacology and
Pharmacognosy
University of Milan
Milan, Italy

A. Magagna
Clinica Medica I
University of Pisa
Pisa, Italy

M. A. Mainardi
Istituto di Clinica Medica II
University of Bologna
40138 Bologna, Italy

M. Mancini
Istituto di Medicina Interna e Malattie
Dismetaboliche
II Facoltà di Medicina e Chirurgia
University of Naples
80131 Naples, Italy

M. Mannelli
Endocrinology Unit
University of Florence
Viale Morgagni, 85
50134 Florence, Italy

S. Manzoni
Clinica Neurologica
University of Padua
Padua, Italy

B. Marino
Department of Cardiac Surgery
University of Rome
Rome, Italy

M. Marzilli
C.N.R. Institute of Clinical Physiology
Istituto di Patologia Medica I
University of Pisa
56100 Pisa, Italy

G. Masotti
Clinica Medica I
University of Florence
Viale Morgagni, 85
50134 Florence, Italy

P. L. Mattioli
Istituto di Medicina Interna e Malattie
  Dismetaboliche
II Facoltà di Medicina e Chirurgia
University of Naples
80131 Naples, Italy

A. Mazza
Istituto di Clinica Medica Generale e
  Terapia Medica I
University of Palermo
Palermo, Italy

Charles N. McCollum
Department of Surgery
Charing Cross Hospital
Fulham Palace Road
London W6 8RF, England

John C. McGiff
Department of Pharmacology
New York Medical College
Valhalla, New York 10595

M. McLaren
University Department of Medicine
Royal Infirmary
10 Alexandra Parade
Glasgow G31 2ER, Scotland

Jawahar Mehta
Department of Medicine
Division of Cardiology
University of Florida College of Medicine
Box J-277, JHMHC
Gainesville, Florida 32610

Edward J. Messina
Department of Physiology
New York Medical College
Valhalla, New York 10595

C. Michelassi
C.N.R. Institute of Clinical Physiology
Istituto di Patologia Medica I
University of Pisa
56100 Pisa, Italy

C. Minelli
Istituto di Clinica Medica II
University of Bologna
40138 Bologna, Italy

P. Minuz
Istituto di Farmacologia
University of Verona
Verona, Italy

J. F. Mustard
Department of Pathology
McMaster University
Hamilton, Ontario L8N3Z5 Canada

Adam K. Myers
Department of Physiology and Biophysics
Georgetown University Medical Center
Washington, D.C. 20007

Alberto Nasjletti
Department of Pharmacology
University of Tennessee Center for the
  Health Sciences
874 Union Avenue—100 Crowe
Memphis, Tennessee 38163

Philip Needleman
Department of Pharmacology
Washington University Medical School
660 South Euclid Avenue
St. Louis, Missouri 63110

Gian Gastone Neri Serneri
Clinica Medica I
University of Florence
Viale Morgagni, 85
50134 Florence, Italy

K. Ogawa
Second Department of Internal Medicine
Nagoya University School of Medicine
Nagoya, Japan

Gordon N. Olinger
Department of Medicine
Medical College of Wisconsin
8700 W. Wisconsin Avenue
Milwaukee, Wisconsin 53226

M. A. Packham
Department of Biochemistry
University of Toronto
Toronto, Ontario M5S 1A8, Canada

M. G. Palumbo
Istituto di Clinica Medica Generale e
*   Terapia Medica I*
University of Palermo
Palermo, Italy

M. Pannain
Istituto di Medicina Interna e Malattie
*   Dismetaboliche*
II Facoltà di Medicina e Chirurgia
University of Naples
80131 Naples, Italy

Maret Panzenbeck
Department of Physiology
New York Medical College
Valhalla, New York 10595

R. Paoletti
Institute of Pharmacology and
*   Pharmacognosy*
University of Milan
Milan, Italy

P. Patrignani
Centro di Studio per la Fisiopatologia
*   dello Shock del C. N. R.*
Catholic University School of Medicine
Via Pineta Sacchetti, 644
00168 Rome, Italy

Carlo Patrono
Department of Pharmacology
Catholic University School of Medicine
Via Pineta Sacchetti, 644
00168 Rome, Italy

H. Patscheke
Institute for Clinical Chemistry
Klinikum Mannheim
University of Heidelberg
Heidelberg, Federal Republic of
*   Germany*

R. Pedrinelli
Clinica Medica I
University of Pisa
Pisa, Italy

Sumer Belbez Pek
Department of Internal Medicine
The University of Michigan
Ann Arbor, Michigan 48109

G. P. Pescarmona
Cattedra di Chimica e Propedeutica
*   Biochimica*
Istituto di Igiene
University of Turin
Turin, Italy

B. A. Peskar
Department of Pharmacology
Ruhr-University Bochum
Im-Lottental
D-4630 Bochum, Federal Republic of
*   Germany*

A. Pezza
Clinica Tisiologica e delle Malattie
*   dell'Apparato Respiratorio*
II Facoltà
University of Naples
Naples, Italy

A. Pierucci
Division of Nephrology
Department of Medicine
University of Rome, "La Sapienza"
Policlinico Umberto I
00100 Rome, Italy

A. Pinto
Istituto di Clinica Medica Generale e
Terapia Medica I
University of Palermo
Palermo, Italy

A. Postiglione
Istituto di Medicina Interna e Malattie
Dismetaboliche
II Facoltà di Medicina e Chirurgia
University of Naples
80131 Naples, Italy

Domenico Prisco
Clinica Medica I
University of Florence
Viale Morgagni, 85
50134 Florence, Italy

M. Prosdocimi
Department of Cytopharmacology
Fidia Research Laboratories
Via Ponte della Fabbrica 3/A
Abano Terme, Italy

F. Pugliese
Division of Nephrology
Department of Medicine
University of Rome, "La Sapienza"
Policlinico Umberto I
00100 Rome, Italy

Antonio Quintana
Departamento de Farmacología
Facultad de Medicina
Universidad del Pais Vasco
Bilbao, Spain

Ewa Raczka
Departamento de Farmacología
Facultad de Medicina
Universidad del Pais Vasco
Bilbao, Spain

E. Ragazzi
Department of Pharmacology
University of Padua
35100 Padua, Italy

Peter W. Ramwell
Department of Physiology and Biophysics
Georgetown University Medical Center
Washington, D.C. 20007

M. L. Randi
Istituto di Semeiotica Medica
University of Padua Medical School
Padua, Italy

G. Razaka
Unité 8 de Cardiologie
INSERM
33600 Pessac, France

Bruno Ricciardelli
Istituto di Clinica Medica I
II Facoltà di Medicina e Chirurgia
Via S. Pansini
University of Naples
80131 Naples, Italy

M. Rigaud
Laboratoire de Biochimie
CHU Dupuytren
87000 Limoges, France

Pier Giorgio Rogasi
Clinica Medica I
University of Florence
Viale Morgagni, 85
50134 Florence, Italy

C. Rostagno
Clinica Medica I
University of Florence
50134 Florence, Italy

Dietrich Rothe
University of Heidelberg Medical School
Bergheimer Strasse 58
6900 Heidelberg, Federal Republic of
Germany

A. Salvetti
Clinica Medica I
University of Pisa
Pisa, Italy

T. Satake
Second Department of Internal Medicine
Nagoya University School of Medicine
Nagoya, Japan

A. Scardi
Istituto di Clinica Medica IV
(Cattedra di Patologia Speciale Medica
II)
University of Florence
Viale Morgagni, 85
50134 Florence, Italy

L. Scarti
Clinica Medica I
University of Florence
Viale Morgagni, 85
50134 Florence, Italy

Gotthard Schettler
University of Heidelberg Medical School
Bergheimer Strasse 58
6900 Heidelberg, Federal Republic of
Germany

Michal Schwartzman
Department of Pharmacology
New York Medical College
Valhalla, New York 10595

R. Sciagrà
Clinica Medica I
University of Florence
Viale Morgagni, 85
50134 Florence, Italy

M. Segni
Department of Pharmacology
Catholic University School of Medicine
Via Pineta Sacchetti 644
00168 Rome, Italy

J. F. L. Shaw
Department of Surgery
Whittington Hospital
London N19 5NF, England

M. Shikano
Second Department of Internal Medicine
Nagoya University School of Medicine
Nagoya, Japan

B. M. Simonetti
Division of Nephrology
Department of Medicine
University of Rome, "La Sapienza"
Policlinico Umberto I
00100 Rome, Italy

I. Simonetti
C. N. R. Institute of Clinical Physiology
Istituto di Patologia Medica I
University of Pisa
56100 Pisa, Italy

C. Sirtori
Institute of Pharmacology and
Pharmacognosy
University of Milan
Milan, Italy

P. Spangenberg
Department of Pathological Biochemistry
Medical Academy
Erfurt, Democratic Republic of Germany

K. Stegmeier
Department of Medical Research
Boehringer Mannheim
University of Heidelberg
Heidelberg, Federal Republic of
Germany

Andrea Stella
Istituto di Clinica Medica IV
University of Milan; and
Centro di Fisiologia Clinica e
Ipertensione
Ospedale Maggiore
Milan, Italy

H. Stern
Department of Physiology
New York Medical College
Valhalla, New York 10595

A. Strano
Istituto di Clinica Medica Generale e
  Terapia Medica I
University of Palermo
Palermo, Italy

G. Strazzulla
Istituto di Clinica Medica IV
(Cattedra di Patologia Speciale Medica
  II)
University of Florence
Viale Morgagni, 85
50134 Florence, Italy

Andrzej Szczeklik
Department of Medicine
Copernicus Academy of Medicine
Skawinska 8
31-066 Cracow, Poland

F. Tessari
Department of Cytopharmacology
Fidia Research Laboratories
Via Ponte della Fabbrica 3/A
Abano Terme, Italy

U. Till
Department of Pathological Biochemistry
Medical Academy
Erfurt, Democratic Republic of Germany

P. Tonin
Clinica Neurologica
University of Padua Medical School
Padua, Italy

M. Toscano
Department of Cardiac Surgery
University of Rome
Rome, Italy

E. Tremoli
Institute of Pharmacology and
  Pharmacognosy
University of Milan
Milan, Italy

S. Treves
Cattedra di Chimica e Propedeutica
  Biochimica
Istituto di Igiene
University of Turin
Turin, Italy

Bruno Trimarco
Istituto di Clinica Medica I
II Facoltà di Medicina e Chirurgia
Via S. Pansini
University of Naples
80131 Naples, Italy

F. Trotta
Clinica Medica I
University of Florence
Viale Morgagni, 85
50134 Florence, Italy

S. Tsutsumi
Second Department of Internal Medicine
Nagoya University School of Medicine
Nagoya, Japan

T. Uno
Second Department of Internal Medicine
Nagoya University School of Medicine
Nagoya, Japan

G. P. Velo
Istituto di Farmacologia
University of Verona
Verona, Italy

C. Ventura
Istituto di Chimica Biologica
University of Bologna
40138 Bologna, Italy

Massimo Volpe
Istituto di Clinica Medica I
II Facoltà di Medicina e Chirurgia
Via S. Pansini
University of Naples
80131 Naples, Italy

L. Wallentin
Department of Internal Medicine
University Hospital
S-581 85 Linköping, Sweden

Mary F. Walsh
Department of Internal Medicine
The University of Michigan
Ann Arbor, Michigan, 48109

P. Weinerowski
Department of Pharmacology
Ruhr-University Bochum
Im-Lottental
D-4630 Bochum, Federal Republic of
  Germany

G. Wittmann
Department of Pharmacology
Ruhr-University Bochum
Im-Lottental
D-4630 Bochum, Federal Republic of
  Germany

D. A. Yardumian
Department of Haematology
Middlesex Hospital and University
  College Hospital
London, England

Alberto Zanchetti
Istituto di Clinica Medica IV
University of Milan; and
Centro di Fisiologia Clinica e
  Ipertensione
Ospedale Maggiore
Milan, Italy

Zofia Zukowska-Grojec
Laboratory of Clinica Science, National
  Institute of Mental Health
Bethesda, Maryland 20205

Advances in Prostaglandin, Thromboxane, and Leukotriene Research, Vol. 13, edited by G. G. Neri Serneri, et al. Raven Press, New York © 1985.

Physiological and Pathological Involvements of Platelets

G. V. R. Born

Department of Pharmacology, King's College, London WC2R 2LS, England

PLATELETS IN HAEMOSTASIS

When blood vessels are injured so that they bleed, circulating platelets adhere to the damaged vessel walls and aggregate, diminishing or arresting the haemorrhage. This interaction between platelets and vessel walls therefore has an easily demonstrable physiological function. There is much clinical and experimental evidence that a deficiency or defect in circulating platelets is associated with "spontaneous" haemorrhages from small vessels. This suggests that platelets are somehow essential for the functional integrity of these vessels, but if there is such a mechanism it has still to be established.

PLATELETS IN ATHEROGENESIS

The old thrombogenic hypothesis of atherosclerosis (19,44) has recently reappeared in modern costume claiming that *platelets* contribute to atherogenesis in three ways: first, through damaging arterial endothelial cells by releasing injurious agents, presumably where circulating platelets adhere (32,33); second, through the release in such situations of a factor responsible for smooth-muscle proliferation in the arterial wall (41); and third, through the formation of persistent mural thrombi, which are organised into intimal thickenings. Such evidence as there is for these propositions fails to establish any of them as relevant to atherosclerosis in animals or human beings (see ref. 45). Underlying all three claims is the assumption that some normal circulating platelets settle on arterial walls long enough to release some of their contents. There is no observational basis for this assumption in normal arteries, although quantitative observations should now be possible with modern imaging techniques.

As the assumption is essential for the various claims just referred to, we have begun an investigation designed to quantify the adhesion of circulating platelets in different types of blood vessels (28). So far, the observations were mainly on small veins. However, some observations were made also on small arteries for comparison. The venous vessels were chosen for quantification in preference to arteries because the comparative slowness of the blood flow made it easier to develop and control the new methods required. The behaviour of platelets *in vivo* is also of interest in itself because of claims that platelets contribute to inflammation (35).

The results showed that the injection of hamster platelets, made fluorescent by *in vitro* labeling with fluorescein isothiocyanate, into the circulation of other hamsters makes it possible to quantify the flowing and sticking of platelets *in vivo*. The experiments provide evidence that there is very little tendency for circulating platelets to stick to the walls of small veins and arterioles, even under conditions in which the adhesion propensities of both platelets and vessel walls might be expected to be increased by preparative manipulations. In venules, such sticking as there was affected only a very small proportion of circulating platelets and those only for very short periods of time. In arterioles, sticking appeared to increase somewhat under conditions in which the blood flow could be assumed to be nonlaminar. If the sticking behaviour of platelets is at all similar in larger arteries, it seems unlikely that it would permit the release of platelet constituents capable of affecting the arterial walls, except just possibly under haemodynamic conditions such as occur at branches or other major unevennesses in the walls. It is assumed further that arterial endothelium is continuously subject to "damage" or "injury" of some kind as a precondition for the adherence of platelets. There is no convincing evidence for this generalisation, especially not in human beings. The first lesions of atherosclerosis, the fatty streaks, commonly begin during childhood or adolescence. It seems most improbable that these could be caused by any conceivable "injury." Specifically, the common assertion that damage is produced by shear stresses in the high-pressure blood system is inherently improbable because of functional adaptations in the course of evolution. The only finding that could conceivably apply to human arteries is that guinea pig aorta has a higher replacement rate of endothelium around the openings of branches than elsewhere (37). This is most simply explained by assuming that endothelial turnover depends, *inter alia*, on haemodynamic effects due to nonlaminar blood flow over such areas. But this should be thought of more correctly as a quasiphysiological effect and, even there, platelets are rarely if ever seen adhering to the walls. The turnover rate of endothelium is increased in experimental hypertension (36). This is compatible with hypertension as a "risk factor" for coronary heart disease. It seems more likely that this is due to an accelerating effect of interendothelial gaps on plasma lipoprotein accumulation (14,43) than to an increase in the indiscriminate or even selective deposition of platelets on arterial walls.

PLATELETS IN THROMBOGENESIS

There is conclusive evidence that occlusive thrombi in arteries damaged by atherosclerosis contain platelets as a major, if not the main, component (17). The formation of platelet thrombi appears so similar to that of haemostatic plugs of platelets that analysis of the mechanism of the latter is likely to provide an understanding of the former. This chapter poses questions about how the thrombogenic mechanism depends on the haemodynamic and chemical environment in which platelets aggregate on acutely damaged vessel walls.

Both the gross and the histological appearance of arterial thrombi establish that their central mass consists mainly of aggregated platelets. What, therefore, is the mechanism responsible for rapid and extensive platelet aggregation in an artery as an apparently random event in time (8)? Close serial sectioning of obstructed coronary arteries has established that the platelet thrombus responsible is invariably associated with recent haemorrhage into an underlying atherosclerotic plaque (15,17,22). The haemorrhages occur through fissures or fractures in the plaque; the sudden appearance of such a fissure or fracture may well be the random, individually unpredictable event affecting coronary arteries that has to be assumed to occur to account for the clinical onset of acute coronary thrombosis (8).

How does haemorrhage into a ruptured plaque initiate platelet thrombogenesis? This can be regarded as part of the general question of how platelets are caused to aggregate through haemorrhage, and most effectively through haemorrhage from arteries. Until recently this question was commonly answered by assuming that the process depends on the adhesion of platelets to collagen, which is exposed where damaged vessel walls are denuded of endothelium. Adhering platelets then release other agents, including thromboxane A_2 and ADP, which in turn are responsible for the adhesion of more platelets as growing aggregates. This explanation is unlikely to be correct, for the following reasons. First, haemostatic and thrombotic aggregates of platelets grow without delay and very rapidly. For example, when an arteriole 200 μm in diameter is cut into laterally, the rate of accession of platelets to the haemostatic plug is of the order of 10^4/sec (10). In contrast, although the adhesion of platelets to collagen itself is almost instantaneous, the subsequent aggregation of platelets, even under optimal conditions for their reactivity, begins only after a delay or lag period of several seconds (46). Second, platelets tend to aggregate as mural thrombi when anticoagulated blood flows through the plastic vessels of artificial organs such as oxygenators or dialysers (40,42) that contain no collagen or anything else capable of activating platelets similarly. This implies that there are conditions under which platelets are activated in the blood by something other than collagen or other constituents of the walls of living vessels.

The plaque on which a thrombus grows has usually narrowed the arterial lumen. At constant blood pressure, the flow of blood is faster through the constriction than elsewhere in the artery. Therefore, high flow and wall shear rates are no hindrance to the aggregation of platelets as thrombi (7). Indeed, the question arises of whether the activation of platelets that precedes their aggregation depends in some way on such abnormal haemodynamic conditions.

The effectiveness of platelet aggregation in plugging a leak is at least as effective in arterioles as in venules. As the haemodynamic situation should be more unfavourable to the formation of aggregates in arterioles than in venules, an explanation of arteriolar haemostasis is likely to account in principle also for that in venules. For that reason, the following considerations are limited to arterioles.

When an arteriole is cut, platelets are seen to adhere with great rapidity to the damaged vessel wall, while the red cells continue to rush by. This high flow velocity in relation to the small size of the vessels implies the presence in the fluid of strong mechanical forces acting normally and tangentially on and near the vessel walls. The cut causes peripheral resistance to the flow to diminish suddenly; if the inflow pressure remains constant, the mean flow velocity increases. Thus the fluid-mechanical forces on platelets adhering and aggregating on the vessel wall become greater still. With increasing size the platelet aggregates tend to constrict the cut, causing a further, although usually temporary, increase in flow velocity.

The blood-flow velocities that would be experienced by platelets closest to the vessel wall and therefore with the highest probability of colliding with the sites of damage can be calculated. Human platelets have a major diameter of about 1.5 μm. In an arteriole of medium size, the flow velocity of plasma and of any cells in it at a distance of 1 μm from the wall is of the order of 10 to 100 μm/msec. Therefore, a platelet flowing within a distance no greater than its own diameter would pass an injury site 100 μm long in at most 10 msec. In the absence of other influences, this would seem to be the time available for such a platelet to adhere to the damaged wall.

The time just calculated as available to circulating platelets "at risk" for adhering to a wall lesion has to be compared with what is known about the time required for platelets to be activated into a condition in which their collision with such a lesion would probably result in adhesion (11). That a process of *activation* is an essential prerequisite for adhesion and aggregation is inferred from the nonreactivity of normal circulating platelets. Presumably, activation consists of a sequence of physical and biochemical events analogous to the activation of muscle (38). The sequence is still being worked out, but several similarities with muscle are already established. Thus, it is known that in platelets an early event is an increased influx of sodium unaccompanied by an equivalent amount of chloride (20) and that activation is associated with an increase of free calcium in platelets (27,30).

As activation is indicated by adhesiveness, the change must involve one or more constituents of the outer surface of platelets. There is evidence that the essence is the exposure of surface receptors for fibrinogen, which has long been known to be an essential and specific plasma co-factor for platelet aggregation (9,16). The activation time of platelets may then be defined as the interval between the encounter of platelets with an activating agent such as ADP and their ability to react with plasma fibrinogen.

That circulating platelets can be activated to adhere in much less time than that required by their gross changes in shape (i.e., $t_{1/2} \approx 1$–2 sec at 37°C) (6) is indicated by direct experimental observations. An arteriole can be irradiated by a laser in such a way that damage is limited to a few square micrometres of endothelium (1). The site of damage is covered almost immediately with platelets that must have been activated in small fractions of a second.

Similar events follow the application of the activating agent ADP by microion-tophoresis to the outside of an arteriole or venule under conditions in which appropriate controls indicate that there is no evidence at all of damage to the endothelial layer (2). Platelet aggregates grow in the vessel exactly opposite the tip of the micropipette, while the blood continues to flow rapidly and without noticeable disturbance over the site. This is explained most simply by assuming that sufficient ADP diffuses between the endothelial cells into the blood to reach platelets passing close to the wall and that this ADP activates them very rapidly indeed.

An extension of this technique has provided a basis for calculating an average activation time for circulating platelets. It was found that the size of platelet aggregates produced by the iontophoretic application of ADP increases exponentially. The rate constant of this increase depended on the mean blood flow velocity, determined in the same vessels at the same time (2). The shape of the experimentally determined curve was simulated closely by a theoretical curve (39) that was derived on the single assumption that platelets require an activation time of about 100 to 200 msec. This time is still one to two orders of magnitude greater than that indicated by the earlier theoretical considerations, so either this experimental derivation overestimates the true activation time or the earlier considerations failed to take something into account that would allow flowing platelets more than a few milliseconds for activation. More time would, for example, be available if the blood flow near the vessel wall were nonlaminar, so that platelets caught up in vortices, however small, might be exposed to localised activating conditions for longer than they would otherwise be. When branching vessels of the microcirculation are observed microscopically, platelets can often be seen trapped in vortices for variable times of up to several seconds. Such delays may occur in the immediate vicinity of major vessel wall lesions, whether caused by disease such as the sudden rupture of an atheromatous plaque (17,23) or by traumatic injury such as a puncture or transection. However, there is no evidence of even the smallest disturbances in the flow of blood in a normal vessel in which platelets are caused to adhere by iontophoretically applied ADP. Moreover, it seems most unlikely that any endothelial unevenness produced by laser injury would give rise to flow disturbances large enough to delay the passage of platelets.

The chemical environment of platelets aggregating *in vivo* has been in doubt until recently. *In vitro* platelets are activated by various chemical agents, and it was uncertain which, if any, of these are responsible for the haemostatic aggregation of platelets in living blood vessels. Recent evidence (47) establishes that ADP is involved in activating platelets *in vivo*.

Novel techniques were developed for the reproducible determination of bleeding times from small arteries of rats and rabbits in the territory supplied by the superior mesenteric artery. One of its main branches was cannulated and infusions were made into the mesenteric circulation of one or other of two enzyme systems that are specific for removing ADP. The reactions catalysed by these enzymes are as follows:

creatine phosphokinase
(CPK)

ADP + creatine phosphate (CP) $\xrightleftharpoons$ ATP + creatine

pyruvate kinase
(PK)

ADP + phosphoenolpyruvate (PEP) $\xrightleftharpoons$ ATP + pyruvate

For both reactions, the equilibrium at physiological pH is far to the right. In both species these infusions increased the bleeding times significantly. It is reasonable to conclude, therefore, that the observed increases in bleeding time are caused by removal from the blood plasma of ADP, the presence of which makes a major contribution to the activation and haemostatic aggregation of arriving platelets. This conclusion is supported by control experiments in which CP was infused alone, without CPK. We have shown this enzyme to be present in blood plasma of both rats and rabbits, in concentrations somewhat higher than in human plasma (21). Completion of the ADP-removing system by the naturally occurring plasma enzymes can therefore account for the observed increases in bleeding time in these control experiments. The validity of our conclusion is supported by the reproducibility of the bleeding times as here determined. In each experiment, control bleeding times were measured before and after infusions of the enzyme systems. Changes in general factors that could be expected to influence bleeding time values, namely the moderate decreases in blood pressure, blood platelet concentration, and haematocrit that were observed, were thereby taken into account. There is other evidence (3) that the bleeding time is not affected by moderate decreases in blood platelet concentrations, that is, as long as they remain above about 5×10^7 platelets/ml.

A reservation about the conclusion arises out of the presence of nucleotide-dephosphorylating enzymes in normal blood, both in plasma (25) and as ectoenzymes on the surfaces of different types of circulating cells (18,31). These enzymes hydrolyse the γ-phosphate of ATP several times more rapidly than β-phosphate of ADP. Both of the infused enzyme systems convert ADP to ATP, which the dephosphorylating enzymes presumably reconvert into ADP. It must be assumed, therefore, that the overall balance between the reaction rates in both directions is such as to diminish the concentration of ADP. Further confirmation of our conclusion about an essential role of ADP in platelet haemostasis will therefore depend on substituting for the above enzyme systems one, such as apyrase, that only dephosphorylates ADP to AMP.

Enzyme systems that remove ADP have been much used to provide evidence for its involvement in reactions of platelets *in vitro* (24,26) or to prevent the activation of platelets during their preparation (34). Apyrase increases the bleeding time from transected vessels in isolated rabbit mesenteries (4) and from punctures or cuts into artificial vessels (12). All this is *in vitro* or *ex vivo* evidence for the dependence of the haemostatic aggregation of platelets on free ADP in the blood. The results reported here are the first to provide similar evidence *in vivo*, as far as the primary physiological function of platelets is concerned. Intravascular coagulation associated with the generalised Schwartzman phenomenon in rabbits can be prevented by the infusion of CP with CPK (48), but that is under pathological conditions in which damaged vascular or blood cells, possibly including platelets, can be expected to release ADP among other agents into the circulating blood.

Our observations increase current interest in the following questions. First, is it possible to demonstrate plasma ADP *directly* in blood at sites of haemostasis or thrombosis at concentrations required to activate platelets? Second, what is the cellular source (or sources) of the ADP? And third, how does this evidence affect therapeutic possibilities for the prevention or reversal of intravascular, particularly arterial, thrombosis?

It has recently become possible to demonstrate free ATP in blood emerging from cuts in small arteries during haemostasis (13,29). On the assumption that this ATP was accompanied by ADP in their normal intracellular proportions, the blood contained enough ADP, at least 10^{-8} M (31a; M. Frojmovic, *personal communication*) to aggregate the platelets. Therefore, the presence of ADP was inferred from that of free ATP, which was quantified by luciferase–luciferin luminescence (10,29) in blood emerging from small arteries punctured with a 100-μm needle. Blood from carotids of anaesthetised rats contained about 3×10^{-7} M ATP within 2 sec; thereafter its concentration decreased and increased again to about 2×10^{-5} M. Heparin (about 15 U/ml) or indomethacin (1 mg/kg) diminished the second increase, suggesting that it represents ATP released from platelets by thrombin. Indomethacin had no significant effect on free ATP present within 2 sec after injury of rabbit ear arteries. The source of this ATP was investigated by perfusing these arteries at 4.5 ml/min with physiological saline containing 1% albumin and 5 U heparin/ml. Each artery was punctured as before. The emerging fluid contained no blood but ATP at about 1.0×10^{-7} M in the first 2 sec, which decreased rapidly thereafter. The results confirm a long-standing proposition (5) that at sites of vascular injury enough ADP is rapidly released from damaged cells into the blood to account for the haemostatic aggregation of platelets. Whatever the source of the plasma ADP, its demonstration suggests novel therapeutic possibilities in the prevention of arterial thrombosis when it is initiated by platelet aggregation (see also ref. 8).

One such possibility would turn on the feasibility of infusing enzyme systems that remove free ADP from the blood. Despite immunological and other problems, it is conceivable that some enzyme with this specificity and a sufficiently long half-life in blood could be investigated for this purpose in appropriate clinical conditions. Furthermore, on the basis of our demonstration that bleeding times were increased also by infusing substrates only, with the implication that the systems are completed by the endogenous plasma enzymes, it is conceivable that therapeutic removal of ADP can be achieved by administering CP or PEP in a way that provides adequate concentrations in the circulating blood.

ACKNOWLEDGMENTS

I wish to thank the British Heart Foundation, the Minna-James-Heineman Foundation of Hanover, and the Fritz Thyssen Foundation of Cologne for generous support.

REFERENCES

1. Arfors, K. E., Cockburn, J. S., and Gross, J. F. (1976): Measurement of growth rate of laser-induced intravascular platelet aggregation, and the influence of blood flow velocity. *Microvasc. Res.*, 11:79–87.
2. Begent, N. A., and Born, G. V. R. (1970): Growth rate *in vivo* of platelet thrombi produced by iontophoresis of ADP, as a function of mean blood flow velocity. *Nature (Lond.)*, 227:926–930.
3. Bergqvist, D., and Arfors, K. E. (1973): Influence of platelet count on haemostatic plug formation and plug stability. An experimental study in rabbits with graded thrombocytopenia. *Thromb. Diath. Haemorr.*, 30:586–596.
4. Bergqvist, D., and Arfors, K. E. (1980): Haemostatic platelet plug formation in the isolated rabbit mesenteric preparation—An analysis of red blood cell participation. *Thromb. Haemostasis*, 4:6–8.
5. Born, G. V. R. (1962): Aggregation of blood platelets by adenosine diphosphate and its reversal. *Nature (Lond.)*, 194:927–929.
6. Born, G. V. R. (1970): Observations on the change in shape of blood platelets brought about by adenosine diphosphate. *J. Physiol.*, 209:487–511.
7. Born, G. V. R. (1977): Fluid-mechanical and biochemical interactions in haemostasis. *Br. Med. Bull.*, 33:193–197.
8. Born, G. V. R. (1979): Arterial thrombosis and its prevention. In: *Proc. VIIIth World Congress of Cardiology*, edited by S. Hayase and S. Murao, pp. 81–91. Excerpta Medica, Amsterdam.
9. Born, G. V. R., and Cross, M. J. (1964): Effects of inorganic ions and of plasma proteins on the aggregation of blood platelets by adenosine diphosphate. *J. Physiol. (Lond.)*, 170:394–414.
10. Born, G. V. R., and Kratzer, M. A. A. (1984): Source and concentration of intracellular adenosine triphosphate during haemostasis in rats, rabbits and man. *J. Physiol. (Lond.)*, 354:419–429.
11. Born, G. V. R., and Richardson, P. D. (1980): Activation time of blood platelets. *J. Membrane Biol.*, 57:87–90.
12. Born, G. V. R., Bergqvist, D., and Arfors, K. E. (1976): Evidence for inhibition of platelet activation in blood by drug effect on erythrocytes. *Nature (Lond.)*, 259:233–235.
13. Born, G. V. R., Görög, P., and Kratzer, M. A. A. (1981): Aggregation of platelets in damaged vessels. *Philos. Trans. R. Soc. B*, 294:241–250.
14. Caro, C. G. (1977): Mechanical factors in atherogenesis. In: *Cardiovascular Flow Dynamics and Measurement*, edited by N. H. C. Hwang and N. A. Normann, pp. 473–487. University Park Press, Baltimore.
15. Constantinides, P. (1966): Plaque fissures in human coronary thrombosis. *J. Atheroscler. Res.*, 6:1–17.
16. Cross, M. J. (1964): Effect of fibrinogen on the aggregation of platelets by adenosine diphosphate. *Thromb. Diath. Haemorrh.*, 12:524–527.
17. Davies, M. J., and Thomas, T. (1981): The pathological basis and microanatomy of occlusive thrombus formation in human coronary arteries. *Philos. Trans. R. Soc. Lond. B*, 294:225–229.
18. De-Pierre, J. W., and Karnovsky, M. L. (1973): Plasma membranes of mammalian cells. A review of methods for their characterisation and isolation. *J. Cell Biol.*, 56:275–303.
19. Duguid, J. B. (1949): Pathogenesis of atherosclerosis. *Lancet*, 2:925.
20. Feinberg, H., Sandler, W. C., Scorer, M., Le Breton, G. C., Grossman, B., and Born, G. V. R. (1977): Movement of sodium into human platelets induced by ADP. *Biochim. Biophys. Acta*, 470:317.
21. Forster, G., Bernt, E., and Bergmeyer, H. V. (1974): Creatine kinase. In: *Methods of Enzymatic Analysis, Vol. 2*, edited by H. V. Bergmeyer, pp. 784–797. Academic Press, New York.
22. Friedman, H. (1970): Pathogenesis of coronary thrombosis, intramural and intraluminal naemorrhage. In: *Thrombosis and Coronary Heart Disease, Vol. 4*, edited by L. A. Halonen, p. 3. Karger, Basel.

23. Friedman, M., and Van den Bovenkamp, G. J. (1966): The pathogenesis of a coronary thrombosis. *Am. J. Pathol.*, 48:19–44.

24. Haslam, R. J. (1964): Role of adenosine diphosphate in the aggregation of human platelets by thrombin and by fatty acids. *Nature (Lond.)*, 202:765–768.

25. Haslam, R. J., and Mills, D. C. B. (1967): The adenylate kinase of human plasma, erythrocytes and platelets in relation to degradation of adenosine diphosphate in plasma. *Biochem. J.*, 103:773–784.

26. Izrael, V., Zawilska, K., Jaisson, F., Levy-Toledano, S., and Caen, J. (1974): Effect of fast removal of plasmatic ADP by the creatine-phosphate and creatine phosphokinase system on human platelet function *in vivo*. In: *Platelets: Production, Function, Transfusion and Storage*, edited by M. G. Baldini and S. Ebbe, pp. 187–195. Grune & Stratton, New York.

27. Kaser-Glanzmann, R., Jakabova, M., George, J. N., and Luscher, E. F. (1977): Stimulation of calcium uptake in platelet membrane vesicles by adenosine 3',5'-cyclic monophosphate and protein kinase. *Biochim. Biophys. Acta*, 466:429.

28. Kortenhaus, H., Schroer, H., and Born, G. V. R. (1982): Quantification of the adhesion of platelets in hamster venules *in vivo*. *Proc. R. Soc. Lond. B*, 215:135–145.

29. Kratzer, M. A. A., and Born, G. V. R. (1981): Free ATP in blood during haemorrhage. *Thromb. Haemostasis*, 46:393.

30. Le Breton, C. G., Sandler, W. C., and Feinberg, H. (1976): The effect of D_2O and chlortetracycline on ADP-induced platelet shape change and aggregation. *Thrombos. Res.*, 8:477.

31. Manery, J. F., and Dryden, E. E. (1979): Ecto-enzymes concerned with nucleotide metabolism. In: *Physiological and Regulatory Functions of Adenosine and Adenine Nucleotides*, edited by H. P. Baer and G. I. Drummond, pp. 323–339. Raven Press, New York.

31a. Milton, J. G., Yung, W., Glushak, C., and Frojmovic, M. M. (1980): Kinetics of ADP-induced human platelet shape change: apparent positive cooperativity. *Can. J. Physiol. Pharmacol.*, 58:45–52.

32. Mustard, J. F., Moore, S., Packham, M. A., and Kinlough Rathbone, R. L. (1977): Platelets, thrombosis and atherosclerosis. *Proc. Biochem. Pharmacol.*, 13:312–325.

33. Mustard, J. F., Packham, M. A., and Kinlough Rathbone, R. L. (1977): Platelets, thrombosis and atherosclerosis. *Adv. Exp. Med. Biol.*, 104:127–144.

34. Mustard, J. F., Perry, D. W., Ardlie, N. G., and Packham, M. A. (1972): Preparation of suspension of washed platelets from humans. *Br. J. Haematol.*, 22:193–204.

35. Nachman, R. L. (1978): The platelet as an inflammatory cell. In: *Platelets: A Multidisciplinary Approach*, edited by G. de Gaetano and S. Garattini, pp. 199–204. Raven Press, New York.

36. Payling-Wright, H. P. (1972): Mitosis patterns in aortic endothelium. *Atherosclerosis*, 15:93–95.

37. Payling-Wright, H. P., and Born, G. V. R. (1971): Possible effect of blood flow on the turnover rate of vascular endothelial cells. In: *Theoretical and Clinical Haemorheology*, edited by H. H. Hartert and A. L. Copley, pp. 220–226. Springer-Verlag, Berlin.

38. Pringle, J. W. S. (1978): Stretch activation of muscle: Function and mechanism. The Croonian Lecture 1977. The Royal Society, London.

39. Richardson, P. D. (1973): Effect of blood flow velocity on growth rate of platelet thrombi. *Nature (Lond.)*, 245:103–104.

40. Richardson, P. D., Galetti, P., and Born, G. V. R. (1976): Regional administration of drugs to control thrombosis in artificial organs. *Trans. Am. Soc. Artif. Intern. Organs*, 22:22–29.

41. Ross, R., and Glomset, J. A. (1973): Atherosclerosis and the arterial smooth muscle cell. Proliferation of smooth muscle is a key event in the genesis of the lesions of atherosclerosis. *Science*, 180:1332–1339.

42. Schmid-Schönbein, H., Rieger, H., and Fischer, T. (1976): Problems arising at the borders of natural and artificial blood vessels. In: *Blood Vessels*, edited by S. Effert and J. Mayer-Erkelenz, pp. 57–63. Springer, Berlin.

43. Stehbens, W. E. (1965): Endothelial cell mitosis and permeability. *J. Exp. Physiol. (Cogn. Med. Sci.)*, 50:90–92.

44. von Rokitansky (1941–46): *Handbuch der Pathologischen Anatomie*. Braumüller & Seidel, Vienna.

45. Walton, K. W. (1975): Pathogenetic mechanisms in atherosclerosis. *Am. J. Cardiol.*, 35:542–558.

46. Wilner, G. D., Nossel, H. L., and LeRoy, E. D. (1969): Aggregation of platelets by collagen. *J. Clin. Invest.*, 47:2616–2621.

47. Zawilska, K. M., Born, G. V. R., and Begent, N. A. (1982): Effect of ADP-utilizing enzymes on the arterial bleeding time in rats and rabbits. *Br. J. Haematol.*, 50:317–325.
48. Zawilska, K., Izrael, V., Chelloul, N., and Caen, J. (1975): Prévention de la coagulation intravasculaire disséminée au course de Phénomenène de Schwartzmann géneralisé chez le lapin par un système enzymatique consommant l'ADP plasmatique. *Actual. Hématol.*, 9:269.

Advances in Prostaglandin, Thromboxane, and Leukotriene Research, Vol. 13, edited by G.G. Neri Serneri, et al. Raven Press, New York © 1985.

Paf-Acether (Platelet-Activating Factor)

Jacques Benveniste

INSERM U 200, Université Paris-Sud, 92140 Clamart, France

In addition to its platelet-activating properties, paf-acether (platelet-activating factor, PAF) is known today to exert a variety of proinflammatory actions, including neutrophil activation. Initially described as originating from basophils in IgE-sensitized rabbits challenged with the specific allergen (8) in a bovine serum albumin-containing medium, it was later obtained from human and hog leukocytes placed for several hours at pH 9.6 (4). It was then shown to be inactivated by phospholipases A_2, C, and D but not by lipase A_1 from *Rhizopus arrhizus* and sphingomyelinase C. The proposed structure was that of a glycerophospholipid devoid of an ester linkage at position 1 and having an acyl group at position 2 (9). This led to the partial synthesis of a platelet-activating component possessing the physicochemical and biological properties of PAF, and the structure 1-*O*-alkyl-2-acetyl-*sn*-glyceryl-3-phosphocholine was proposed (10,17). From that time we have named this mediator paf-acether, therefore emphasizing the chemical originality of the molecule having an ether linkage at position 1 and an acetyl group at position 2 (Fig. 1). This structure was confirmed by the total synthesis of 1-*O*-octadecyl-2-*O*-acetyl-*sn*-glyceryl-3-phosphorylcholine (21). The final proof for the structure of paf-acether was given by the structural elucidation of its natural biologically inactive derivative, 2-lyso paf-acether, which after acetylation shared the same biological and physicochemical properties with paf-acether. By chemical and spectral means, particularly by chemical ionization mass spectrometry, 2-lyso paf-acether was shown to be a mixture of 1-*O*-alkyl-glyceryl-3-phosphorylcholine with an octadecyl or hexadecyl alkyl chain (35). Similarly, naturally occurring paf-acether (AGEPC) contained a mixture of 18:0 (90%) and 16:0 (10%) alkyl ether residues (22).

Paf-acether is routinely assayed in an aggregometer on rabbit platelets, purified by differential centrifugations and washings (8). Platelets are treated with 0.1 mM aspirin between the first and second washing, and aggregation is performed in the presence of the ADP scavenger complex, creatine phosphate/creatine phosphokinase (CP/CPK). Under these conditions, the height of the recorded aggregation is directly proportional, within certain limits, to the amount of the agonist. By using standard amounts of synthetic paf-acether, the activity is expressed in weight or in concentration. Another method is based on the release of radiolabeled serotonin previously incorporated into platelets before the first washings.

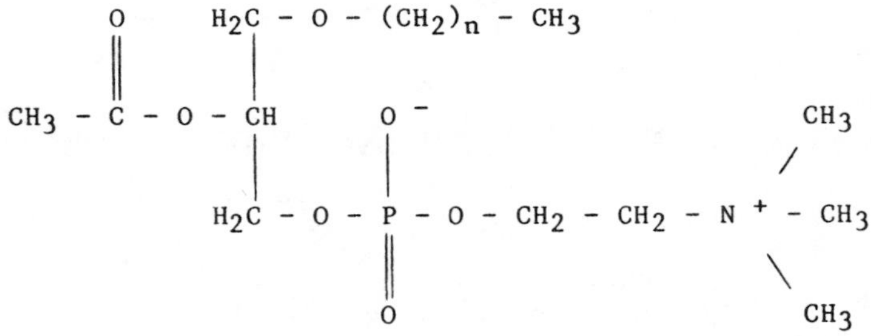

FIG. 1. Structure of paf-acether: 1-*O*-alkyl-2-acetyl-*sn*-glyceryl-3-phosphorylcholine, where $n = 15, 17$.

Given the numerous substances present in biological fluids and cell supernatants that can activate platelets, it was necessary to strictly define paf-acether. Even before the knowledge of its molecular structure, we have used the following criteria to precisely identify it from, for example, arachidonic acid, thrombin, ADP, and prostanoids. These are (a) aggregation of platelets in the presence of aspirin or indomethacin and of ADP scavengers, (b) elution pattern identical to that of hog leukocyte (and now synthetic) paf-acether on silicic acid thin-layer or high-pressure liquid chromatography, and (c) inactivation by phospholipases A_2, C, and D, and insensitivity to lipase from *R. arrhizus*.

SOURCES OF PAF-ACETHER

Early and more recent results have clearly established that paf-acether originated from rabbit basophils (8,11,40). The release from human basophils was also observed (12), a result contradicted by other investigators (11,39). The first nonbasophil identified source was the peritoneal macrophage from rat and mouse (27). It was shown later that the level of formation and release of paf-acether by these cells depended on their state of activation, since inflammatory macrophages synthesize less paf-acether than the resident ones (19,36). Paf-acether was released on stimulation of alveolar macrophages from rat, rabbit, baboon, and human normal volunteers by the ionophore A 23187. In contrast, the release of paf-acether by opsonized zymosan was observed in rat and rabbit but not in monkey or human. Alveolar macrophages from asthmatic patients released paf-acether when stimulated with the specific pneumallergen. The allergens used were those inducing a positive prick test or a human basophil degranulation test in asthmatic patients. Such allergens were unable to induce the release of paf-acether from alveolar macrophages from normal donors. The specific release of paf-acether by alveolar macrophages from asthmatic patients induced by sensitizing allergens may represent a new pathway in the physiopathology of human asthma disease (see below).

Paf-acether was shown to originate from rabbit and human neutrophils stimulated with opsonized zymosan or the ionophore A 23187 (26). A potent aggregating substance was found in the supernatants of rabbit and human platelets stimulated by the Ca^{2+} ionophore A 23187. This substance met all the biological and physicochemical characteristics of paf-acether just described. Formation of paf-acether was altered neither by aspirin nor indomethacin nor by CP/CPK (16). Stimulation of rabbit platelets with collagen or thrombin also led to the formation of paf-acether. The kinetics and the amounts of paf-acether formed were compatible with its hypothesized role as the mediator of the third pathway of platelet aggregation, at least in the rabbit.

PAF-ACETHER METABOLISM

The release of paf-acether from macrophages (as well as from all the other cell types) is abolished by EDTA, bromophenacyl bromide, mepacrine, and 874 CB (Clin-Midy), indicating the intervention of a phospholipase A_2 in paf-acether formation. This result suggested (a) the activation of a phospholipase A_2 leading both to the release from membrane ether phospholipids of 2-lyso paf-acether and paf-acether (see below), and (b) the existence of an enzyme capable of acetylating 2-lyso paf-acether into paf-acether or of hydrolyzing paf-acether into 2-lyso paf-acether (Fig. 2). It is quite clear that 2-lyso paf-acether is the metabolic precursor of paf-acether. It is biologically transformed into the active substance by incorporation of an acetyl group, linked to coenzyme A. Radiolabeling experiment demonstrated the reality of this deacylation-reacylation mechanism. Platelets incubated with tritiated acetyl-CoA formed labeled paf-acether (14). The acetyltransferase was evidenced in microsomes from various tissues (44), then in paf-acether-producing cells, peritoneal and alveolar macrophages, neutrophils, and platelets (1,2,24,25,28,32). The same biosynthetic pathway was also described in rabbit neutrophils (29). However, this pathway is different from the *de novo* synthesis of the alkyl chain or transfer of CDP-choline on alkyl acetyl glycerol that do not occur on cell stimulation. When macrophages are stimulated by calcium ionophore or zymosan, acetyltransferase activity increases more than three times over control (31). Such a modulation of acetyltransferase activity may represent one of the regulatory mechanisms of paf-acether production. 2-Lyso paf-acether also results from deacylation of paf-acether by an acetylhydrolase evidenced by workers from Snyder's group (3,25). This is a cytosolic enzyme that might play a key regulating role on the biological activity of the molecule. Similar enzymatic activity was recently described in human serum (20). However, 2-lyso paf-acether does not accumulate in cells, since it is reacylated in position 2 to yield 1-*O*-alkyl-2-*O*-acyl-*sn*-glyceryl-3-phosphorylcholine. This was shown to occur in human and rabbit neutrophils, in rat alveolar macrophages, and in rabbit platelets (1,15,42). Alkyl ether analogs of phosphatidylcholine are sources for arachidonic acid release on cell activation (1,15). The impaired formation of paf-acether by inflammatory macrophages has been explained by a defect in a biosynthetic step. Substrate limitation and/or lower enzyme activities were thus envisioned. Resident and inflammatory macrophages synthesized comparable amounts of 2-lyso paf-acether, indicating that the phospholipase A_2-dependent step in paf-acether biosynthesis was

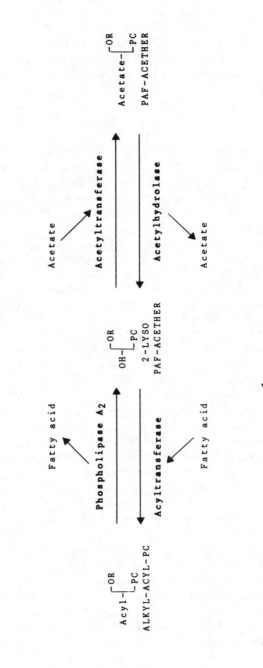

FIG. 2. Metabolism of paf-acether [PC: phosphocholine, R: $(CH_2)_nCH_3$].

intact in these cells, whereas the acetylation step was impaired. Determination of the acetyltransferase activity in each population indicated that it was comparable, except in thioglycollate macrophages where it was reduced by 10-fold (37), explaining the impaired formation of paf-acether by these cells (36). By contrast, the formation of paf-acether by activated macrophages was restored by incubating the cells with 100 μM acetyl-CoA, indicating that in the latter cells a low availability in acetate donors might be responsible for the defect in paf-acether formation. These data exemplify the regulation of paf-acether formation by substrate and/or enzyme limitation.

PATHOBIOLOGICAL EFFECTS OF PAF-ACETHER

References on this topic are too numerous to cite, but for an overview see refs. 6 and 38.

Paf-acether is the most potent aggregating agent so far described; concentrations of 10 to 100 pM can trigger activation of rabbit washed platelets, but 60 times more is needed to trigger aggregation of rabbit platelets suspended in plasma. There are also variations in sensitivity in different species, the most responsive platelets being those of guinea pigs, followed by those of rabbits, dogs, and humans. Rat platelets in plasma are unresponsive to paf-acether. Platelet aggregation induced by paf-acether is also inhibited by the so-called membrane-active drugs (e.g., reserpine).

Neutrophil activation by paf-acether was suggested by experiments showing that its intravenous injection causes thrombocytopenia but also neutropenia with formation of neutrophil aggregates (reviewed in ref. 23). Thereafter, *in vitro* neutrophil aggregation was described with concentration of paf-acether as low as 100 pM (13). Since then, a number of reports described the role of paf-acether as a neutrophil-activating factor. At concentrations varying between 0.1 and 1 μM, it induces lysosomal enzyme release, chemotaxis, and release of superoxide anions (23).

Alveolar macrophages and monocytes are capable of releasing paf-acether, so experiments were performed to evaluate the paf-acether effect on lung tissue. Intravenous injection of paf-acether induced acute and reversible pulmonary and circulatory alterations. The modifications observed were similar to those observed during IgE anaphylactic shock in rabbits. The pulmonary effect of an intravenous injection of paf-acether was first described in the guinea pig (43). Injection of 60 ng/kg induced a bronchoconstriction that was platelet-dependent, since it was inhibited by a prior injection of goat antiplatelet globulin. This bronchoconstriction was observed in animals pretreated with aspirin or eicosatetraynoic acid, therefore excluding the participation of arachidonic acid metabolites. The bronchomotor effect was accompanied by a decrease in circulating platelets. Paf-acether is the most powerful bronchoconstricting agent so far described, acting in guinea pigs at 60 ng/kg, as compared to arachidonic acid at 0.2 mg/kg, serotonin at 5 mg/kg, or histamine at 10 to 20 mg/kg. Similar effects were observed in rabbits. Intratracheal administration of paf-acether (60 μg/kg) to premedicated baboons provoked an immediate bronchomotor effect determined as an increase of the peak inspiratory pressure. Oxygen blood tension decreased a few minutes after injection. A decrease in circulating platelets and neutrophils occurred. The bronchomotor effect was not inhibited by a pretreatment with aspirin or atropine but was partially inhibited by intravenous injection of a β-adrenergic drug (salbutamol, 0.5 mg i.v.) (18).

All these pulmonary and circulatory modifications mimic human asthma disease. In keeping with the release of paf-acether by human alveolar macrophages and particularly on stimulation with the sensitizing allergen in asthmatic patients, our results suggest that paf-acether might play a role in the pathogenesis of human asthma.

The structure of paf-acether turned out to be exactly that of antihypertensive polar renomedullary lipid (APRL) (30). We have repeatedly observed the hypotensive effect of paf-acether in guinea pigs, baboons, and rats. The platelets of the latter are refractory to paf-acether, so the hypotensive effect appears to be independent from platelet aggregation. Also, PGI_2 (prostacyclin), which suppresses platelet aggregation in guinea pigs, does not influence hypotension (43). Moreover, given orally to rabbits, APRL or paf-acether does not affect platelet (or leukocyte) counts but is still active on hypertension (30). We have described a dramatic negative inotropic effect and decrease in coronary flow induced by paf-acether administered in the nanomolar range in guinea pig isolated perfused heart (7).

Intradermal administration of nanomolar doses of paf-acether to humans and rats induced edema and hyperalgesia (33,34,41), which was not inhibited by indomethacin or aspirin.

The contribution of paf-acether to the inflammatory process seems considerable in the light of its *in vitro* effects. Such an implication is difficult to assess *in vivo* because this mediator is rapidly destroyed in the circulating blood (5,20). Nevertheless, the effects produced by paf-acether are observed within minutes after injection. The bulk of the knowledge accumulated on this mediator justifies the important efforts now made in searching for molecules capable of inhibiting the metabolism, release, and biological effects of paf-acether.

REFERENCES

1. Albert, D. J., and Snyder, F. (1983): Biosynthesis of 1-alkyl-2-acetyl-*sn*-glycero-3-phosphocholine (platelet-activating factor). *J. Biol. Chem.*, 258:97–102.
2. Alonso, F., Garcia Gil, M., Sanchez-Crespo, L., and Mato, J. M. (1982): Activation of 1-alkyl-2-lysoglycero-3-phosphocholine-acetyl-CoA transferase. *J. Biol. Chem.*, 257:3376–3378.
3. Blank, M. E., Lee, T. C., Fitzgerald, V., and Snyder, F. (1981): A specific acetyl-hydrolase for 1-alkyl-2-acetyl-sn-glycero-3-phosphocholine (a hypotensive and platelet-activating lipid). *J. Biol. Chem.*, 256:175–178.
4. Benveniste, J. (1974): Platelet-activating factor, a new mediator of anaphylaxis and immune complex deposition from rabbit and human basophils. *Nature (Lond.)*, 249:581–583.
5. Benveniste, J. (1974): A possible role for IgE in immune complex disease. In: *The Biological Role of the IgE System*, edited by K. Ishizaka and D. H. Dayton, pp. 187–205. Department of Health, Education and Welfare, Washington.
6. Benveniste, B., and Arnoux, A., editors (1983): *Platelet-Activating Factor and Structurally Related Ether-Lipids. INSERM Symposium no. 23*. Elsevier Science, Amsterdam.

7. Benveniste, J., Boullet, C., Brink, C., and Labat, C. (1983): The actions of paf-acether (platelet-activating factor) on guinea-pig isolated heart preparations. *Br. J. Pharmacol.*, 80:81–83.
8. Benveniste, J., Henson, P. M., and Cochrane, C. G. (1972): Leukocyte-dependent histamine release from rabbit platelets: The role of IgE, basophils, and a platelet-activating factor. *J. Exp. Med.*, 136:1356–1377.
9. Benveniste, J., Le Couedic, J. P., Polonsky, J., and Tencé, M. (1977): Structural analysis of purified platelet-activating factor by lipases. *Nature (Lond.)*, 269:170–171.
10. Benveniste, J., Tencé, M., Varenne, P., Bidault, J., Boullet, C., and Polonsky, J. (1979): *C. R. Acad. Sci. Paris*, 289D:1037–1040.
11. Betz, S. J., Lotner, G. A., and Henson, P. M. (1980): Generation and release of platelet-activating factor (PAF) from enriched preparations of rabbit basophils; Failure of human basophils to release PAF. *J. Immunol.*, 125:2749–2755.
12. Camussi, G., Aglieta, M., Coda, R., Bussolino, F., Piacibello, W., and Tetta, C. (1981): Release of platelet-activating factor (PAF) and histamine. II. The cellular origin of human PAF: Monocytes, polymorphonuclear neutrophils and basophils. *Immunology*, 33:523–534.
13. Camussi, G., Tetta, C., Bussolino, F., Caligaris-Cappio, F., Coda, R., Masera, C., and Segoloni, (1981): Mediators of immune-complex-induced aggregation of polymorphonuclear neutrophils. II. Platelet-activating factor as the effector substance of immune-induced aggregation. *Int. Arch. Allergy Appl. Immunol.*, 64:25–41.
14. Chap, H., Mauco, G., Simon, M. F., Benveniste, J., and Douste-Blazy, L. (1981): Biosynthetic labelling of platelet-activating factor (PAF-acether) from radioactive acetate by stimulated platelets. *Nature (Lond.)*, 289:312–314.
15. Chignard, M., Le Couedic, J. P., Tencé, M., Vargaftig, B. B., and Benveniste, J. (1979): The role of platelet-activating factor in platelet aggregation. *Nature (Lond.)*, 279:799–800.
16. Chilton, F. H., O'Flaherty, J., Marshall Ellis, J., Swendsen, C. L., and Wykle, R. L. (1983): Selective acylation of lyso platelet activating factor by arachidonate in human neutrophils. *J. Biol. Chem.*, 258:7268–7271.
17. Demopoulos, C. A., Pinckard, R. N., and Hanahan, D. J. (1979): Platelet-activating factor. Evidence for 1-*O*-alkyl-2-acetyl-*sn*-glyceryl-3-phosphorylcholine as the active component (a new class of lipid chemical mediators). *J. Biol. Chem.*, 254:9355–9358.
18. Denjean, A., Arnoux, B., Masse, R., Lockhart, A., and Benveniste, J. (1983): Acute effects of intratracheal administration of platelet-activating factor (paf-acether) in baboons. *J. Appl. Physiol.*, 55:799–804.
19. Drapier, J. C., Roubin, R., Petit, J. F., and Benveniste, J. (1983): Lipid mediator synthesis in peritoneal macrophages from mice injected with immunostimulants. *Biochim. Biophys. Acta*, 751:90–98.
20. Farr, R. S., Wardlow, M. L., Cox, C. P., Meng, K. E., and Greene, D. E. (1983): Human serum acid-labile factor is an acylhydrolase that inactivates platelet-activating factor. *Fed. Proc.*, 42:3120–3122.
21. Godfroid, J. J., Heymans, F., Michel, E., Redeuilh, H. C., Steiner, E., and Benveniste, J. (1980): Platelet-activating factor (PAF-acether): Total synthesis of 1-*O*-octadecyl 2-*O*-acetyl-*sn*-glycero-3-phosphorylcholine. *FEBS Lett.*, 116:161–164.
22. Hanahan, D. J., Demopoulos, C. A., Liehr, J., and Pinckard, R. N. (1980): Identification of platelet-activating factor isolated from rabbit basophils as acetyl glyceryl ether phosphorylcholine. *J. Biol. Chem.*, 225:5514–5516.
23. Henson, P. M. (1981): Cellular sources of platelet-activating factor. In: *Pharmacology of Inflammation and Allergy*, edited by F. Russo-Marie, B. B. Vargaftig, and J. Benveniste, *Vol. 100*, pp. 63–81. INSERM, Paris.
24. Jouvin-Marche, E., Ninio, E., Beaurain, G., Tencé, M., Niaudet, P., and Benveniste, J. (1984): Biosynthesis of paf-acether (platelet-activating factor). VII. Precursors of paf-acether and acetyltransferase activity in human leukocytes. *J. Immunol.*, 133:892–898.
25. Lee, T. C., Malone, B., Wasserman, S. I., Fitzgerald, V., and Snyder, F. (1982): Activities of enzymes that metabolize platelet-activating factor (1-alkyl-2-acetyl-*sn*-glycero-3-phosphocholine) in neutrophils and eosinophils from humans and the effect of a calcium ionophore. *Biochem. Biophys. Res. Commun.*, 105:1303–1308.
26. Lotner, G. Z., Lynch, J. M., Betz, S. J., and Henson, P. M. (1980): Human neutrophil-derived platelet-activating factor. *J. Immunol.*, 124:676–684.
27. Mencia-Huerta, J. M., and Benveniste, J. (1979): Platelet-activating factor (PAF) and macrophages.

I. Evidence for the release from rat and mouse peritoneal macrophages and not from mastocytes. *Eur. J. Immunol.*, 9:409–415.

28. Mencia-Huerta, J. M., Roubin, R., Morgat, J., and Benveniste, J. (1982): Biosynthesis of platelet-activating factor (PAF-acether). III. Formation of PAF-acether from synthetic substrates by stimulated murine macrophages. *J. Immunol.*, 129:809–813.

29. Mueller, H. W., O'Flaherty, J. T., and Wykle, R. L. (1983): Biosynthesis of platelet-activating factor in rabbit polymorphonuclear neutrophils. *J. Biol. Chem.*, 258:6213–6218.

30. Muirhead, E. E., Byers, L. W., Desiderio, D. M., Brooks, B., and Brosius, W. M. (1981): Antihypertensive lipids from the kidney: Alkyl ether analogs of phosphatidylcholine. *Fed. Proc.*, 40:2285–2290.

31. Ninio, E., Mencia-Huerta, J. M., and Benveniste, J. (1982): Biosynthesis of platelet-activating factor (Paf-acether). V. Enhancement of acetyl-transferase activity in murine peritoneal cells by the calcium ionophore A 23187. *Biochim. Biophys. Acta*, 751:298–304.

32. Ninio, E., Mencia-Huerta, J. M., Heymans, F., and Benveniste, J. (1982): Biosynthesis of platelet-activating factor (PAF-acether). I. Evidence for an acetyl-transferase activity in murine macrophages. *Biochim. Biophys. Acta*, 710:23–31.

33. Pinckard, R. N., Kniker, W. T., Lee, L., Hanahan, D. J., and McManus, L. M. (1980): Vasoactive effects of 1-*O*-alkyl-2-acetyl-*sn*-glyceryl-3-phosphorylcholine (AcGEPC) in human skin. *J. Allergy Clin. Immunol.*, 65:196.

34. Pirotzky, E., Page, C. P., Roubin, R., Pfister, A., Paul, W., Bonnet, J., and Benveniste, J. (1984): Paf-acether-induced plasma exudation in rat skin is independent of platelets and neutrophils. *Microcirculation*, in press.

35. Polonsky, J., Tencé, M., Varenne, P., Das, B. C., Lunel, J., and Benveniste, J. (1980): Release of 1-*O*-alkylglyceryl 3-phosphorylcholine, *O*-deacetyl platelet-activating factor, from leukocytes: Chemical ionization mass spectrometry of phospholipids. *Proc. Natl. Acad. Sci. U.S.A.*, 12:7019–7023.

36. Roubin, R., Mencia-Huerta, J. M., and Benveniste, J. (1982): Release of platelet-activating factor (PAF-acether) and leukotrienes C and D from inflammatory macrophages. *Eur. J. Immunol.*, 12:141–146.

37. Roubin, R., Mencia-Huerta, J. M., Landes, A., and Benveniste, J. (1982): Biosynthesis of platelet-activating factor (PAF-acether). IV. Impairment of acetyl-transferase and not of phospholipase A_2 activity in thioglycollate-elicited mouse macrophages. *J. Immunol.*, 129:809–813.

38. Roubin, R., Tencé, M., Mencia-Huerta, J. M., Arnoux, B., Ninio, E., and Benveniste, J. (1983): A chemically defined monokine-macrophage-defined platelet-activating factor. In: *Lymphokines*, edited by E. Pick, *Vol. 8*, pp. 249–276. Academic Press, New York.

39. Sanchez-Crespo, M., Alonso, F., and Egido, J. (1980): Platelet-activating factor in anaphylaxis and phagocytosis. I. Release from human peripheral polymorphonuclears and monocytes during the stimulation by ionophore A 23187 and phagocytosis but not from degranulating basophils. *Immunology*, 40:645–655.

40. Siraganian, R. P., and Osler, A. G. (1971): Destruction of rabbit platelets in the allergic response of sensitized leukocytes. I. Demonstration of a fluid phase intermediate. *J. Immunol.*, 106:1244–1251.

41. Stimler, N. P., Bloor, C. M., Hugli, T. E., Wykle, R. L., McCall, C. E., and O'Flaherty, J. T. (1981): Anaphylactic actions of platelet-activating factor. *Am. J. Pathol.*, 105:64–69.

42. Touqui, L., Jacquemin, C., and Vargaftig, B. B. (1983): Conversion of ^{3}H-Paf-acether by rabbit platelets is independent from aggregation: Evidences for a novel metabolite. *Biochem. Biophys. Res. Commun.*, 110:890–893.

43. Vargaftig, B. B., Lefort, J., Chignard, M., and Benveniste, J. (1980): Platelet-activating factor induces a platelet dependent bronchoconstriction unrelated to the formation of prostaglandin derivatives. *Eur. J. Pharmacol.*, 65:185–192.

44. Wykle, R. L., Malone, B., and Snyder, F. (1980): Enzymatic synthesis of 1-alkyl-2-acetyl-*sn*-glycero-3-phosphocholine, a hypotensive and platelet-aggregating lipid. *J. Biol. Chem.*, 255:10256–10260.

Advances in Prostaglandin, Thromboxane, and
Leukotriene Research, Vol. 13, edited by G. G. Neri
Serneri, et al. Raven Press, New York © 1985.

Effects of Platelet-Activating Factor on Coronary Hemodynamics and Coronary Venous Plasma Levels of TXB$_2$, 6-Keto-PGF$_{1\alpha}$, and Leukotriene C$_4$ Immunoreactivity in the Intact Domestic Pig Heart

*David Ezra, *Giora Feuerstein, **Peter W. Ramwell,
†Edward Hayes, and *Robert E. Goldstein

*Neurobiology Research Unit and Departments of Pharmacology and Medicine,
Uniformed Services University of the Health Sciences, Bethesda, Maryland 20814;
**Department of Physiology and Biophysics, Georgetown University, Washington, D.C.
20007; and †Merck Sharp & Dohme, Rahway, New Jersey 07065

Activated white blood cells (WBC) and platelets have been implicated in the pathogenesis of anaphylactic shock and may figure in ischemic heart disease and other cardiovascular disorders. Platelet-activating factor [1-O-hexadecyl-2-acetyl-sn-glycero-3-phosphorylcholine (AGEPC)], a phospholipid produced by WBC and platelets (1), seemed a likely mediator of cardiac abnormalities accompanying anaphylaxis or other immune responses, since its production is stimulated by IgE-mediated mechanisms. Moreover, AGEPC has been shown to release thromboxane (TX) A$_2$ and leukotrienes (3), all potent constrictors of coronary arteries (2). For these reasons, we postulated that direct intracoronary administration of AGEPC may have significant deleterious effects on myocardial perfusion.

To examine this hypothesis, domestic pigs weighing 20 to 30 kg were anesthetized with ketamine and sodium pentobarbital and subjected to thoracotomy. Instruments were introduced for continuous measurement of left anterior descending (LAD) coronary blood flow (CBF, electromagnetic flow probe), systemic blood pressure (BP), heart rate, and lead II of the electrocardiogram. Intracoronary (i.c.) administration of AGEPC (kindly provided by Dr. F. Snyder, Oak Ridge Associated Universities, Oak Ridge, Tennessee), 0.3 to 10 nmol, was performed by 0.1-ml bolus injection with saline flush via a Herd–Barger catheter introduced distal to the coronary flow probe.

In 10 pigs, AGEPC produced dose-dependent, biphasic changes in CBF with an initial rise (11–50%) followed by a more prolonged fall (6–92%) below baseline CBF (baseline mean ± standard error: 39 ± 2 ml/min). Similar changes occurred in coronary vascular resistance. More severe CBF decreases were accompanied by electrocardiographic signs of regional myocardial ischemia. The leukotriene antagonist FPL-55712 (1–3 mg i.c.) attenuated the AGEPC-induced CBF decrement: $54 \pm 13\%$ fall after AGEPC, 1 nmol, was reduced to a fall of $34 \pm 15\%$ when AGEPC followed FPL-55712 ($n = 8$). Also, AGEPC reduced CBF by $15 \pm 7\%$ 60 min after intravenous indomethacin, 6 mg/kg, compared with $79 \pm 10\%$ before indomethacin ($n = 5$). These data suggested that the decrease in CBF caused by AGEPC was mediated by lipoxygenase metabolites and, particularly, cyclooxygenase metabolites of arachidonate.

To further clarify biochemical changes accompanying the coronary actions of AGEPC, we gave continuous i.c. infusions of AGEPC, 0.3 to 3 nmol/min, to 4 pigs prepared as just described. Coronary venous blood from myocardium perfused by the LAD was sampled for TXB_2, 6-keto-$PGF_{1\alpha}$, and leukotriene C_4 immunoreactivity (LTC_4-ir) (radioimmunoassay, RIA). Hemodynamic responses were qualitatively similar to those described for bolus AGEPC administration. At maximal reduction in CBF (after 2–4 min of AGEPC infusion), plasma TXB_2 was significantly elevated to an equal degree in arterial and coronary venous samples (Table 1). Plasma 6-keto-prostaglandin $F_{1\alpha}$ tended to be somewhat higher in the coronary vein, and arteriovenous difference for this substance tended to increase with AGEPC administration. Plasma LTC_4-ir levels were low prior to AGEPC and did not change significantly in response to AGEPC infusion.

The data presented here indicate that AGEPC is a potent vasoactive substance that affects the coronary circulation in a complex manner. The initial coronary vasodilation that we observed was not significantly affected by FPL-55712 or indomethacin and thus seems unrelated to arachidonate metabolism. Of particular interest is the ability of AGEPC to cause later reduction in CBF, reaching the point of regional myocardial ischemia in high doses. Marked attenuation of AGEPC-mediated CBF reduction by indomethacin and rises in plasma TXB_2 associated with AGEPC administration suggest that AGEPC-induced increase in TXA_2 release may play an important role in coronary constriction due to AGEPC. Enhanced prostacyclin release into coronary vessels may also modulate AGEPC responses. Effects of FPL-55712 and data relating to LTC_4-ir suggest that leukotrienes play a lesser role in the coronary actions of AGEPC.

TABLE 1. *Effects of AGEPC on coronary eicosanoid levels (ng/ml)*

	TXB_2		6-Keto-prostaglandin $F_{1\alpha}$		LTC_4-ir	
	A	V	A	V	A	V
Baseline	0.72 ± 0.30	0.73 ± 0.18	0.48 ± 0.09	0.87 ± 0.41	1.2 ± 1.2	0.2 ± 0.2
AGEPC[b]	2.15 ± 0.69^a	2.78 ± 0.48^a	0.92 ± 0.34	2.88 ± 1.22	0.9 ± 0.1	0.6 ± 0.2

[a]Significant at $p < 0.05$ compared with pre-AGEPC baseline values (Student's t-test for paired data).
[b]At 0.3–3 nmol/min, i.c.
These results were obtained in 4 pigs. Data are given as mean $\pm$ standard error.
Abbreviations: A = arterial plasma concentration; V = venous plasma concentration.

In conclusion, our findings support the possibility that AGEPC released from activated WBC or platelets aggregating on injured coronary vessels or, alternatively, responding to IgE-mediated immune mechanisms may severely compromise myocardial perfusion with important deleterious consequences for electrical stability and mechanical performance of the heart.

REFERENCES

1. Demopoulous, C. A., Pinckard R. N., and Hanahan, D. J. (1979): Platelet-activating factor. Evidence for 1-*O*-alkyl-2-acetyl-*sn*-glyceryl-3-phosphorylcholine as the active component (a new class of lipid chemical mediators). *J. Biol. Chem.*, 254:9355–9358.
2. Ezra, D., Boyd, L. M., Feuerstein, G., and Goldstein, R. E. (1983): Coronary constriction by leukotriene C_4, D_4, and E_4 in the intact pig heart. *Am. J. Cardiol.*, 51:1451–1454.
3. Voelkel, N. G., Worthen, J. T., Henson, P. M., and Murphy, R. C. (1982): Nonimmunologic production of leukotrienes induced by platelet-activating factor. *Science*, 218:286–288.

Advances in Prostaglandin, Thromboxane, and
Leukotriene Research, Vol. 13, edited by G. G. Neri
Serneri, et al. Raven Press, New York © 1985.

Redox Metabolism Regulation in Normal and Metabolically Altered Human Platelets

*A. Bosia, *D. Ghigo, *F. Bussolino, *S. Treves,
*G. P. Pescarmona, **P. Spangenberg, and **U. Till

*Cattedra di Chimica e Propedeutica Biochimica, Istituto di Igiene, Università di Torino,
10126 Torino, Italy; and **Department of Pathological Biochemistry, Medical Academy,
Erfurt, Democratic Republic of Germany

Two distinct enzymatic pathways exist for the oxygenation of arachidonic acid (AA) in platelets. AA is converted into thromboxane A_2 by the cyclooxygenase pathway, and into 12-HETE (12-hydroxy-5,8,10,14-eicosatetraenoic acid) by the lipoxygenase pathway.

The membrane-bound prostaglandin (PG) endoperoxide synthetase displays both cyclooxygenase $(20:4 + 2O_2 \rightarrow PGG_2)$ and peroxidase $(PGG_2 + AH_2 \rightarrow PGH_2 + A + H_2O)$ activity. The enzyme displays maximal oxygenase activity within seconds after substrate addition and is then irreversibly inactivated after a few minutes. This self-catalyzed inactivation represents a negative control mechanism (4). Enzyme self-destruction is enhanced under conditions that permit the accumulation of the 15-hydroperoxy intermediate PGG_2, and, conversely, is diminished if rapid PGG_2 reduction occurs (5). The reducing cofactor in the PG–peroxidase reaction has not yet been identified, while glutathione (GSH) is the reducing agent of 12-hydroperoxy-5,8,10,14-eicosatetraenoic acid (12-HPETE) to 12-hydroxy-5,8,10,14-eicosatetraenoic acid (12-HETE) in the lipoxygenase pathway (1).

Our previous results showed that during AA-induced aggregation a fast and reversible decrease in GSH and NADPH levels and a powerful activation of the hexosemonophosphate (HMP) shunt occur (6): GSH is regenerated via the NADPH-dependent GSH-reductase, and NADPH is formed by the HMP shunt.

The results of the present work indicate that NADPH may provide the reducing power for the peroxidase activity of prostaglandin endoperoxide synthetase.

HMP SHUNT REGULATION IN PLATELETS

Two steps in AA catabolism are potentially NADPH-consuming, namely, the peroxidase activity of the prostaglandin endoperoxide synthetase and the GSH-dependent 12-HPETE peroxidase in the 12-lipoxygenase pathway. Addition of AA to platelets lowers NADPH levels (6). This is immediately opposed by stimulation of glucose-6-phosphate dehydrogenase (G6PD) and 6-phosphogluconate dehydrogenase, the NADPH-producing steps of HMP shunt.

In order to check the dependence of G6PD on NADP⁺/NADPH ratio, we incubated platelet-rich plasma at different methylene blue concentrations, which led to a dose-dependent oxidation of NADPH (Fig. 1). Under these conditions the NADP⁺/NADPH ratio increases and a stimulation of HMP shunt occurs. The rate of platelet intracellular G6PD, as determined by HMP shunt rates at different concentrations of methylene blue, varies with the observed NADP⁺/NADPH ratio in a linear manner. These results show that G6PD is the rate-limiting enzyme of HMP shunt, and the NADP⁺/NADPH ratio is the major modulator of G6PD activity in platelets. Resting platelets use only 0,5‰ of V_{max} of G6PD, and this is sufficient to maintain the NADP pool 99% reduced: the cells have a large potential for stepping up the G6PD rate in case of need, for instance in case of AA oxidative metabolism. AA-induced aggregation was measured after 10 min preincubation with different methylene blue concentrations (Fig. 1). The extent of aggregation decreases with decreasing NADPH levels: the rate of AA consumption appears to be limited by the availability of the electron donor.

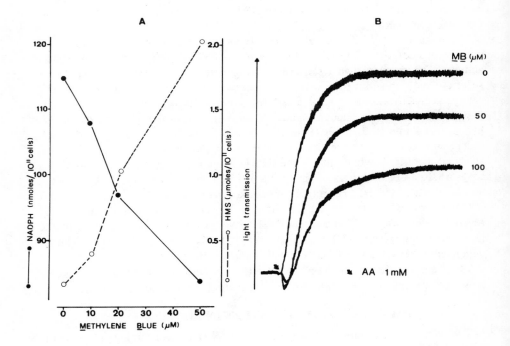

FIG. 1.   A: NADPH levels (nmoles/10¹¹ cells) and hexose monophosphate shunt (HMS) activity (μmoles glucose/10¹¹ cells) in human platelet-rich plasma after 15 min incubation at different methylene blue (MB) concentrations. NADPH was estimated by enzymatic recycling (6). Activity of the HMS was determined from the amount of ¹⁴CO₂ evolved during incubation of the platelet-rich plasma with [1-¹⁴C]glucose (6).   **B:** Arachidonic acid (AA, 1 mM) induced aggregation after 10 min preincubation of platelet-rich plasma with different methylene blue (MB) concentrations.

ROLE OF NADPH IN ARACHIDONIC ACID
OXIDATIVE METABOLISM

The role of NADPH as a reducing cofactor in the cyclooxygenase pathway is stressed by the results shown in Fig. 2. In the range 0.3 to 2.0 mM, AA stimulates HMP shunt in a dose-dependent manner. A large portion of the AA-mediated stimulation of the HMP shunt is inhibited by 0.4 mM acetylsalicylic acid (ASA), a concentration that selectively blocks the oxygenase activity of the prostaglandin endoperoxide synthetase. ASA had no effect on the stimulation of HMP shunt following the oxidation of GSH by diamide and *t*-butyl hydroperoxide (data not shown). The ASA-sensitive and the ASA-insensitive HMP shunt fluxes show a

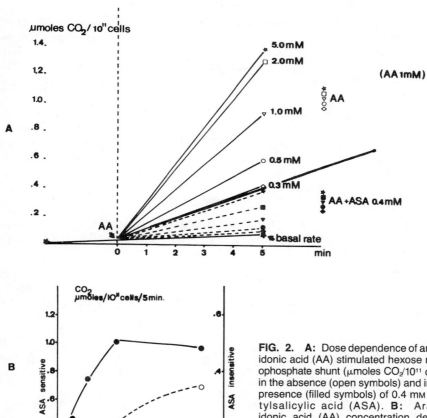

FIG. 2. A: Dose dependence of arachidonic acid (AA) stimulated hexose monophosphate shunt (μmoles $CO_2/10^{11}$ cells) in the absence (open symbols) and in the presence (filled symbols) of 0.4 mM acetylsalicylic acid (ASA). **B:** Arachidonic acid (AA) concentration dependence of ASA-sensitive and ASA-insensitive hexose monophosphate shunt fluxes.

different behavior in front of AA concentrations (Fig. 2), pointing to different NADPH-consuming enzymes (PG-peroxidase and GSH-dependent peroxidase activity of lipoxygenase). These results indicate that NADPH may provide the reducing power for the peroxidase-catalyzed conversion of PGG_2 to PGH_2.

The role of GSH as a cosubstrate for the PG-peroxidase activity of prostaglandin endoperoxide synthetase is not clear, since PG-peroxidase has no GSH-peroxidase activity, although PGG_2 can be an active acceptor for the GSH-peroxidase (2).

As far as GSH is concerned, we demonstrated (3) that aggregation can be modulated by compounds that oxidize cellular GSH, e.g., diamide, divicine, cumene, and t-butyl hydroperoxide. When added simultaneously with one of the inducers (AA, ADP, thrombin), an accelerated and reversible aggregation is observed: the accelerating effect on aggregation can be explained by stimulation of cyclooxygenase from the hydroperoxides that accumulate under these conditions in the lipoxygenase pathway. These observations are of importance in order to interpret the enhanced dose response to ADP and AA in G6PD-deficient platelets and (b) the increased responsiveness to ADP and thrombin and the higher production of thromboxane B_2 in diabetic platelets. In both conditions, intracellular GSH level is significantly lowered.

The oxidation of GSH and NADPH by hydroperoxides in the endoplasmic reticulum was shown to release Ca^{2+} from the hepatocyte (7): this observation stresses the importance of $NADPH/NADP^+$ and GSH/GSSG redox state during AA-induced aggregation and their relevance in the Ca^{2+}-dependent mechanism of platelet activation.

ACKNOWLEDGMENTS

This study was supported by grants from National Project on Platelet Metabolism and Function, Ministero Pubblica Istruzione, Rome, Italy and from Regione Piemonte.

REFERENCES

1. Bryant, R. W., Simon, T. C., and Bailey, J. M. (1982): Role of glutathione peroxidase and hexose monophosphate shunt in the platelet lipoxygenase pathway. *J. Biol. Chem.*, 257:14937–14943.
2. Cadenas, E., Sies, H., Nastainczyk, W., and Ullrich, V. (1983): Singlet oxygen formation detected by low-level chemiluminescence during enzymatic reduction of prostaglandin G_2 to H_2. *Hoppe-Seyler's Z. Physiol. Chem.*, 364:519–528.
3. Hofmann, J., Lösche, W., Hofmann, B., Arese, P., Bosia, A., Pescarmona, G. P., and Till, U. (1983): Effect of compounds causing reversible perturbation of the cellular thiol-disulfide status on the aggregation of human blood platelets. *Biomed. Biochim. Acta*, 42:479–487.
4. Lands, W. E. M. (1981): Control of prostaglandin biosynthesis. *Prog. Lipid Res.*, 20:875–883.
5. Ohki, S., Ogino, N., Yamamoto, S., and Hayaishi, O. (1979): Prostaglandin hydroperoxidase, an integral part of prostaglandin endoperoxide synthetase from bovine vesicular gland microsomes. *J. Biol. Chem.*, 254:829–836.
6. Pescarmona, G. P., Bosia, A., Hofmann, J., Lösche, W., Arese, P., and Till, U. (1981): Effect of arachidonic acid on the hexose monophosphate shunt and related coenzymes in human blood platelets. *Acta Biol. Med. Germ.*, 40:7–14.
7. Sies, H., Graf, P., and Estrela, J. M. (1981): Hepatic calcium efflux during cytochrome P-450-dependent drug oxidations at the endoplasmic reticulum in intact liver. *Proc. Natl. Acad. Sci. U.S.A.*, 78:3358–3362.

Advances in Prostaglandin, Thromboxane, and Leukotriene Research, Vol. 13, edited by G.G. Neri Serneri, et al. Raven Press, New York © 1985.

Role of Prostaglandins in Microcirculatory Function

Gabor Kaley, Thomas H. Hintze, Maret Panzenbeck, and Edward J. Messina

Department of Physiology, New York Medical College, Valhalla, New York 10595

The concept that prostaglandins and related metabolites of arachidonic acid are local regulators of the microcirculation is one that has been investigated extensively for the past fifteen years. It is based on the observations that the administration of both locally synthesized prostaglandins or prostaglandin synthesis inhibitors is capable of profoundly changing microvascular tone and reactivity in various vascular beds and species (23,25,37). Since little, if any, prostaglandin is detected in arterial blood, largely because of efficient pulmonary destruction (34), prostaglandins must be considered local hormones that are synthesized at, or near, their site of action (19). Although a variety of hormones and pharmacologic agents will cause an increase in the synthesis of prostaglandins, precisely what concentrations of vaso-active prostaglandins must be achieved in and around small blood vessels to affect local blood flow is a question that has not yet been answered. The wealth of evidence that has accumulated within the past few years, however, strongly suggests that the release of prostaglandins from small blood vessels is perhaps a universal feature of the response of these tissues to different stimuli and interventions and might constitute an important aspect of the regulation of microvascular function (13,14). Thus, alterations in intrinsic prostaglandin synthesis have been implicated in the mediation of a variety of physiological and pathophysiological responses of the microvasculature and in the pathogenesis of some common disorders (Table 1). For example, a reduction in the synthesis and/or responsiveness to the dilator prostaglandin E_2 and prostacyclin has been suggested to have a primary role in the development of essential hypertension (16). Similarly, increased platelet thromboxane synthesis (8) and decreased vascular prostacyclin synthesis (1) have been found in patients with diabetes mellitus.

PROSTAGLANDINS AND REGULATION OF LOCAL BLOOD FLOW

Circulating prostaglandins (PG) [primarily prostacyclin (PGI_2)] and prostaglandins synthesized within endothelial cells of small blood vessels (primarily PGI_2 and PGE_2) are powerful vasodilator agents in the heart (28), kidney (20), and skeletal muscle (25) of most species examined. The increase in blood flow after

TABLE 1. *Role of metabolites of arachidonic acid in the regulation of the microcirculation*

Physiological role	Pathological role
Vascular tone	Hypertension
Vascular reactivity	Vascular spasm
Autoregulation	Diabetes
Sympathetic nerve activity	Circulatory shock
Vasomotion	Peripheral vascular disease
Exchange	Inflammation
Lymphatic vessels	
Blood viscosity	Thrombotic disorders
Platelet-vessel wall interactions	

their administration or the administration of their precursor, arachidonic acid, is due principally to a dilation of arterioles (Fig. 1). Furthermore, it was shown that in mesenteric and cremasteric circulation of rats PGE_1 and PGE_2 antagonize, and in some instances completely inhibit, the constrictor action of a variety of pressor hormones, including norepinephrine, angiotensin, and vasopressin. This reduction in vascular responsiveness to constrictor agents often lasts long after the abating of the vasodilation to E-prostaglandins (25). It is important to emphasize that this unique modulating effect of PGE_1 and PGE_2 is not exerted by PGI_2 (21), even though the threshold concentration for dilation of third and fourth order arterioles (10–25 μm internal diameter) in rat skeletal muscle is significantly lower for PGI_2 than for PGE_2 (4,21). It is also possible that in certain organs dilator prostaglandins contribute to the maintenance of basal blood flow. For example, in skeletal muscle, inhibitors of prostaglandin synthesis reduce significantly resting arteriolar diameters and increase arteriolar vasomotion frequency, influencing tissue blood flow directly (3). Also, prostaglandin synthesis blockade enhances the responses to norepinephrine (24,39) and angiotensin (24) substantiating the hypothesis that vasodilator prostaglandins contribute, especially in the skeletal muscle circulation, to the regulation of vascular tone. There seems to be general agreement that resistance vessels of experimentally hypertensive animals possess a decreased threshold as well as an exaggerated constrictor responsiveness to sympathetic stimulation and vasopressor agents. On the basis of all of the above, one could postulate that either a decreased response to or a reduced capacity of blood vessels to synthesize vasodepressor prostaglandins is, at least partially, responsible for the increased vascular resistance characteristic of hypertensive states (17). A change in the reactivity of arterioles of experimentally diabetic rats to norepinephrine is also likely to be related to an altered vascular prostaglandin metabolism (27).

The interaction between prostaglandins and the sympathetic nervous system, however, goes far beyond the postjunctional modulation of responsiveness of blood vessels to norepinephrine. There is also considerable evidence to indicate that in a variety of tissues prostaglandins are formed when sympathetic nerves are activated

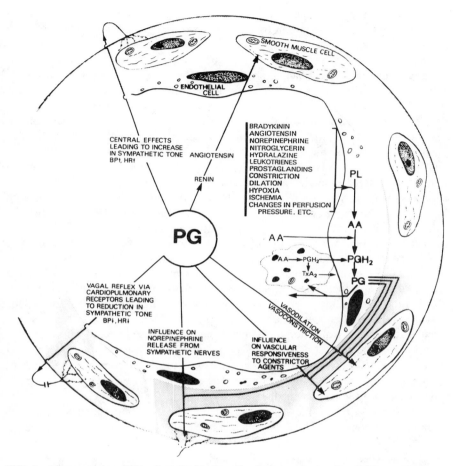

FIG. 1. Microvascular effects of prostaglandins. Circulating prostaglandins (PG) as well as those synthesized from arachidonic acid (AA) in platelets, endothelial cells, and underlying structures can influence arteriolar smooth muscle directly or indirectly resulting in changes in vascular tone and reactivity. PL = phospholipid.

and that, in turn, they inhibit norepinephrine release (9). For example, in the isolated, perfused kidney of the rabbit, PGE_2 attenuates, and inhibition of prostaglandin synthesis enhances, the vasoconstrictor responses to sympathetic nerve stimulation (18). Interestingly, the concentration of PGE_2 needed to inhibit the vasoconstriction is at least an order of magnitude lower than that which causes vasodilation. This suggests that the physiological role of prostaglandins in the regulation of microcirculatory blood flow might reside primarily in their capacity to reduce sympathetically-mediated vasoconstriction, rather than in their ability to relax vascular smooth muscle directly. Additional support for the latter is provided by recent studies showing that in skeletal muscle of rats both arteriolar constriction and augmentation of vasomotion by indomethacin were significantly blunted by α-adrenergic blockade (3).

Prostaglandins are synthesized in all types of blood vessels, primarily in endothelial cells (38). The principal prostaglandin made in large conduit-type vessels including the aorta, of most species examined thus far, is PGI_2. In contrast, microvessels and microvascular endothelial cells (e.g., those derived from myocardium of rabbit or cerebral cortex of cow) exhibit pathways of arachidonate metabolism that are quite different; thus from small vessels, both under basal and stimulated conditions, the release of PGE exceeds that of 6-keto-$PGF_{1\alpha}$ (the principal hydrolytic product of PGI_2) (6). Based on all of the foregoing, it is tempting to speculate that the regulation of vascular tone and blood flow by small blood vessels is under the control of locally released PGE_2, rather than PGI_2. In line with this concept, the major actions of circulating and locally formed PGI_2 are directed primarily, but not exclusively, toward platelet aggregation and platelet-vessel wall interactions (2,19), whereas those of PGE_2 are directed toward the modulation of vascular tone and reactivity to and release of norepinephrine (9,10,25).

Local release of prostaglandins from blood vessels occurs in response to a large variety of stimuli, including hormones, diverse pharmacologic agents, and changes in physiological conditions (Fig. 1) via stimulation of phospholipases. Whether the increase in the local concentration of prostaglandins has any relevance to the actual vascular response is a question that cannot, in all cases, be answered with certainty. Bradykinin-induced dilator responses of skeletal muscle arterioles (24) or renal blood vessels (20) are antagonized, and in some instances completely abolished, by inhibitors of prostaglandin synthesis. These results can be interpreted to mean that dilator prostaglandins mediate, in large part, the response to bradykinin. However, this is not a universal phenomenon since within the heart no such mediation is discernible (11). Prostaglandin release has also been shown to modulate the vascular response to angiotensin (24) and norepinephrine (18), and to mediate the renal blood flow response to hydralazine (36). However, the increase in prostaglandin synthesis after the local, intracoronary administration of nitroglycerin is of questionable significance since indomethacin does not affect the response of the coronary circulation to the drug (32). Nonspecific stimulation of phospholipase(s) by physical forces (e.g., changes in intramural tension), through perturbation of cell membranes or changes in the ionic or biochemical milieu, can also significantly influence microvascular function. Thus, the increase in blood flow following occlusion of single arterioles in rat skeletal muscle is considerably attenuated by inhibitors of prostaglandin synthesis (26). In contrast, in the heart, reactive hyperemic responses are not mediated by prostaglandins (11,28). Evidently, the involvement of prostaglandins in the regulation of local blood flow is tissue specific.

Recent studies also implicated some products of the lipoxygenase pathway of arachidonate metabolism as having an influence on microvascular function. Leukotriene (LT) B_4 was shown to stimulate leukocyte migration, and LTC_4 and LTD_4 to increase microvascular permeability (35). In addition, LTC_4 and LTD_4 were reported to have considerable effects on vascular tone. Unlike PGE_2 and PGI_2, however, they constrict rat skeletal muscle arterioles (22) and reduce coronary blood flow in dogs (33). To what extent these lipoxygenase products are produced in resistance vessels and to what extent they participate in the moment-to-moment regulation of vascular tone are yet to be determined. There is also little, if any, information available concerning the existence of a nonprostaglandin, "endothelium-dependent" relaxation or dilation in resistance vessels. There is considerable evidence to indicate that dilation of large blood vessels *in vitro*, to a variety of endogenously-produced hormones and drugs, requires an intact endothelium (5). Even the relaxation to arachidonic acid of some vessels was shown to be endothelium dependent. Interestingly, however, none of these responses is blocked by indomethacin, indicating that prostaglandins are not involved in the response. However, the data are consistent with the idea that stimulated endothelial cells release a labile, oxidation product of arachidonic acid that then relaxes vascular smooth muscle via stimulation of guanylate cyclase (5). If the endothelium-dependent relaxing factor(s) (EDRF) is a product of arachidonic acid, and if, in fact, it has a role in the regulation of resistance vessels *in vivo*, then one would expect that it would be formed in endothelial cells and have a role in the vasodilation that follows the administration of arachidonic acid. However, in the microcirculation of heart or skeletal muscle blockade of cyclooxygenase completely abolishes the arachidonic acid-induced vasodilation (11,12). This argues against the existence of nonprostaglandin, endothelium-dependent vasodilation in resistance vessels or a significant role for arachidonic acid in the generation of EDRF. In summary, it is unlikely that products of arachidonic acid metabolism, other than those synthesized via cyclooxygenase, have a major role in the physiological regulation of local blood flow.

CONTROL OF BLOOD PRESSURE BY PROSTAGLANDINS

Considerable progress has been achieved since the discovery that blood vessels synthesize and release vasoactive prostaglandins. Quite aside from their local function they have also been implicated in the control of cardiovascular reflex activity and systemic blood pressure (Fig. 1). For example, the cardiopulmonary administration of relatively small doses of PGI_2 (and PGE_2 in somewhat larger amounts) or the increase in myocardial prostaglandin synthesis after the intracoronary administration of arachidonic acid causes reflex hypotension and bradycardia in dogs (12), effects that are eliminated by sectioning afferent vagal fibers. The reflex hypotension results primarily from vasodilation in kidney and skeletal muscle. Furthermore, the slowing of the heart and the reduction in peripheral resistance are accompanied by an increase in cardiac output and a decrease in left ventricular *dP/dt*. The chemically-sensitive receptors that are responsible for these reflex effects are found in the posterior wall of the left ventricle. It is tempting to speculate that in certain physiologic or pathophysiologic conditions in various species, including humans, sufficiently high concentrations of prostaglandins could be produced in the vicinity of these receptors to cause modulation of blood flow in skeletal muscle and kidney. Reports in the literature also indicate that in a variety of species central (intracarotid) administration of PGE_2 causes a paradoxical pressor response. The PGE_2 pressor effect occurs primarily through increased sympathetic outflow resulting in an elevation of regional vascular resistances, but depending on the species may also have a renin–angiotensin or vasopressin component (31). Critical investigations are still necessary to determine whether the effects of PGE_2 on the central nervous system regulation of blood pressure are of any importance in animals or humans. There is also considerable evidence that implicates prostaglandins in the regulation of renal renin release. It is likely that PGI_2 and/or its active, more stable metabolite, 6-keto-PGE_1, is responsible for the renin release following administration, *in vitro* or *in vivo*, of arachidonic acid (19). However, it is uncertain which specific signal, among the many that control renin release, is affected by prostaglandins; nor is it known whether the role of prostaglandins is direct or indirect (30). Nonetheless, one cannot preclude the possibility that a prostaglandin-induced increase in the activity of the renin–angiotensin system contributes to the regulation of vascular tone and blood pressure.

Because prostaglandins, especially PGE_2, play an important role in the functioning of the sympathetic nervous system and in the control of local vascular reactivity to norepinephrine (7), it was of considerable interest to ascertain whether they might not also participate in the control of systemic blood pressure induced by a generalized increase in sympathetic activity. To this end, we recently investigated the effects of inhibitors of prostaglandin synthesis (indomethacin and meclofenamate) on the increase in sympathetic tone caused by carotid sinus hypotension by bilateral carotid occlusion (BCO) in anesthetized dogs. Results of our studies show that inhibition of prostaglandin synthesis causes a significant enhancement of the increases in arterial pressures and peripheral resistance to BCO normally seen (Fig. 2). Prostaglandins, therefore, may play a role in the control of systemic arterial pressure by the regulation of carotid baroreflex sensitivity. Further, it has been demonstrated that in humans, following sympathetic stimulation by the application of cold indomethacin, while decreasing PGE_2 levels, significantly increased plasma norepinephrine concentration and forearm vascular resistance, compared with control periods (29). These findings suggest that in humans PGE_2 may be involved in the modulation of sympathetic responses of resistance vessels. In other experiments, blockade of prostaglandin synthesis with indomethacin in dogs significantly attenuated vasodepressor responses to infusions of nitroglycerin. However, in dogs with α-receptor blockade, indomethacin actually intensified the fall in blood pressure to the drug (15). All of these findings are consistent with the notion that prostaglandins (primarily PGE_2) contribute to the reflex control of blood pressure. Inhibition of prostaglandin synthesis could enhance neuronal release of norepinephrine and at the same time increase the sensitivity of vascular smooth muscle to the released norepinephrine and other vasoconstrictor hormones. Thus, it is possible that modulation of sympathetic nervous system function is the primary avenue through which prostaglandins control cardiovascular responses.

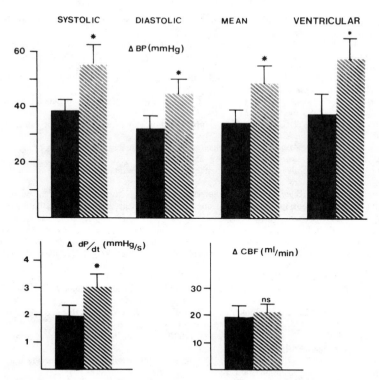

FIG. 2. Effects of inhibition of prostaglandin synthesis on cardiovascular function. In anesthetized dogs with heart rate kept constant by pacing, changes in blood pressure (BP), ventricular pressure, LV *dP/dt*, and coronary blood flow (CBF) are shown during bilateral carotid artery occlusion before *(solid bars)* and after *(striped bars)* inhibition of prostaglandin synthesis with indomethacin. With the exception of CBF, the actual increases in BP and *dP/dt* in response to carotid artery occlusion are significantly greater after indomethacin than before. Units of *dP/dt* in 1000 mm Hg/sec. *$p = <0.05$; ns = not significant.

ACKNOWLEDGMENTS

This work was supported in part by grants from the NHLBI, the American Heart Association and the Westchester Heart Association. We thank Dr. John Pike of the Upjohn Company for the continuous and generous supply of prostaglandins.

REFERENCES

1. Dollery, C. T., Freidman, L. A., Hensby, C. N., et al. (1979): Circulating prostacyclin may be reduced in diabetes. *Lancet*, 2:1365.
2. Dusting, G. J., Moncada, S., Mullane, K. M., and Vane, J. R. (1978): Implications of prostacyclin generation for modulation of vascular tone. *Clin. Sci. Mol. Med.*, 55(Suppl.):195–198.
3. Faber, J. E., Harris, P. D., and Joshua, I. G. (1982): Microvascular response to blockade of prostaglandin synthesis in rat skeletal muscle. *Am. J. Physiol.*, 243:H51–60.
4. Faber, J. E., Harris, P. D., and Miller, F. N. (1982): Microvascular sensitivity to PGE$_2$ and PGI$_2$ in skeletal muscle of decerebrate rat. *Am. J. Physiol.*, 243:H844–851.

5. Furchgott, R. F. (1984): The role of endothelium in the responses of vascular smooth muscle to drugs. *Ann. Rev. Pharmacol. Toxicol.*, 24:175–197.
6. Gerritsen, M. E., and Cheli, C. D. (1983): Arachidonic acid and prostaglandin endoperoxide metabolism in isolated rabbit and coronary microvessels and isolated and cultivated coronary microvessel endothelial cells. *J. Clin. Invest.*, 72:1658–1671.
7. Güllner, H.-G. (1983): The interactions of prostaglandins with the sympathetic nervous system—a review. *J. Autonomic Nervous System*, 8:1–12.
8. Halushka, P. V., Rogers, R. C., Loadholt, C. B., et al. (1981): Increased platelet thromboxane synthesis in diabetes mellitus. *J. Lab. Clin. Med.*, 97:87–96.
9. Hedqvist, P. (1977): Basic mechanisms of prostaglandin action on autonomic neurotransmission. *Ann. Rev. Pharmacol. Toxicol.*, 17:259–279.
10. Hedqvist, P. (1979): Actions of prostaglandin (PGI_2) on adrenergic neuroeffector transmission in the rabbit kidney. *Prostaglandins*, 17:249–250.
11. Hintze, T. H., and Kaley, G. (1977): Prostaglandins and the control of blood flow in the canine myocardium. *Circ. Res.*, 40:313–320.
12. Hintze, T. H., and Kaley, G. (1984): Ventricular receptors activated following myocardial prostaglandin synthesis initiate reflex hypotension, reduction in heart rate, and redistribution of cardiac output in the dog. *Circ. Res.*, 54:239–247.
13. Kaley, G. (1976): The role of prostaglandins in vascular hemeostasis. *Fed. Proc.*, 35:2358–2359.
14. Kaley, G. (1979): Microcirculatory-endocrine interactions: Role of prostaglandins. In: *Microcirculation, Volume 3*, edited by G. Kaley and B. M. Altura, pp. 503–529. University Park Press, Baltimore.
15. Kaley, G., Panzenbeck, M. J., and Baez, A. (1983): Prostaglandin contribution to the vasodepressor response to nitrates is abolished by alpha-receptor blockade in dogs. *Fed. Proc.*, (Abstr.) 42:500.
16. Lee, J. B., Patak, R. V., and Mookerjee, B. K. (1976): Renal prostaglandins and the regulation of blood pressure and sodium and water hemeostasis. *Am. J. Med.*, 70:798–816.
17. Lukacsko, P., Messina, E. J., and Kaley, G. (1980): Reduced hypotensive action of arachidonic acid in the spontaneously hypertensive rat. *Hypertension*, 2:657–663.
18. Malik, K. U., and McGiff, J. C. (1975): Modulation by prostaglandins of adrenergic transmission in the isolated perfused rabbit and rat kidney. *Circ. Res.*, 36:599–609.
19. McGiff, J. C. (1981): Prostaglandins, prostacyclin, and thromboxanes. *Ann. Rev. Pharmacol. Toxicol.*, 21:479–509.
20. McGiff, J. C., Malik, K. U., and Terragno, N. A. (1976): Prostaglandins as determinants of vascular reactivity. *Fed. Proc.*, 35:2382–2387.
21. Messina, E. J., and Kaley, G. (1980): Microcirculatory responses to prostacycline (PGI_2) and PGE_2 in the rat cremaster muscle. In: *Advances in Prostaglandin and Thromboxane Research, Volume 7*, edited by B. Samuelsson, P. W. Ramwell, and R. Paoletti, pp. 719–722. Raven Press, New York.
22. Messina, E. J., Rodenberg, J., and Kaley, G. (1984): Leukotrienes constrict rat cremaster arterioles. *Microvasc. Res.* (Abstr.), 27:256.
23. Messina, E. J., Weiner, R., and Kaley, G. (1974): Microcirculatory effects of prostaglandins E_1, E_2 and A_2 in the rat mesentery and cremaster muscle. *Microvasc. Res.*, 8:77–89.
24. Messina, E. J., Weiner, R., and Kaley, G. (1975): Inhibition of bradykinin vasodilation and potentiation of norepinephrine and angiotensin vasoconstriction by inhibition of prostaglandin synthesis in skeletal muscle of the rat. *Circ. Res.*, 37:430–437.
25. Messina, E. J., Weiner, R., and Kaley, G. (1976): Prostaglandins and local circulatory control. *Fed. Proc.*, 35:2357–2375.
26. Messina, E. J., Weiner, R. and Kaley, G. (1977): Arteriolar reactive hyperemia: Modification by inhibitors of prostaglandin synthesis. *Am. J. Physiol.*, 232:H571–575.
27. Myers, T. O., and Messina, E. J., (1982): Altered microcirculatory reactivity to norepinephrine in diabetes. *Microvasc. Res.* (Abstr.), 41:1760.
28. Needleman, P. J. and Kaley, G. (1978): Cardiac and coronary prostaglandin synthesis and function. *N. Engl. J. Med.*, 298:1122–1128.
29. Neri-Serneri, G. G., Masotti, G., Castellani, S., Scarti, L., Trotta, F., and Manelli, M. (1983): Role of PGE_2 in the modulation of the adrenergic response in man. *Cardiovasc. Res.*, 17:662–670.

30. Oates, J. A., Whorton, A. R., Gerkens, J. F., Branch, R. A., Hollifield, S. W., and Frölich, J. C. (1979): The participation of prostaglandins in the control of renin release. *Fed. Proc.*, 38:72–74.
31. Okuno, T., Lindheimer, M. D., and Oparil, S. (1982): Central effects of prostaglandin E_2 on blood pressure and plasma renin activity. *Hypertension*, 4:809–816.
32. Panzenbeck, M. J., Baez, A., and Kaley, G. (1984): Nitroglycerin and nitroprusside increase coronary blood flow in dogs by a mechanism independent of prostaglandin release. *Am. J. Cardiol.*, 53:936–940.
33. Panzenbeck, M. J., and Kaley, G. (1983): Leukotriene D_4 reduces coronary blood flow in the anesthetized dog. *Prostaglandins*, 25:661–670.
34. Piper, P., and Vane, J. (1971): The release of prostaglandins from lung and other tissues. *Ann. NY Acad. Sci.*, 180:363–385.
35. Samuelsson, B. (1982): The leukotrienes: An introduction. In: *Leukotrienes and Other Lipoxygenase Products*, edited by B. Samuelsson and R. Paoletti, pp. 1–17. Raven Press, New York.
36. Spokas, E. G., and Wang. H. H. (1980): Regional blood flow and cardiac responses to hydralazine. *J. Pharmacol. Exp. Ther.*, 212:294–303.
37. Vane, J. R., and McGiff, J. C. (1975): Possible contribution of endogenous prostaglandins to the control of blood pressure. *Circ. Res.*, 36–37(Suppl. I):168–176.
38. Weksler, B. B., Marcus, A. J., and Jaffe, E. A. (1977): Synthesis of prostaglandin I_2 (prostacyclin) by cultured human and bovine endothelial cells. *Proc. Natl. Acad. Sci. U.S.A.*, 74:3922–3926.
39. Zimmerman, B. G., Ryan, M. J., Gomez, S., and Kraft, E. (1973): Effect of the prostaglandin synthesis inhibitors indomethacin and eicosa 5-8-11-14 tetraynoic acid on adrenergic responses in dog cutaneous vasculature. *J. Pharmacol. Exp. Ther.*, 187:315–323.

Advances in Prostaglandin, Thromboxane, and Leukotriene Research, Vol. 13, edited by G. G. Neri Serneri, et al. Raven Press, New York © 1985.

The Phospholipase C Diglyceride Lipase Pathway Contributes to Arachidonic Acid Release and Prostaglandin E_2 Formation in Platelet-Derived Growth Factor Stimulated Swiss 3T3 Cells

Andreas J. R. Habenicht, Matthias Goerig, Jürgen Grulich, Dietrich Rothe, Rainer Gronwald, Gotthard Schettler, and Burkhard Kommerell

University of Heidelberg, Medical School, 6900 Heidelberg, Federal Republic of Germany

There is considerable uncertainty about the relative contribution of the phospholipase C diglyceride lipase pathway versus phospholipase A_2 for arachidonic acid (AA) release from membrane phospholipids (1–3). We have previously demonstrated a platelet-derived growth factor (PDGF) sensitive phospholipase C diglyceride lipase pathway in cultured Swiss 3T3 cells (2). In order to obtain further evidence for a role of this pathway in prostaglandin (PG) synthesis, we looked for ways to pharmacologically activate phospholipase C.

Swiss 3T3 cells were cultured as described (2). Before incubation of the quiescent cells with PDGF, cellular lipids were biosynthetically prelabeled with either [^{3}H]glycerol or [^{14}C]arachidonic acid (AA). NaF at concentrations between 0.5 and 5 mM enhanced the effect of PDGF on 1,2-diglyceride accumulation by 80 to 100% (Fig. 1). Concomitantly, NaF stimulated release of monoacylglycerol and AA, the two hydrolytic products of diglyceride lipase (Fig. 2, A and B). Furthermore, NaF stimulated formation of PGE_2 as determined by radioimmunoassay (RIA) (Fig. 2C). While no effect of NaF on hydrolysis of phosphatidylcholine, phosphatidylethanolamine, lysophosphatidylcholine, or phosphatidic acid and only a small effect on triglyceride in [^{3}H]glycerol-prelabeled cells could be detected, NaF greatly stimulated phosphatidylinositol hydrolysis. Direct evidence of diglyceride lipase activity in Swiss 3T3 cell homogenates was obtained by the demonstration of generation of the two hydrolytic products of diglyceride lipase *in vitro* using 1-palmitoyl-[2-^{14}C]-arachidonoyl-diglyceride, as shown in Fig. 3.

In summary, our results indicate that the phospholipase C diglyceride lipase pathway contributes to AA release and PGE_2 biosynthesis in PDGF-stimulated Swiss 3T3 cells.

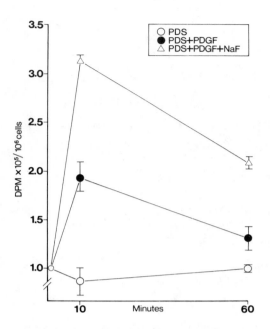

FIG. 1. Effect of NaF on 1,2-diglyceride formation in PDGF-stimulated Swiss 3T3 cells. Swiss 3T3 cells were cultured as described (2). At 48 hr before the beginning of the experiment, cellular lipids were prelabeled by incubating the cultures with [³H]glycerol at 6 μCi/ml (New England Nuclear, Boston, Mass.). Before addition of the growth factor and NaF, the culture medium was removed and the cell monolayer was washed three times with 2 ml phosphate buffered saline. At the beginning of the experiment the cultures were divided into three groups and either received PDGF at 15 ng/ml dissolved in 50 μl 10 mM acetic acid (●) or PDGF at 15 ng/ml and 5 mM NaF (△) or 50 μl 10 mM acetic acid (○). At the time points indicated in the figure, radioactivity in cellular diglyceride was determined as described (2). Data points represent means of three parallel cultures ± SD. PDS = plasma-derived serum.

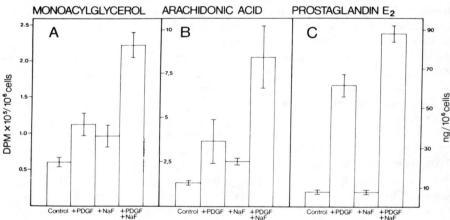

FIG. 2. Effect of NaF on monoacylglycerol and AA release and PGE₂ formation in Swiss 3T3 cells stimulated by PDGF. Swiss 3T3 cells were cultured as described (2). **A:** At 48 hr before the beginning of the experiment, cellular lipids were biosynthetically labeled with [³H]glycerol as described in Fig. 1. **B:** At 24 hr before the beginning of the experiment, cellular lipids were labeled with 1 μCi [¹⁴C] AA (New England Nuclear, Boston, Mass.). **C:** PGE₂ levels in the culture medium were determined by RIA after reversed-phase extraction and thin-layer chromatography. On day 3, the cultures were divided into four groups and either received 50 μl 10 mM acetic acid (control), PDGF at 12 ng/ml dissolved in 50 μl 10 mM acetic acid or 5 mM NaF dissolved in phosphate buffered saline, or PDGF at 12 ng/ml and NaF. At 10 min after addition of the growth factor, radioactivity in monoacylglycerol **(A)**, AA **(B)**, or the levels of PGE₂ **(C)** were determined in the culture medium. Data represent means of three parallel cultures ± SD.

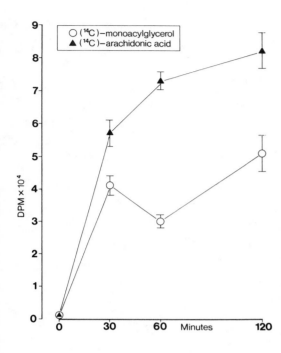

FIG. 3. Demonstration of diglyceride lipase in Swiss 3T3 cells *in vitro.* Swiss 3T3 cells were cultured as described (2). Homogenates were prepared by disruption of cells in buffer containing 10 mM Tris-HCl (pH 7.4, 0.25% sucrose, 1 mM EDTA) using a Tekmar homogenizer (Janke und Kuntzel, Staufen, FRG) at 2×10^4 rpm, six times 10 sec. Diglyceride lipase was assayed in buffer containing 300 μg 3T3 cell homogenate, 1 mg/ml bovine serum albumin (free fatty acid free, Sigma, München, FRG), 125 mM Tris-HCl, pH7.4, 10 mM $MgCl_2$, and 10.3 μM 1-palmitoyl-[2-^{14}C]arachidonoyl diglyceride in a total volume of 600 μl. The diglyceride was prepared by phospholipase C treatment (*Bacterium cereus*, Sigma Chemie, München, FRG) of 1-palmitoyl-[2-^{14}C]arachidonoyl phosphatidylcholine (New England Nuclear, Boston, Mass.). At the indicated time points, the reaction was stopped by addition of chloroform/methanol and lipids were separated by thin-layer chromatography as described (2). Data represent means of three parallel samples $\pm$ SD.

ACKNOWLEDGMENT

This work was supported by the Deutsche Forschungsgemeinschaft.

REFERENCES

1. Bell, R. L., and Majerus, P. W. (1980): Thrombin-induced hydrolysis of phosphatidylinositol in human platelets. *J. Biol. Chem.*, 255:1790–1792.
2. Habenicht, A. J. R., Glomset, J. A., King, W. C., Nist, C., Mitchell, C. D., and Ross, R. (1981): Early changes in phosphatidylinositol and arachidonic acid metabolism in quiescent Swiss 3T3 cells stimulated to divide by platelet-derived growth factor. *J. Biol. Chem.*, 256:12329–12335.
3. Lapetina, E. G., Billah, M. M., and Cuatrecasas, P. C. (1981): The phosphatidylinositol cycle and the regulation of arachidonic acid production. *Nature (Lond.)*, 292:367–369.

Advances in Prostaglandin, Thromboxane, and Leukotriene Research, Vol. 13, edited by G. G. Neri Serneri, et al. Raven Press, New York © 1985.

Development of a Radioimmunoassay for the Measurement of Prostacyclin Metabolites in Unextracted Plasma

M. McLaren, J. J. F. Belch, and C. D. Forbes

University Department of Medicine, Royal Infirmary, Glasgow, G31 2ER, Scotland

Published "normal" values of 6-keto-prostaglandin $F_{1\alpha}$ (6-keto-$PGF_{1\alpha}$) measured by radioimmunoassay (RIA) still show wide variations (2–4), making it difficult to compare work from different groups. Extraction of the test sample is an important step and, unless extensive purification is carried out after extraction, leads to a detectable level of 6-keto-$PGF_{1\alpha}$ being obtained from a distilled water blank. Because of the impracticability of this, we examined the variables involved in radioimmunoassay—incubation time and temperature, quantities of tracer and antibody used, and separation method—to try to find a sensitive and reproducible method for use in unextracted plasma. We found that only by reducing the total counts to 3,000 cpm and lowering the final dilution of antibody from 1:17,500 to 1:35,000 could we bring the normal pool plasma within the limits of detection of the assay.

Using gas chromatography–mass spectometry (GC-MS), very low levels (<2 pg/ml) of 6-keto-$PGF_{1\alpha}$ have been reported (1), and as this is generally undetectable using radioimmunoassay the method is currently receiving much criticism. However, only $<50\%$ of prostacyclin (PGI_2) is metabolised into 6-keto-$PGF_{1\alpha}$, with little work being published on the remainder.

We suggest that a method that measures PGI_2 metabolites on unextracted plasma may be the best method to give an overall picture. Using our methodology we have obtained a sensitivity of 10 pg/ml using a tritiated tracer. Our normal range is 10 to 22 pg/ml ($\bar{x} = 11.7 \pm 7.0$), and the recovery of added 6-keto-$PGF_{1\alpha}$ is $95 \pm 9\%$. Interassay and intraassay variations are 4.9 and 4%, respectively.

In order to confirm that our assay is measuring metabolites of PGI_2, we carried out two studies. In the first, known quantities of PGI_2 were allowed to hydrolyse in phosphate buffer and were assayed along with the same amounts of 6-keto-$PGF_{1\alpha}$ standards (Fig. 1).

In the second, levels of PGI_2 metabolites were measured during an infusion of PGI_2 (Fig. 2).

If the object is to measure absolute values of 6-keto-$PGF_{1\alpha}$, the best method is GC–MS. However, this may give a misleading picture when examining variations in PGI_2 production. For clinical work we suggest that RIA is the method of choice.

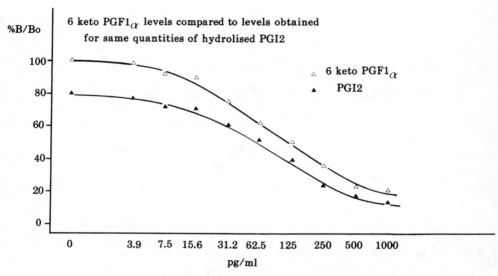

FIG. 1. Prostacyclin metabolite assay.

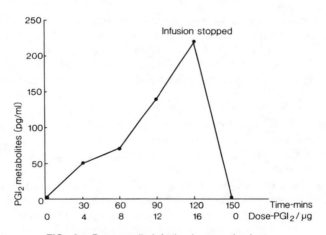

FIG. 2. Prostacyclin infusion in normal volunteer.

REFERENCES

1. Blair, I. A., Barrow, S. E., Waddel, K. A., Lewis, P. J., and Dollery, C. T. (1982): Prostacyclin is not a circulating hormone in man. *Prostaglandins*, 23:379–389.
2. Lewis, P. J., Boylan, P., Friedman, L. A., Hensby, C. N., and Downing, I. (1980): Prostacyclin in pregnancy. *Br. Med. J.*, 280:1581–1582.
3. Viinikka, L., and Yukorkala, O. (1982): Different results of plasma 6-keto-prostaglandin F_1 utilizing two antisera with apparently similar specificity. *Prostaglandins Leukotrienes Med.*, 9:1–7.
4. Yukorkala, O., and Viinikka, L. (1981): Maternal levels of 6-keto-prostaglandin F_1 during pregnancy and puerperium. *Prostaglandins Med.*, 7:95–99.

*Advances in Prostaglandin, Thromboxane, and
Leukotriene Research, Vol. 13*, edited by G. G. Neri
Serneri, et al. Raven Press, New York © 1985.

Is Prostacyclin Effective on Transmembrane Calcium Movements?

G. Fassina, L. Caparrotta, M. Floreani, and E. Ragazzi

Department of Pharmacology, University of Padua, 35100 Padua, Italy

Prostacyclin (PGI_2) protects the myocardium *in vivo* and *in vitro* from acute ischemic damage (11,13). Schrör et al. (13) predicted a stabilizing effect on cell membranes by PGI_2 to prevent the ischemia-induced destruction of adrenergic nerve endings, which suggests that factors other than platelets and coronary vasodilatation may be involved in protection of the myocardium by PGI_2. Prostacyclin is the main prostaglandin derivative released from rat, rabbit, guinea pig, cat, and dog heart (2,6,8).

In a previous study we found that PGI_2 elicited a concentration-dependent increase (3×10^{-8} to 10^{-5} M) of contractile tension on spontaneously beating guinea pig atria, as well as on electrically driven left atria (4). The heart rate was also stimulated by PGI_2, but the chronotropic effect was low and not directly dose-dependent. Endogenous catecholamines do not seem to be involved in the positive inotropic effect of PGI_2, since this effect is still evident after chemical sympathectomy. Beta and alpha blocking agents and H_2 and H_1 antihistaminic drugs did not antagonize PGI_2-induced myocardial stimulation (4).

The next step of our investigation was to study the influence of PGI_2 on ion movements, mainly Ca^{2+} and Na^+, by using drugs known to block fast Na^+ channels, slow Ca^{2+} channels, and other ion currents (3). The most interesting result was that the PGI_2-induced inotropic effect was not antagonized by low concentrations of either verapamil (2×10^{-8} M) or nifedipine (3×10^{-9} M). Prostacyclin, however, was able to restore cardiac functionality when higher concentrations of verapamil (4×10^{-7} M) or nifedipine (5×10^{-8} M) reduced myocardial functionality to slow and irregular contraction. However, PGI_2 was no longer effective when contractility was totally abolished by verapamil at 10^{-6} M or nifedipine at 5×10^{-7} M. These data suggest that extracellular Ca^{2+} influx, even when it occurs at very low rates, is required so that PGI_2 is able to exert its positive inotropic effect.

Our study investigated the possibility that PGI_2 might influence two membrane enzyme systems, Na^+/K^+ ATPase and adenylate cyclase, that are related to transmembrane calcium fluxes and intracellular calcium kinetics.

Na^+/K^+ ATPase, partially purified from beef heart according to Matsui and Schwartz (10), was measured in the presence of PGI_2 in concentrations of 10^{-8} to 10^{-6} M (Table 1). PGI_2, at any of the concentrations tested, did not modify the enzyme-specific activity, thus excluding an ouabain-like mechanism of action.

The action of PGI_2 was studied on isolated guinea pig atria in the presence of forskolin, the most potent activator of the catalytic subunit of adenylate cyclase, which provides a unique and invaluable tool for assessing the role of cyclic AMP in cellular responses and for studying the mechanisms involved (14). Forskolin exerts a positive inotropic and chronotropic effect on heart muscle (9). The percent variation of contractile tension induced by PGI_2 alone (5×10^{-8} to 10^{-6} M) and in the presence of forskolin (5×10^{-8} and 10^{-7} M) is illustrated in Fig. 1. The concentration-effect curves clearly indicate an additive effect by forskolin and PGI_2 on stimulation of myocardial contraction, since the percent increase on tension development by PGI_2 is not modified by forskolin addition. This suggests that the mechanism of action involved in the positive inotropic effect by forskolin and PGI_2 might be independent from one another. These data also stand in accordance with the ineffectiveness of PGI_2 on myocardial cyclic nucleotide levels in dogs (7) and with the limited elevation of cyclic AMP content that PGI_2 produced in rat atria at very high concentration levels (10^{-5} M) (1).

In summary, the results indicate that there is (a) no interaction by prostacyclin with adrenergic or histaminergic systems, (b) a mechanism of action different from that of digitalis glycosides and probably independent of cyclic AMP, and (c) a permissive role of calcium ion, as evidenced by PGI_2 interaction with calcium influx inhibitors.

We found from these data that advancing the hypothesis that PGI_2 might act on the excitation–contraction coupling process seems reasonable. It remains to be investigated whether tubular T-system or sarcoplasmic reticulum calcium release are involved, even though preliminary studies at subcellular level, on highly purified sarcoplasmic reticulum vesicles, seem to sustain our hypothesis (12).

TABLE 1. *Effect of prostacyclin on beef heart Na^+/K^+ ATPase activity[a]*

Drug	Na^+/K^+ ATPase activity (μmoles P_i formed/mg/hr)
—	7.87 ± 0.34
PGI_2, 10^{-8} M	7.54 ± 0.28
PGI_2, 10^{-7} M	7.32 ± 0.17
PGI_2, 10^{-6} M	7.30 ± 0.10

[a]Incubation medium (1 ml final volume): 50 ml Tris-HCl, pH 7.4, 100 mM NaCl, 200 mM KCl, 2 mM $MgCl_2$, 3 mM ATP, 150 μg protein, and 0.2 mM ouabain where present. Na^+/K^+ ATPase activity was calculated as the difference between the activities in the presence and in the absence of ouabain. P_i was determined according to Fiske and Subbarow (5).

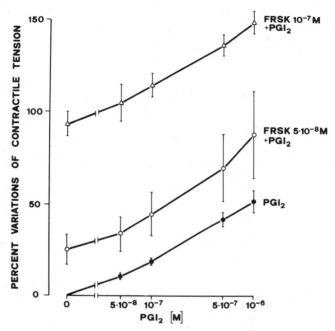

FIG. 1. Guinea pig atria were incubated in a solution of the following composition: (mM): NaCl 120, KCl 2.7, $MgCl_2$ 0.09, NaH_2PO_4 0.4, $CaCl_2$ 1.36, $NaHCO_3$ 11.9, glucose 5.5, pH 7.4 at 29°C, gassed with a mixture of 95% O_2-5% CO_2. The preparations were subjected to a constant resting tension of 1 g. The atrial contraction was recorded isometrically by a highly sensitive transducer (Basile, type DYO for isolated auricles). Concentration–response curves were determined by adding single doses. Contractile force of the atria was expressed as a percentage of the initial value prior to treatment with PGI_2. Data are the mean ± SE of eight different hearts.

REFERENCES

1. Collins, G. A., MacLeod, B. A., and Walker, M. J. A. (1982): Blood pressure and cardiac tissue responses to prostacyclin (PGI_2) in various species. *Can. J. Physiol. Pharmacol.*, 60:134–139.
2. De Deckere, E. A. M., Nugteren, D. H., and Ten Hoor, F. (1977): Prostacyclin is the major prostaglandin released from the isolated perfused rabbit and rat heart. *Nature (Lond.)*, 268:160–163.
3. Fassina, G., Perissinotto, L., and Caparrotta, L. (1984): Positive inotropic effect of prostacyclin on isolated guinea pig atria. Mechanism of action. In: *Prostaglandins and Membrane Ion Transport*, edited by P. Braquet, S. Nicosia, J. C. Frölich, and R. Garay, pp. 201–207. Raven Press, New York.
4. Fassina, G., Tessari, F., and Dorigo, P. (1983): Positive ionotropic effect of a stable analogue of PGI_2 and PGI_2 on isolated guinea pig atria. *Pharmacol. Res. Commun.*, 15:735–749.
5. Fisk, C. H., and Subbarow, J. (1925): The colorimetric determination of phosphorus. *J. Biol. Chem.*, 66:375–400.
6. Isackson, P. C., Raz, A., Denny, S. E., Pure, E., and Needleman, P. A. (1977): A novel prostaglandin is the major product of arachidonic acid metabolism in rabbit heart. *Proc. Natl. Acad. Sci. U.S.A.*, 74:101–105.
7. Ito, T., Ogawa, K., and Enomoto, I. (1980): Prostaglandins and cyclic nucleotides: Effects of PGI_2 and PGE_1 on cardiac hemodynamic and coronary arterial and myocardial cyclic nucleotide levels in dogs. *Jpn. Circ. J.*, 44:755–761.

8. Lefer, A. M., Messenger, M., and Okamatsu, S. (1982): Salutary actions of thromboxane synthetase inhibition during global myocardial ischemia. *Arch. Pharm. (Weinheim)*, 321:130–134.

9. Lindner, E., and Metzger, H. (1983): The action of forskolin on muscle cells is modified by hormones, calcium ions and calcium antagonists. *Arzneim-Forsch.*, 33:1436–1441.

10. Matsui, H., and Schwartz, A. (1966): Purification and properties of a highly active ouabain-sensitive Na^+,K^+-dependent adenosinetriphophatase from cardiac tissue. *Biochim. Biophys. Acta*, 128:380–390.

11. Ogletree, M. L., Lefer, A. M., Smith, J. B., and Nicolau, K. C. (1979): Studies on the protective effect of prostacyclin in acute myocardial ischemia. *Eur. J. Pharmacol.*, 56:95–103.

12. Salvatori, S., Damiani, E., Margreth, A., Fassina, G., and Caparrotta, L. (1984): Effect of prostacyclins on sarcoplasmic reticulum Ca^{2+}-pump. In: *Prostaglandins and Membrane Ion Transport*, edited by P. Braquet, S. Nicosia, S. C. Frölich, and R. Garay, pp. 209–216. Raven Press, New York.

13. Schrör, K., Darius, H., Addicks, K., Köster, R., and Smith, E. F. (1982): PGI_2 prevents ischemia-induced alterations in cardiac catecholamines without influencing nerve-stimulation-induced catecholamine release in nonischemic conditions. *J. Cardiac Pharmacol.*, 4:741–748.

14. Seamon, K. B., and Daly, J. W. (1983): Forskolin, cyclic AMP and cellular physiology. *Trends Pharmacol. Sci.*, 4:120–123.

Advances in Prostaglandin, Thromboxane, and
Leukotriene Research, Vol. 13, edited by G. G. Neri
Serneri, et al. Raven Press, New York © 1985.

Pharmacological Modification of Leukotriene Release and Coronary Constrictor Effect in Cardiac Anaphylaxis

P. Weinerowski, G. Wittmann, U. Aehringhaus, and B. A. Peskar

Department of Pharmacology, Ruhr-University Bochum,
D-4630 Bochum, Federal Republic of Germany

The modification of anaphylactic release of leukotriene (LT) C_4-like immuno-reactivity from isolated guinea pig hearts and of LT-induced coronary constriction by the muscarinic receptor agonist methacholine and by various exogenous prostaglandins (PG) was investigated. The vasodilators PGI_2 and PGE_2 as well as the vasoconstrictors PGD_2, $PGF_{2\alpha}$, and 11,9-epoxymethano-PGH_2, a PG endoperoxide analogue with biological properties similar to thromboxane (TX) A_2, inhibited the anaphylactic coronary constriction without affecting release of LTC_4-like immuno-reactivity. On the other hand, the increased anaphylactic LT release in the presence of methacholine was not paralleled by more pronounced coronary constriction after challenge. These results suggest that the coronary constrictor effect of endogenous LT is modified by the drugs used by direct vascular effects and/or effects on other anaphylactic mediators.

INTRODUCTION

The most striking symptom of the anaphylactic reaction of isolated perfused sensitized guinea pig hearts is coronary constriction, which typically occurs with an early more severe phase followed by a long-lasting, less pronounced reduction of coronary flow (2). The possible clinical importance of the antigen-induced coronary reaction is emphasized by a recent report of suspected coronary arterial spasm in a patient during an acute allergic response (6). Various mediators like histamine (3,13), PG (11), TXB_2 (2), the stable degradation product of the biologically active TXA_2 (5) and LT (1) have been demonstrated to be released during guinea pig cardiac anaphylaxis. Sulfidopeptide-containing LT are now known to be constituents of a slow-reacting substance of anaphylaxis (SRS-A) (12). LTC_4 and LTD_4 have been shown to be particularly potent coronary vasoconstrictors (9). We have now investigated the modification of cardiac anaphylactic LT release and LT-induced coronary constriction by the muscarinic receptor agonist methacholine and by various exogenous PG.

METHODS

Hearts of ovalbumin-sensitized guinea pigs were perfused and challenged with antigen, as described previously (1). In experiments with indomethacin (Sigma, 1×10^{-5} g/min) or methacholine (Sigma, 1×10^{-5} g/min and 3×10^{-5} g/min), drug infusions were started 15 min before antigen injection. When the methacholine effects were antagonized by atropine (Sigma, 3.75×10^{-5} g/min), the antagonist was added to the perfusion medium 7 min before challenge. Similarly, infusions of exogenous PGE_2, prostacyclin (PGI_2) (both PGE_2 and PGI_2 at 1×10^{-7} and 5×10^{-7} g/min), PGD_2, $PGF_{2\alpha}$, and 11,9-epoxymethano-PGH_2, a stable endoperoxide analogue with biological properties similar to TXA_2 (4) (all at 1×10^{-7} g/min), into indomethacin-treated hearts were started 7 min before antigen injection. Coronary flow was measured by direct determination of the perfusate volume per collection period. Release of LTC_4-like immunoreactivity, 6-keto-$PGF_{1\alpha}$, and TXB_2 from the hearts into the perfusates was determined using radioimmunoassays as described previously (1). All PG used were a generous gift of Dr. J. Pike, Upjohn Co., Kalamazoo, Michigan.

RESULTS AND DISCUSSION

Isolated perfused anaphylactic guinea pig hearts released considerable amounts of arachidonic acid-derived mediators. Thus, in the perfusate collection period 1 to 5 min after antigen injection, the hearts released (means $\pm$ SEM, $n = 9$) 7.25 ± 2.20 ng immunoreactive LTC_4, 80.06 ± 14.71 ng TXB_2, and 24.70 ± 6.98 ng 6-keto-$PGF_{1\alpha}$. In the presence of indomethacin (1×10^{-5} g/min), release of the cyclooxygenase products 6-keto-$PGF_{1\alpha}$ and TXB_2 was almost completely abolished ($p < 0.001$ as compared to controls), while release of LTC_4-like immunoreactivity was simultaneously significantly enhanced ($p < 0.025$). Infusion of indomethacin resulted in a delay of the onset of the early phase of anaphylactic coronary constriction but did not influence the late less pronounced phase. These results suggest that endogenous vasoconstrictor cyclooxygenase products like TXA_2 contribute to the early phase, while LT may be involved in the late phase of anaphylactic coronary constriction. While exogenous PGD_2, $PGF_{2\alpha}$, and 11,9-epoxymethano-PGH_2 (all at 1×10^{-7} g/min), infused into indomethacin-treated hearts, caused vasoconstriction, PGI_2 and PGE_2 (both at either 1×10^{-7} g/min or 5×10^{-7} g/min) induced significant vasodilatation. The typical antigen-induced coronary constriction was, however, inhibited in the presence of either vasoconstrictor PG or vasodilator PG. On the other hand, the various PG in the concentrations used did not significantly affect anaphylactic release of LTC_4-like immunoreactivity. These results suggest that the PG effects on anaphylactic coronary constriction are due to direct effects on vascular smooth-muscle tone and/or effects on the release of other mediators like histamine and platelet-activating factor.

In the presence of the cholinergic receptor agonist methacholine (1×10^{-5} g/min and 3×10^{-5} g/min), a significant and dose-dependent increase in the release of LTC_4-like immunoreactivity from anaphylactic guinea pig hearts was observed.

Atropine (3.75×10^{-5} g/min) effectively antagonized the methacholine effect on release of LTC_4-like immunoreactivity, indicating that the cholinergic receptors involved are of the muscarinic type. The enhanced release of immunoreactive LTC_4 during infusion of methacholine was not paralleled by a more pronounced anaphylactic coronary constriction, probably because of the direct vasodilator effect of the cholinergic agonist. Cholinergic enhancement of the immunologic release of SRS-A has also been observed in passively sensitized rats (7) and in human lung tissue *in vitro* (8). LT released from the heart during an acute allergic reaction reaches the lungs quickly via the bloodstream and may thus aggravate pulmonary symptoms elicited by LT generated locally. Furthermore, while muscarinic receptor stimulation has an effect opposite to that induced by LTC_4 and LTD_4 in the coronary vascular bed, increased vagal tone and sulfidopeptide-containing LT act synergistically at the bronchial smooth muscle. This is in contrast to the effects of β-sympathomimetic drugs, which inhibit bronchial smooth-muscle contraction and simultaneously inhibit release of anaphylactic mediators including SRS-A (10).

ACKNOWLEDGMENT

This work was supported by the Deutsche Forschungsgemeinschaft.

REFERENCES

1. Aehringhaus, U., Peskar B. A., Wittenberg, H. R., and Wölbling, R. H. (1983): Effect of inhibition of synthesis and receptor antagonism of SRS-A in cardiac anaphylaxis. *Br. J. Pharmacol.*, 80:73–80.
2. Anhut, H., Bernauer, W., and Peskar, B. A. (1977): Radioimmunological determination of thromboxane release in cardiac anaphylaxis. *Eur. J. Pharmacol.*, 44:85–88.
3. Brocklehurst, W. E. (1960): The release of histamine and formation of slow-reacting substance (SRS-A) during anaphylactic shock. *J. Physiol.*, 151:416–435.
4. Coleman, R. A., Humphrey, P. P. A., Kennedy, I., Levi, G. P., and Lumley, P. (1981): Comparison of the actions of U46619, a prostaglandin H_2-analogue, with those of prostaglandin H_2 and thromboxane A_2 on some isolated smooth muscle preparations. *Br. J. Pharmacol.*, 73:773–778.
5. Hamberg, M., Svensson, J., and Samuelsson, B. (1975): Thromboxanes: A new group of biologically active compounds derived from prostaglandin endoperoxides. *Proc. Natl. Acad. Sci. U.S.A.*, 72:2994–2998.
6. Hirsch, S. A. (1982): Acute allergic reaction with coronary vasospasm. *Am. Heart J.*, 193:928–932.
7. Kaliner, M. A., Orange, R. P., Koopman, W. J., and Austen, K. F. (1972): Pathopharmacologic enhancement of the IgE-mediated release of histamine and slow-reacting substance of anaphylaxis in the rat. In: *Inflammation, Mechanisms and Control*, edited by J. A. Lepow and P. A. Ward, pp. 139–145. Academic Press, New York.
8. Kaliner, M. A., Orange, R. P., La Raia, P. J., and Austen, K. F. (1972): Cholinergic enhancement of the immunologic release of histamine and slow reacting substance of anaphylaxis (SRS-A) from human lung tissue. *Fed. Proc.*, 31:748.
9. Letts, L. G., and Piper, P. J. (1982): The actions of leukotrienes C_4 and D_4 on guinea-pig isolated hearts. *Br. J. Pharmacol.*, 76:169–176.
10. Liebig, R., Bernauer, W., and Peskar, B. A. (1974): Release of prostaglandins, a prostaglandin metabolite, slow reacting substance and histamine from anaphylactic lungs, and its modification by catecholamines. *Naunyn-Schmiedeberg's Arch. Pharmakol.*, 284:279–293.

11. Liebig, R., Bernauer, W., and Peskar, B. A. (1975): Prostaglandin, slow reacting substance and histamine release from anaphylactic guinea-pig hearts and its pharmacological modification. *Naunyn-Schmiedeberg's Arch. Pharmakol.*, 289:65–76.
12. Murphy, R. C., Hammarström, S., and Samuelsson, B. (1979): Leukotriene C: A slow-reacting substance from murine mastocytoma cells. *Proc. Natl. Acad. Sci. U.S.A.*, 76:4275–4279.
13. Schild, H. O. (1937): Release of histamine-like substance in anaphylactic shock from various organs of the guinea-pig. *J. Physiol.*, 90:34P.

Advances in Prostaglandin, Thromboxane, and Leukotriene Research, Vol. 13, edited by G. G. Neri Serneri, et al. Raven Press, New York © 1985.

Leukotriene D₄ Reduces Pressor Responses to Sympathetic Stimulation, Angiotensin, and Vasopressin

*Mohamed A. Bayorh, **Zofia Zukowska-Grojec, *David Ezra, **Irwin J. Kopin, and *Giora Feuerstein

*Neurobiology Research Division, Uniformed Services University of the Health Sciences, Bethesda, Maryland 20814; and **Laboratory of Clinical Science, National Institute of Mental Health, Bethesda, Maryland 20205*

Leukotriene D_4 (LTD_4), a constituent of slow-reacting substance of anaphylaxis (SRS-A), produces hemodynamic and cardiovascular changes that are akin to those seen in acute anaphylactic shock (5,7,9). Systemic administration of LTD_4 to conscious as well as pithed SHR rats elicits an initial pressor response followed by long-lasting hypotension (9), whereas in normotensive Wistar-Kyoto rats only the pressor phase and benign bradycardia were present. The relative bradycardia that attends the prolonged hypotension induced by LTD_4 seems to be a direct cardiac effect of LTD_4, since it occurred in pithed rats which are devoid of reflexes (9).

To investigate the peripheral cardiovascular derangements induced by LTD_4, we studied the interaction between LTD_4 and the major pressor systems—the sympathetic nervous system, vasopressin, and angiotensin II—in pithed SHR rats.

MATERIALS AND METHODS

Male SHR rats were anesthetized with 2% halothane in oxygen; the right jugular vein was cannulated and bilateral vagotomy was performed at midcervical level. Both carotid arteries were cannulated: one for recording blood pressure and heart rate, and the other for collecting blood samples. After tracheal cannulation, rats were pithed (6) by insertion of a steel rod down the spinal cord to the first sacral vertebra. Beginning at least 15 min after the injection of gallamine, the sympathetic nervous outflow from the spinal cord was stimulated for 1 min using a monophasic squarewave pulse (50 V, 1 msec duration) at 0.3 and 3.0 Hz at 10-min intervals before and 10 min after LTD_4 (20 μg/kg, i.v.). To evaluate the cardiovascular responses to other pressor agents, animals were prepared as described above. Two doses of either vasopressin (0.3 and 3.0 μg/kg) or angiotensin II (0.1 and 1.0 μg/kg) were administered i.v. before and 10 min after LTD_4. Blood samples were collected by free flow from the carotid cannulae before and during the last 15 sec

TABLE 1. Changes in blood pressure (BP) and heart rate (HR) in response to different pressors before and after LTD$_4$[a]

Change	Stimulation (Hz)		Angiotensin (μg/kg)		Vasopressin (μg/kg)	
	0.3	3.0	0.1	1.0	0.03	0.1
ΔBP before LTD$_4$ (mmHg)	30 ± 4	115 ± 9	29 ± 6	85 ± 12	48 ± 6	143 ± 2
ΔBP after LTD$_4$ (mmHg)	11 ± 1***	34 ± 4***	8 ± 1**	26 ± 1**	8 ± 2**	29 ± 3***
ΔHR before LTD$_4$ (beats/min)	72 ± 16	97 ± 13	39 ± 9	81 ± 11	−19 ± 6	−25 ± 9
ΔHR after LTD$_4$ (beats/min)	42 ± 2	65 ± 7*	38 ± 11	66 ± 9	−72 ± 10**	−62 ± 10*

[a]Values are expressed as mean ± SEM for 5 to 7 rats. Asterisks denote level of statistical significance (Student's t-test) as follows: * $p < 0.05$; ** $p < 0.01$; *** $p < 0.001$.

TABLE 2. *Plasma catecholamine levels in response to sympathetic stimulation at 3.0 Hz before and after LTD₄*[a]

Time	NE (pg/ml)	EPI (pg/ml)
Before LTD$_4$	1674 ± 86	1805 ± 153
After LTD$_4$	1208 ± 201*	4319 ± 827*

[a]Results are mean ± SEM for 7 rats. The basal plasma NE (norepinephrine) and EPI (epinephrine) were 52 ± 12 and 17 ± 2 pg/ml, respectively. Asterisk denotes level of statistical significance: *$p < 0.05$.

of the 1-min interval stimulation at 3.0 Hz. Plasma norepinephrine and epinephrine were assayed by a radioenzymatic procedure (8).

RESULTS

Blood Pressure and Heart Rate Responses to LTD₄ in Pithed Rats

The basal blood pressure and heart rate of the pithed rats were $57 ± 5$ mmHg and $301 ± 11$ beats/min, respectively; there was no significant difference between the groups. LTD$_4$ suppressed the pressor responses to stimulation (50 V, 1 msec for 1 min) at 0.3 and 3.0 Hz by 64% ($p < 0.001$) and 71% ($p < 0.001$), respectively. Plasma norepinephrine response to stimulation at 3.0 Hz was significantly ($p < 0.05$) reduced in the presence of LTD$_4$. The evoked release of epinephrine secretion from the adrenal medulla was enhanced ($+ 139\%$, $p < 0.05$) by LTD$_4$, but the tachycardia was blocked. The pressor responses to 0.1 and 1.0 µg/kg angiotensin II were blocked by 73% ($p < 0.05$) and 70% ($p < 0.01$), respectively. The pressor effects seen after vasopressin (0.03 and 0.1 µg/kg) were also blocked (by 83 and 80%, respectively) by previous administration of LTD$_4$ (Tables 1 and 2).

DISCUSSION

The present study provides data that indicate that diminished peripheral vascular reactivity to pressor stimuli is also a major cause of the hypotension produced by LTD$_4$. Thus, the pressor responses to three different vasoconstrictors—endogenously released norepinephrine, vasopressin, and angiotensin II—were significantly reduced in rats treated with LTD$_4$. Cardiac responses to stimulation-induced catecholamine release and to vasopressin were also markedly diminished.

The diminished vascular and cardiac responses to different pressor stimuli given during the hypotensive shock syndrome induced by LTD$_4$ may be the result of several factors. LTD$_4$ may act indirectly by releasing vasodilator substances (including prostaglandins), since both LTC$_4$ and LTD$_4$ have been shown to dose-dependently increase the release of prostacyclin (PGI$_2$) and prostaglandin (PG) E$_2$

(4), which are vasodilators. Acute infusions of cyclooxygenase metabolites of arachidonate (AA), PGE, and PGI (3) were shown to be associated with reduced responsiveness of the peripheral vasculature to different pressor stimuli. Furthermore, chronic administration of AA (precursor of various prostaglandins and leukotrienes) diminished the pressor responses to sympathetic stimulation from the spinal cord of pithed SHR rats and to other pressor agents (1,2).

In conclusion, the results presented in this study demonstrate that LTD_4 causes severe derangements of vascular smooth-muscle constriction. Since LTD_4 is the major constituent of SRS-A, its effects on vascular and myocardial contractility may play a major role in anaphylactic shock.

ACKNOWLEDGMENT

This study was supported in part by USAMRDC contract #No 02018-83.

REFERENCES

1. Bayorh, M.A., Zukowska-Grojec, Z., Ezra, D., Feuerstein, G., and Kopin, I. J. (1983): Cardiovascular and sympathetic responses to chronic arachidonate in spontaneously hypertensive (SHR) and wistar kyoto (WKY) rats. *Hypertension*, 5:172–179.
2. Ezra, D., Bayorh, M. A., Zukowska-Grojec, Z., Lazar, J. D., Kopin, I. J., and Feuerstein, G. (1983): Effect of chronic arachidonate on blood pressure of spontaneously hypertensive rats. *Clin. Exp. Hypertens.*, 9:1485–1499.
3. Feuerstein, G., and Kopin, I. J. (1981): Effect of PGD_2, PGE_2, $PGF_{2\alpha}$ and PGI_2 on blood pressure, heart rate and plasma catecholamine responses to spinal cord stimulation in the rat. *Prostaglandins*, 21:189–206.
4. Feuerstein, N., Foegh, M., and Ramwell, P. W. (1981): Leukotrienes C_4 and D_4 induce prostaglandin and thromboxane from rat peritoneal macrophages. *Br. J. Pharmacol.*, 72:391–398.
5. Feuerstein, G., Zukowska-Grojec, Z., and Kopin, I. J. (1981): Cardiovascular effects of leukotriene D_4 in SHR and WKY rats. *Eur. J. Pharmacol.*, 76:107–110.
6. Gillespie, J. A., and Muir, T. C. (1967): A method of stimulating the complete sympathetic outflow from the spinal cord to blood vessels in the pithed rat. *Br. J. Pharmacol. Chemother.*, 10:78–87.
7. Lewis, R. A., and Austin, F. K. (1981): Mediation of local homeostasis and inflammation by leukotrienes and other mast cell-dependent compounds. *Nature (Lond.)*, 293:103–108.
8. Weise, V., and Kopin, I. J. (1976): Assay of catecholamines in human plasma: Studies of a single isotope radioenzymatic procedure. *Life Sci.*, 19:1673–1686.
9. Zukowska-Grojec, Z., Bayorh, M. A., Kopin, I. J., and Feuerstein, G. (1982): Leukotriene D_4: Cardiovascular and sympathetic effects in SHR and WKY rats. *J. Pharmacol. Exp. Ther.*, 223:183–189.

Advances in Prostaglandin, Thromboxane, and Leukotriene Research, Vol. 13, edited by G.G. Neri Serneri, et al. Raven Press, New York © 1985.

Lipoxygenase-Derived Products in Cultured Human Aortic Smooth Muscle Cells

*J. Larrue, *G. Razaka, *D. Daret,
*J. Henri, **M. Rigaud, and *H. Bricaud

*Unité 8 de Cardiologie, INSERM, 33600 Pessac, and
**Laboratoire de Biochimie, CHU Dupuytren, 87000 Limoges, France

Aortas are very active in converting arachidonic acid (AA) to prostanoids, with the major product being prostacyclin (PGI_2) (4). In addition, the formation of the lipoxygenase product 12-HETE (hydroxyeicosaenoic acid) has been recognized (2).

In this chapter we present evidence that cultured smooth muscle cells (SMCs) from adult human aortas possess, in addition to their cyclooxygenase activity, the ability to metabolize AA via lipoxygenase enzymes.

MATERIAL AND METHODS

Human tissues were derived from biopsies of ascending aortas obtained during valvular surgery in informed patients who were known to be free of atherosclerosis. SMCs were obtained from explants as previously described (3). All experiments were done with just confluent cells in secondary cultures before passage five. SMCs (1 mg/ml) were incubated at 37°C in a Krebs-Ringer (pH 7.4) medium with 10 μM [14C]AA for 20 min. Alternatively, [14C]AA-prelabeled SMCs were treated with 10 μM calcium ionophore A23187. When inhibitors [aspirin, indomethacin, nordihydroguaiaretic acid (NDGA)] were used, they were added 10 min prior to the beginning of incubation. The incubations were terminated by the addition of 1.5 vol ice-cold methanol and the extraction was performed as described (3).

Aliquots of the extracted material were submitted either to thin-layer chromatography (TLC) or high-performance liquid chromatography (HPLC) and gas chromatrography—mass spectroscopy (GC-MS) (3). The separated radioactive products were counted with liquid scintillation.

RESULTS

The homogenates of cultured SMCs converted 6.4 ± 1.4 (mean $\pm$ SEM, $n = 6$) of the added [14C]AA to radioactive products. The predominant cyclooxygenase metabolites formed as characterized by their chromatographic mobility on TLC were 6-keto prostaglandin (PG) $F_{1\alpha} > PGF_{2\alpha} > PGE_2$. Indomethacin (30 μM) and aspirin (100 μM) inhibited by 60% the formation of these products. The predominant lipoxygenase products characterized using both TLC and HPLC had a chromatographic mobility corresponding to 15-, 12-, and 5-HETE, respectively. Indomethacin (30 μM) significantly reduced the formation of 15-HETE (− 38%) and, by contrast, stimulated the production of 12-HETE by 50% without any significant effect on 5-HETE (Fig. 1). Smaller amounts of other products were also separated on TLC and HPLC. Among them were 12 hydroxy-5,8,10 heptadecatrienoic acid (HHT) ($0.9 \pm 0.2\%$), whose synthesis was inhibited by cyclooxygenase inhibitors, and products ($0.4 \pm 0.1\%$) with the chromatographic mobility of leukotriene B_4 (LTB_4) on TLC with a solvent system consisting of ether:hexane:acetic acid (60:40:1, v/v/v).

When [^{14}C]AA-prelabeled smooth muscle cells were incubated with the Ca^{2+} ionophore A 23187, prostaglandins represented 28% and monohydroxy acids represented 4.5% of the total radioactivity released in the incubation medium. This latter percentage was greatly enhanced (+ 16.4%) by adding unlabeled platelets in the incubation medium (platelet/SMCs ratio of 10:1) and was raised further in the presence of 100 μM aspirin (+ 24.7%). As previously shown for cell homogenates, the formation of 15-HETE was inhibited under aspirin treatment. By contrast, 12-HETE synthesis was significantly enhanced (16 versus 9.6%). Dihydroxy acids (2.2% of the total radioactivity released) were not significantly modified, as expressed in percent, by platelet activation with or without aspirin treatment. The composition of this fraction was further resolved using HPLC techniques (Fig. 2).

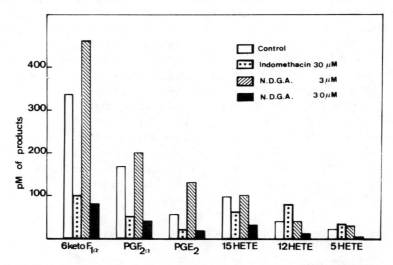

FIG. 1.   [^{14}C]AA transformation by homogenates of human aortic SMC. Cells (1 mg/protein) were preincubated 15 min with inhibitors, then 10 nmol [^{14}C]AA was added in a final volume of 1 ml.

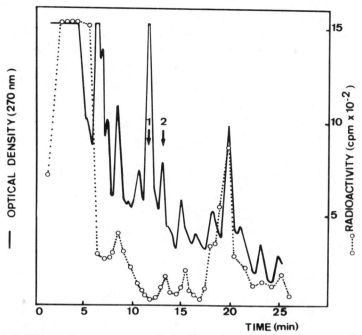

FIG. 2. HPLC separation of dihydroxylated products obtained from A 23187-stimulated [^{14}C]AA-labeled cells in the presence of unlabeled platelets: 3×10^6 prelabeled cells were incubated with unlabeled platelets in the ratio of 1:10 in the presence of 10 μM A23187. Approximately one-tenth of the sample was applied to HPLC, resolved on 5 μC$_{18}$, mobile phase methanol:water:acetic acid (67:33,0.01), pH 4.7, flow rate 1 ml/min. Authentic standards were run prior to injection of sample. The radioactive peak at 16 min was not characterized. The 20-min peak represented HHT. 1 = 5s,12s-diHETE, all trans; 2 = LTB$_4$ + 5,12-diHETE.

The major peak of radioactivity coeluted with authentic LTB$_4$ standard, and spectral characteristics were in a good agreement with the presence of hydrolyzed products of the labile intermediate LTA$_4$, but the formation of the double lipoxygenase product 5s,12s-diHETE cannot be excluded and the exact nature of dihydroxylated compounds requires further investigations.

DISCUSSION

The present data show that arachidonate products of the lipoxygenase metabolic pathway can be formed from both exogenous and endogenous substrates in human cultured aortic SMCs. Monohydroxy acids have been characterized by their chromatographic mobility using TLC and reverse phase HPLC (RP-HPLC) techniques and by GC-MS. Additionally, the presence of diHETE has been recognized. Since nonsteroidal antiinflammatory drugs (NSAID) such as indomethacin (30 μM) or aspirin (100 μM) partially inhibited the formation of 15-HETE, the origin of this product remains uncertain; by contrast, NSAID did not modify 5-HETE formation and significantly enhanced 12-HETE synthesis.

The biological activity of these monohydroxy acids remains to be defined clearly, but it is of importance that their hydroxy precursors inhibit both cyclooxygenase and PGI_2 synthetase activities (6). In addition, these compounds have been recently recognized as potent inhibitors of platelet aggregation (1). These data support the hypothesis that these products have the potential to modulate the inflammatory process in the vascular wall and point to their importance in the atherosclerotic process (5).

REFERENCES

1. Croset, M., and Lagarde, M. (1983): Stereospecific inhibition of PGH_2-induced platelet aggregation by lipoxygenase products of icosanoic acids. *Biochem. Biophys. Res. Commun.*, 112:878–883.
2. Greenwald, J. E., Bianchine, J. R., and Wong, L. K. (1979): The production of the arachidonate metabolite HETE in vascular tissue. *Nature (Lond.)*, 281:588–589.
3. Larrue, J., Rigaud, M., Razaka, G., Daret, D., Demond-Henri, J., and Bricaud, H. (1983): Formation of monohydroxy eicosatetraenoic acids from arachidonic acid by cultured rabbit aortic smooth muscle cells. *Biochem. Biophys. Res. Commun.*, 112:242–249.
4. Moncada, S., Gryglewski, R. J., Bunting, S., and Vane, J. R. (1976): An enzyme isolated from arteries transforms prostaglandins endoperoxides to an unstable substance that inhibits platelet aggregation. *Nature (Lond).*, 263:663–665.
5. Nakao, J., Ooyama, T., Ito, M., Chang, W. C., and Murota, S. (1982): Comparative effect of lipoxygenase products of arachidonic acid on rat aortic smooth muscle cell migration. *Atherosclerosis*, 44:339–342.
6. Salmon, J. A., Smith, D. R., Flower, R. J., Moncada, S., and Vane, J. R. (1978): Further studies on the enzymatic conversion of prostaglandin endoperoxide into prostacyclin by porcine microsomes. *Biochim. Biophys. Acta*, 523:250–262.

Advances in Prostaglandin, Thromboxane, and Leukotriene Research, Vol. 13, edited by G. G. Neri Serneri, et al. Raven Press, New York © 1985.

Cardiac Prostaglandin Synthesis in Spontaneous and in Effort Angina

Gian Gastone Neri Serneri, Domenico Prisco, Pier Giorgio Rogasi, Gian Carlo Casolo, and Sergio Castellani

Clinica Medica I, University of Florence, 50134 Florence, Italy

A large number of investigations on isolated hearts have shown that the heart synthesizes prostaglandins (PGs) of D, E, and F series and especially prostacyclin (PGI_2) (1,2,25,30,32,33,45–47,65,70,72).

Studies performed on coronary artery rings and isolated coronary microvessels indicate that PGI_2 is formed especially by the large coronary arteries, whereas PGE_2 is the major product of coronary microvessels (15,16). Thromboxane A_2 (TXA_2) synthesis by normal coronary vasculature could not be demonstrated (15,65,70).

Much evidence indicates that the primary site of PG biosynthesis is the coronary vasculature and not the cardiac myocytes (48,72,78). Biosynthesis and release of PGs by the heart and the isolated coronary arteries can be elicited by hypoxia (27,45,77) and myocardial ischemia (6,29,48,71,74).

Studies on cardiac PGs have special importance for patients with ischemic heart disease (IHD) because cardiac PGs, and especially PGI_2, influence coronary tone in isolated coronary arterial strips (26,68,69) and coronary vascular resistance in isolated perfused hearts (22,48,68). Moreover, of the various endogenous vasoactive substances that act through a receptor mechanism, PGs appear to be the only class of compounds that influence basal tone of human isolated coronary arteries (18). Administration of aspirin or indomethacin to patients with coronary artery disease aggravates variant and exercise-induced angina (19,37–39) and significantly reduces coronary blood flow (14). In addition, TXA_2 and PGI_2 seem to be related to the occurrence of reperfusion arrhythmias in dogs (7). TXA_2 contributes to the occurrence of arrhythmias (5,8), whereas PGI_2 seems to prevent them (5).

Investigations on cardiac PG synthesis in humans are lacking, with the exception of that of Novack et al. (60), who reported that the constant rate infusion of ^{14}C-labeled arachidonic acid into the aortic root resulted in production of 6-keto-$PGF_{1\alpha}$, the stable metabolite of PGI_2, and to a lesser extent in the formation of ^{14}C-PGs of D, E, and F series. However, there is evidence that prostaglandins can be involved in the occurrence of myocardial ischemic attacks (23,49,50,67,75). The potential role of prostaglandins in the pathogenesis of myocardial ischemia has found further support in the findings that human arteries and veins produce TXA_2 (52) in addition to PGI_2 and PGE_2 and that PGI_2 and PGE_2 modulate the vascular response to sympathetic stimulation (52,55,58). Sympathetic stimulation is also able to induce TXA_2 formation by the human vessel wall (56,58).

Thus, a more definite knowledge of cardiac prostaglandin biosynthesis appears to be crucial for a more profound comprehension of coronary physiology and of IHD pathophysiology.

CARDIAC PROSTAGLANDIN SYNTHESIS IN MAN

Application of cold has been demonstrated to be a stimulus able to induce PG synthesis in man, probably via sympathetic stimulation. More precisely, 2-min cold application (cold pressor test slightly modified) results in a significant elevation of PGE_2, PGI_2, and TXA_2 (as TXB_2) plasma levels associated with an increase of forearm vascular resistance (51). Moreover, simultaneous determination of PGs in arterial and venous blood withdrawn from the radial artery and brachial vein demonstrated the occurrence of a significant venous–arterial gradient following cold application, thus indicating that the distal vascular bed of the arm is the primary site of PG formation following sympathetic stimulation. Finally, it is worth stressing that aspirin administration is able to inhibit PGI_2 but not PGE_2 and TXA_2 formation by the vessel wall (56,58).

Thus we used cold application and the consequent sympathetic stimulation in order to investigate prostaglandin synthesis by the heart in man. Prostaglandins were assayed by radioimmunoassay in blood drawn from the peripheral vein, the coronary sinus, and the aorta. PGI_2 was assayed as 6-keto-$PGF_{1\alpha}$ according to Patrono et al. (63), TXA_2 as TXB_2 according to Granstrom et al. (20), and PGE_2 and $PGF_{2\alpha}$ were measured according to Patrono et al. (62). $PGF_{2\alpha}$ was undetectable in all samples processed.

In control subjects (patients not suffering from ischemic heart disease who underwent coronary angiography and ventriculography for diagnostic purposes), 6-keto-$PGF_{1\alpha}$ concentration in coronary sinus blood was not different from that of aortic and peripheral venous blood (Fig. 1). Similarly, no significant differences in plasma PGE_2 and TXB_2 concentration between coronary sinus, aorta, and peripheral venous blood could be found (Fig. 1).

Sympathetic stimulation was associated with a significant increase of 6-keto-$PGF_{1\alpha}$ levels in peripheral venous, in coronary sinus, and in aortic blood (Fig. 2). The elevation in coronary sinus blood was significantly higher than in aortic blood, and thus a transcardiac gradient of 6-keto-$PGF_{1\alpha}$ concentration could be observed. Therefore, synthesis of PGI_2 by coronary vasculature occurs following sympathetic stimulation (Fig. 2).

Sympathetic stimulation was also able to induce a significant increase in PGE_2 concentration in peripheral venous, coronary sinus, and aortic blood (Fig. 3). However, the increase in peripheral venous blood was remarkable, whereas the increase in coronary sinus and in aortic blood was much lower. In all the subjects,

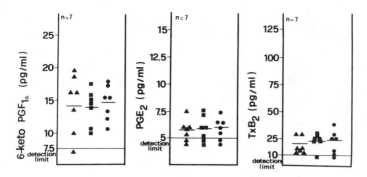

FIG. 1. Control subjects. Baseline levels of 6-keto-PGF$_{1\alpha}$, PGE$_2$, and TXB$_2$ in different vascular beds (▲ = vein; ■ = aorta; ● = coronary sinus).

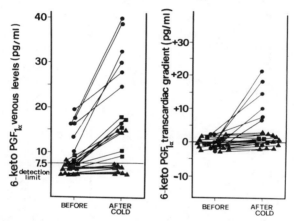

FIG. 2. 6-Keto-PGF$_{1\alpha}$ levels in blood from peripheral vein *(left)* and 6-keto-PGF$_{1\alpha}$ transcardiac gradient *(right)* following sympathetic stimulation in different groups of patients (● = controls; ■ = stable effort angina; ▲ = spontaneous angina).

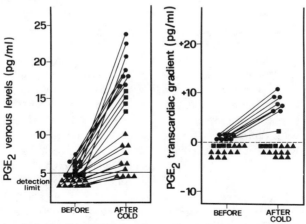

FIG. 3. PGE$_2$ levels in blood from peripheral vein *(left)* and PGE$_2$ transcardiac gradient *(right)* following sympathetic stimulation in different groups of patients (● = controls; ■ = stable effort angina; ▲ = spontaneous angina).

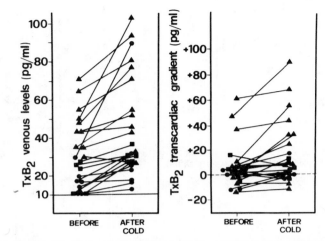

FIG. 4. TXB$_2$ levels in blood from peripheral vein *(left)* and TXB$_2$ transcardiac gradient *(right)* following sympathetic stimulation in different groups of patients ($\bullet$ = controls; $\blacksquare$ = stable effort angina; $\blacktriangle$ = spontaneous angina).

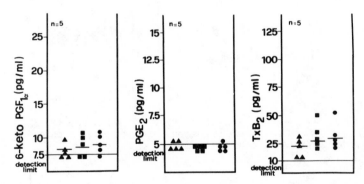

FIG. 5. Stable effort angina. Baseline levels of 6-keto-PGF$_{1\alpha}$, PGE$_2$, and TXB$_2$ in different vascular beds ($\blacktriangle$ = vein; $\blacksquare$ = aorta; $\bullet$ = coronary sinus).

PGE$_2$ levels in coronary sinus were higher than in the aorta, thus indicating the formation of PGE$_2$ in coronary vasculature after sympathetic stimulation (Fig. 3).

TXB$_2$ levels significantly increased after sympathetic stimulation in peripheral venous blood, but unlike 6-keto-PGF$_{1\alpha}$ and PGE$_2$, TXB$_2$ did not significantly increase following sympathetic stimulation either in coronary sinus or in aorta (Fig. 4). In conclusion, these results indicate that resting cardiocoronary biosynthesis of PGI$_2$ and PGE$_2$ is very low. However, it significantly increases, especially prostacyclin biosynthesis, following sympathetic stimulation. This fact can obviously be of physiological importance. In normal subjects, cold application induces an early alpha-mediated vasoconstriction with increase of coronary vascular resistance (10,28). This vasoconstriction is short-lasting and quickly overwhelmed by the metabolic beta-mediated arteriolar vasodilatation (11,12,17,40) induced by the increase of arterial blood pressure and myocardial activity (21,64). Thus the final result of cold application in normal subjects is an increase in coronary blood flow with a decrease in coronary vascular resistance (13,43,44). PGI_2 and PGE_2 have been shown to modulate vasoconstrictor response to sympathetic stimulation, and the inhibition of prostaglandin synthesis results in an inappropriate and long-lasting vasoconstriction of the forearm vasculature (56,58) as well as of coronary vasculature in patients with coronary artery disease (14).

The absence of a transcardiac TXB_2 gradient both at rest and after sympathetic stimulation strongly indicates that normal coronary vasculature and normal myocytes do not synthesize TXA_2.

PROSTAGLANDIN SYNTHESIS IN PATIENTS WITH ISCHEMIC HEART DISEASE

The influence of prostaglandins on vascular coronary resistance (47,48) and the powerful coronary vasoconstrictor activity of TXA_2 (9,76) has prompted many investigators to study the possible role of prostaglandins in the pathogenesis of IHD. Significant reduction of PGI_2-like activity in plasma has been reported in patients with IHD (59), and elevated levels of TXB_2 have been found in peripheral blood (50,75) and in coronary sinus blood (23,67,75) during ischemic spontaneous attacks and during myocardial ischemia induced by atrial pacing (24,31,75). However, in all these investigations but one (50), no precaution was taken to prevent TXA_2 generation by platelets as a consequence of myocardial ischemia (66) or by aggregating platelets during the passage through the sampling catheters. Thus TXB_2 elevation in the blood withdrawn from coronary sinus could not be primarily related to the occurrence of myocardial ischemia. On the other hand, TXB_2 plasma levels in peripheral venous blood at rest and after sympathetic stimulation have been found to be different in patients with different clinical forms of angina (57). Patients with spontaneous active angina showed higher TXB_2 levels at rest and following sympathetic stimulation associated with an increased and longer lasting vascular response than controls and patients with effort stable angina. In all these patients platelets were blocked by a previous aspirin administration, so that the increase in TXA_2 following sympathetic stimulation could not be related to platelet synthesis. Therefore these findings seem to suggest an altered PG production in patients with different forms of angina and especially in patients with active spontaneous angina.

PROSTAGLANDIN SYNTHESIS IN PATIENTS WITH STABLE EFFORT ANGINA

In patients with stable effort angina (EA), 6-keto-$PGF_{1\alpha}$ levels in peripheral venous and in coronary sinus blood are lower than in controls (Figs. 1 and 5). No significant differences can be found between coronary sinus and aortic blood (Fig. 5). Similarly, no transcardiac gradient in 6-keto-$PGF_{1\alpha}$ levels is observed following sympathetic stimulation. Thus patients with EA show significantly lower PGI_2 coronary formation than controls (Fig. 2).

PGE_2 levels in coronary sinus blood are usually undetectable in these patients, both at rest and after sympathetic stimulation (Figs. 3 and 5).

In EA patients as well as in controls, no difference in plasma TXB_2 concentration between coronary sinus and aorta is usually found either at rest or after sympathetic stimulation, thus indicating no significant TXA_2 synthesis by coronary vasculature or myocytes.

In conclusion, in EA patients a reduced coronary synthesis of PGI_2 and PGE_2 exists, but no cardiocoronary synthesis of TXA_2 can be found.

PROSTAGLANDIN SYNTHESIS IN PATIENTS WITH
SPONTANEOUS ANGINA

In all patients but one with spontaneous angina, 6-keto-$PGF_{1\alpha}$ was undetectable in blood from peripheral vein, coronary sinus, and aorta (Figs. 1, 5, and 6). Unlike in the controls, sympathetic stimulation does not induce significant elevation in 6-keto-$PGF_{1\alpha}$ concentration in coronary sinus blood, and no transcardiac concentration gradient can be found (Fig. 2). Thus these findings indicate that prostacyclin synthesis by coronary vasculature is significantly decreased both at rest and following sympathetic stimulation in patients with spontaneous angina as well as in patients with stable effort angina.

PGE_2 synthesis is also reduced, because baseline PGE_2 levels in coronary sinus blood and after cold application are undetectable in all patients when platelets are completely blocked by a previous aspirin administration (Figs. 3 and 6).

Unlike controls and EA patients, patients with spontaneous angina have TXB_2 levels in coronary sinus blood significantly higher than in aortic blood, thus indicating an abnormal transcardiac gradient of TXB_2 concentration (Fig. 6). The differences in TXB_2 levels between the coronary sinus and the aorta significantly increase following sympathetic stimulation (Fig. 4), thus confirming the abnormal

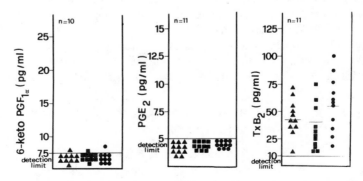

FIG. 6.   Spontaneous angina. Baseline levels of 6-keto-$PGF_{1\alpha}$, PGE_2, and TXB_2 in different vascular beds (▲ = vein; ■ = aorta; ● = coronary sinus).

cardiocoronary TXA_2 synthesis in patients with spontaneous angina. Therefore a marked difference does exist between patients with spontaneous angina and patients with stable EA.

The higher levels of TXB_2 in coronary sinus blood and the increased formation following sympathetic stimulation observed in patients with spontaneous angina are unrelated to the presence and severity of coronary angiographic lesions. Patients with similar degrees of coronary artery disease, like patients with stable EA, do not show a transcardiac gradient in TXB_2 concentration at rest or after cold application.

Moreover, patients with spontaneous angina differ from controls and EA patients in having higher TXB_2 levels in peripheral venous blood at rest and higher TXB_2 increases after sympathetic stimulation, even if platelets are completely blocked by a previous aspirin administration. Patients with inactive spontaneous angina and patients with active angina investigated again in the inactive phase do not show the increased capacity to synthesize TXA_2, and they do not differ from patients with stable EA (50).

Thus abnormal cardiac or coronary capacity to synthesize TXA_2 seems to be a property of the acute phase of angina and not of the coronary artery disease.

MEANING OF THE ALTERED PROSTAGLANDIN SYNTHESIS

Present findings and the results from other investigations (60) demonstrate that the normal human heart synthesizes PGI_2 and PGE_2 whereas it is not able to synthesize appreciable amounts of TXA_2. Moreover, PG synthesis is significantly increased by sympathetic stimulation. In IHD patients an abnormal cardiac PG synthesis occurs. Two different kinds of altered PG formation can be found: (a) a reduced synthesis of vasodilating PGI_2 and PGE_2, and (b) an abnormal synthesis of TXA_2. The reduced formation of PGI_2 and PGE_2 can be found in most of the patients with IHD, independently of the different clinical manifestation of the angina. Thus it seems to be a common feature of the IHD. On the other hand, the abnormal cardiac or coronary capacity to synthesize TXA_2 can be found only in patients with spontaneous angina in the active phase, so that it seems to be a peculiar property of the instability of the angina and not a feature of the coronary artery disease. This opinion is also suggested by the absence of relationship between the abnormal TXA_2 formation and the presence and severity of the coronary angiographic lesions.

It is intriguing to speculate about the functional meaning of the reduced coronary synthesis of PGI_2 and PGE_2. Unfortunately we could not measure coronary blood flow and coronary vascular resistance during sympathetic activation. PGs have been found to influence basal tone of human coronary arteries (18) and coronary vascular resistance in isolated perfused hearts (22,27,48,68,69). Moreover, the inhibition of PG synthesis in man by indomethacin administration resulted in an increase of coronary vascular resistance (14). Therefore these findings seem to indicate that cardiac PGs participate in the modulation of coronary vascular resistance, just as they do in peripheral (forearm and leg) vascular resistance (56,58).

Patients with spontaneous angina in the active phase are particularly prone to coronary vasospasm, both spontaneous and induced (3,4,34,35)—i.e., they are prone to an exaggerated, long-lasting vasoconstriction. These patients have been found to differ from EA patients and from patients with spontaneous angina in the inactive phase for the abnormal cardiocoronary synthesis of TXA_2, in addition to the reduced PGI_2 and PGE_2 synthesis. Moreover, in these patients an abnormal, exaggerated, long-lasting increase of forearm vascular resistance has been reported (57). Thus the inappropriate, often vasospastic, coronary response to different vasoconstrictor stimuli peculiar to the unstable angina (57) might reflect at the coronary level the increased and long-lasting vasoconstrictor response found in the peripheral vascular bed. The association of the exaggerated and long-lasting vascular response with the abnormally elevated TXA_2 synthesis seems to suggest (but it does not prove) that the abnormal cardiocoronary TXA_2 biosynthesis, in addition to the reduced vasodilator PG formation, can be responsible for the occurrence of coronary vasospasm in patients with spontaneous angina.

The mechanism of the abnormal cardiocoronary TXA_2 synthesis is unknown. This abnormal capacity of the heart to synthesize TXA_2 might be similar to the abnormal capacity that the rabbit kidney acquires in the unilateral ureter obstruction (41,42,61) when the idronephrotic kidney becomes able to synthesize marked amounts of TXA_2.

In this condition the increased synthesis of TXA_2 seems to be due to the proliferation of fibroblast-like cells and to the critical presence of mononuclear cells (61) induced by ureter obstruction. At this time there are no known factors or conditions capable of rendering unstable the silent or clinically quiescient coronary artery disease. However, it is worth stressing that patients with active spontaneous angina differ from EA patients and from patients with inactive spontaneous angina for other transient, not permanent, features, such as the elevated plasma levels of fibrinopeptide A (53,54), the increased TXA_2 formation by platelets (36,54,73), and the increased TXA_2 production in the forearm vascular bed (57). Thus the instability of coronary artery disease might be due to both local and general factors.

ACKNOWLEDGMENT

This investigation has been supported by grant 82.01082.83 from the Italian National Research Council, Project Atherosclerosis.

REFERENCES

1. Alexander, R. W., Kent, K. M., and Pisano, J. I. (1975): Regulation of postocclusive hyperemia by endogenously synthesized prostaglandins in the dog heart. *J. Clin. Invest.*, 55:1174–1181.
2. Belo, S. E., and Talesni, J. K. (1982): Coronary vasoconstrictor and vasodilator actions of arachidonic and in the isolated perfused heart of the rat. *Br. J. Pharmacol.*, 76:269–286.
3. Bertrand, M. E., La Blanche, J. M., Tilmont, P. Y., Thienleux, F. A., Delforge, M. R., Cerve, A. G., and Asseman, P. (1982): Frequency of provoked coronary arterial spasm in 1089 consecutive patients undergoing coronary arteriography. *Circulation*, 65:1299–1306.

4. Chahine, R. A. (1982): La part du spasm en pathologie coronaire. *Ann. Cardiol. Angiol.*, 31:563–570.

5. Coker, S. J., and Parratt, J. R. (1983): Effects of dazoxiben on arrhythmias and ventricular fibrillation induced by coronary artery occlusion and reperfusion in anaesthetised grey hounds. *Br. J. Clin. Pharmacol.*, 15:875–955.

6. Coker, S. J., Marshall, R. J., Parratt, J. R., and Zeitlin, I. J. (1981): Does the local myocardial release of prostaglandin E_2 or F_{2alpha} contribute to the early consequences of acute myocardial ischaemia? *J. Mol. Cell. Cardiol.*, 13:425–434.

7. Coker, S. J., Parratt, J. R., Ledingham, M., and Zeitlin, I. J. (1981): Thromboxane and prostacyclin release from ischaemic myocardium in relation to arrhythmias. *Nature (Lond.)*, 291:323–324.

8. Coker, S. J., Parratt, J. R., Ledingham, M., and Zeitlin, I. J. (1982): Evidence that thromboxane contributes to ventricular fibrillation induced by reperfusion of the ischaemic myocardium. *J. Mol. Cell. Cardiol.*, 14:483–485.

9. Ellis, E. S., Oez, O., and Roberts, L. J. (1976): Coronary arterial smooth muscle contraction by a substance released from platelets: Evidence that it is thromboxane A_2. *Science* 193:1135–1147.

10. Ertl, G., and Fuchs, M. (1980): Alpha-adrenergic vasoconstriction in arterial and arteriolar sections of the canine coronary circulation. *Basic Res. Cardiol.*, 75:600–614.

11. Feigl, E. O. (1967): Sympathetic control of coronary circulation. *Circ. Res.*, 20:262–271.

12. Feigl, E. O. (1983): Coronary physiology. *Physiol. Rev.*, 63:1–205.

13. Feldman, R. L., Whittle, J. L., Marx, J. D., Pepine, C. J., and Conti, C. R. (1982): Regional coronary hemodynamic responses to cold stimulation in patients without variant angina. *Am. J. Cardiol.*, 49:665–673.

14. Friedman, P. L., Brown, E. J., Gunther, S., Alexander, R. W., Barry, W. H., Mudge, G. H., and Rossman, W. (1981): Coronary vasoconstrictor effect of indomethacin in patients with coronary-artery disease. *N. Engl. J. Med.*, 305:1171–1175.

15. Gerritsen, M. E., and Printz, M. P. (1981): Sites of prostaglandin synthesis in the bovine heart and isolated bovine microvessels. *Circ. Res.*, 49:1152–1163.

16. Gerritsen, M. E., and Cheli, C. D. (1983): Arachidonic acid and prostaglandin endoperoxide metabolism in isolated rabbit and coronary microvessels and isolated and cultivated coronary microvessel endothelial cells. *J. Clin. Invest.*, 72:1658–1672.

17. Gewirtz, H., Most, A. S., and Williams, D. O. (1982): The effect of generalized alpha-receptor stimulation on regional myocardial blood flow distal to a severe coronary artery stenosis. *Circulation*, 65:1329–1336.

18. Ginsburg, R., Bristow, M. R., Harrison, D. C., and Stinson, E. B. (1980): Studies with isolated human coronary arteries. Some general observations, potential mediators of spasm, role of calcium antagonists. *Chest*, 78(suppl.):180–186.

19. Golding, D. (1970): Angina and indomethacin. *Br. Med. J.*, 4:622–624.

20. Granström, E., Kindahl, H., and Samuelsson, B. (1976): Radioimmunoassay for thromboxane B_2. *Anal. Lett.*, 9:611–627.

21. Greene, M. A., Goltax, A. J., Lustig, G. A., and Roglow, E. (1965): Circulatory dynamics during the cold pressor test. *Am. J. Cardiol.*, 16:54–60.

22. Gunther, S., and Cannon, P. J. (1980): Modulation of angiotensin II coronary vasoconstriction by cardiac prostaglandin synthesis. *Am. J. Physiol.*, 7:H895–H901.

23. Hirsh, P. D., Hills, L. D., Campbell, W. B., Firth, B. G., and Willerson, J. T. (1981): Release of prostaglandins and thromboxane into the coronary circulation in patients with ischemic heart disease. *N. Engl. J. Med.*, 304:685–691.

24. Hirsh, P. D., Firth, B. G., Campbell, W. B., Dehmer, G. J., and Willerson, J. T. (1983): Effects of provocation on transcardiac thromboxane in patients with coronary artery disease. *Am. J. Cardiol.*, 51:727–733.

25. Isakson, P. C., Raz, A., Danny, S. E., Pure, E., and Needleman, P. (1977): A novel prostaglandin is the major product of arachidonic and metabolism in rabbit heart. *Proc. Natl. Acad. Sci. U.S.A.*, 74:101–105.

26. Kalsner, S. (1975): Endogenous prostaglandin release contributes directly to coronary artery tone. *Can. J. Physiol. Pharmacol.*, 53:560–565.

27. Kalsner, S. (1976): The effect of hypoxia on prostaglandin output and tone in isolated coronary arteries. *Can. J. Physiol. Pharmacol.*, 55:882–887.

28. Kelley, K. O., and Feigl, E. O. (1978): Segmental alpha-receptor-mediated vasoconstriction in the canine coronary circulation. *Circ. Res.*, 43:908–917.
29. Kraemer, R. J., and Folts, J. D. (1973): Release of prostaglandins following temporary occlusion of the coronary artery. *Fed. Proc.*, 32:454–456.
30. Levi, R., Allan, G., and Zavecz, J. H. (1976): Prostaglandins and cardiac anaphylaxis. *Life Sci.*, 18:1255–1264.
31. Lewy, R. I., Wiener, L., Walinsky, P., Lefer, A. M., Silver, M. J., and Smith, J. B. (1980): Thromboxane release during pacing-induced angina pectoris: Possible vasoconstrictor influence on the coronary vasculature. *Circulation*, 61:1165–1171.
32. Liebig, R., Bernauer, W., and Peskar, B. A. (1975): Prostaglandin, slow reacting substance and histamine release from anaphilactic guinea pig hearts and its pharmacological modification. *Naunyn Schmiedeberg's Arch. Pharmakol.*, 289:65–76.
33. Limas, C. J., and Cohn, J. N. (1973): Isolation and properties of myocardial prostaglandin synthetase. *Cardiovasc. Res.*, 7:623–628.
34. Maseri, A. (1980): Coronary vasospasm in ischemic heart disease. *Chest*, 78(suppl. 1):210–215.
35. Maseri, A., Chierchia, S., L'Abbate, A., Biagini, A., Distante, A., Parodi, O., Brunelli, G., and Severi, S. (1982): Role du spasm dans l'angine de poitrine l'infarctus du myocarde et la morte subite. *Arch. Med. Coeur*, 75:701–716.
36. Mehta, J., Mehta, P., and Conti, C. R. (1980): Platelet function studies in coronary heart disease. IX. Increased prostaglandin generation and abnormal platelet sensitivity to prostacyclin and endoperoxide analog in angina pectoris. *Am. J. Cardiol.*, 46:943–947.
37. Miwa, K., Kambara, H., and Kawai, C. (1979): Variant angina aggravated by aspirin. *Lancet*, 2:1382.
38. Miwa, K., Kambara, H., and Kawai, C. (1981): Exercise induced angina provoked by aspirin administration in patient with variant angina. *Am. J. Cardiol.*, 47:1210–1214.
39. Miwa, K., Kambara, H., and Kawai, C. (1983): Effect of aspirin in large doses on attacks of variant angina. *Am. Heart J.*, 105:351–355.
40. Mohrman, D. E., and Feigl, E. O. (1978): Competition between sympathetic vasoconstriction and metabolic vasodilatation in the canine coronary circulation. *Circ. Res.*, 42:79–86.
41. Morrison, A. R., Nishikawa, K., and Needleman, P. (1977): Unmasking of thromboxane A synthesis by ureteral obstruction in the rabbit kidney. *Nature (Lond.)*, 267:259–260.
42. Morrison, A. R., Nishikawa, K., and Needleman, P. (1978): Thromboxane A biosynthesis in the ureter obstructed isolated perfused kidney of the rabbit. *J. Pharmacol. Exp. Ther.*, 205:1–8.
43. Mudge, G. H., Crossman, W., Mills, R. M., Lesch, H., and Braunwald, E. (1976): Reflex increase in coronary vascular resistance in patients with ischemic heart disease. *N. Engl. J. Med.*, 295:1333–1336.
44. Mudge, G. H., Goldberg, S., Günther, S., Mann, T., and Brossman, W. (1979): Comparison of metabolic and vasoconstrictor stimuli on coronary vascular resistance in man. *Circulation*, 59:544–550.
45. Needleman, P., Bronson, S. D., Whyche, A., Sivakoff, M., and Nicolaou, K. C. (1978): Cardiac and renal prostaglandin I_2. Biosynthesis and biological effects in isolated perfused rabbit tissue. *J. Clin. Invest.*, 61:839–849.
46. Needleman, P., Kay, S. L., and Isakson, P. C. (1975): Relationship between oxygen tension, coronary vasodilatation and prostaglandin biosynthesis in the isolated rabbit heart. *Prostaglandins*, 9:123–134.
47. Needleman, P., Kulkarni, P. S., and Raz, A. (1977): Coronary tone modulation: Formation and actions of prostaglandins, endoperoxides and thromboxanes. *Science*, 195:409–412.
48. Needleman, P. N., and Kaley, G. (1978): Cardiac and coronary prostaglandin synthesis and function. *N. Engl. J. Med.*, 298:1122–1128.
49. Neri Serneri, G. G. (1979): Prostacyclin, thromboxane and ischemic heart disease. In: *Myocardial Infarction*, edited by D. T. Mason, G. G. Neri Serneri, and M. T. Oliver, pp. 299–311. Excerpta Medica, Amsterdam.
50. Neri Serneri, G. G. (1982): Prostaglandins in patients with ischemic heart disease. In: *Cardiovascular Pharmacology of the Prostaglandins*, edited by A. G. Herman, P. M. Vanhoutte, H. Denolin, and A. Goossens, pp. 361–374. Raven Press, New York.
51. Neri Serneri, G. G., Abbate, R., Gensini, G. F., Galanti, G., Paoli, G., and Laureano, R. (1982): Platelet aggregation and thromboxane A_2 production after adrenergic stimulation in young healthy humans. *Haemostasis*, 11:40–48.

52. Neri Serneri, G. G., Abbate, R., Gensini, G. F., Panetta, A., Casolo, G. C., and Carini, M. (1983): Thromboxane A₂ production by human arteries and veins. *Prostaglandins*, 25:753–766.

53. Neri Serneri, G. G., Gensini, G. F., Abbate, R., Laureano, R., and Parodi, O. (1980): Is raised plasma fibrinopeptide A a marker of acute coronary insufficiency? *Lancet*, 2:982–983.

54. Neri Serneri, G. G., Gensini, G. F., Abbate, R., Mugnaini, C., Favilla, S., Mannelli, C., Chierchia, S., and Parodi, O. (1981): Increased fibrinopeptide A TXA₂ formation in patients with ischemic heart disease: Relationships to coronary pathoanatomy, risk factors and clinical manifestations. *Am. Heart J.*, 101:185–194.

55. Neri Serneri, G. G., Masotti, G., Castellani, S., Scarti, L., Morettini, A., Sciagrà, R., and Mannelli, M. (1983): Effects of PGE₂ inhibition on norepinephrine plasma levels after adrenergic stimulation in man. In: *Advances in Prostaglandins, Thromboxane, and Leukotriene Research, Vol. 12*, edited by B. Samuelsson, R. Paoletti, and P. W. Ramwell, pp. 365–371. Raven Press, New York.

56. Neri Serneri, G. G., Masotti, G., Castellani, S., Scarti, L., Trotta, F., and Mannelli, M. (1983): Role of PGE₂ in the modulation of the adrenergic response in man. *Cardiovasc. Res.*, 17:662–670.

57. Neri Serneri, G. G., Masotti, G., Gensini, G. F., Abbate, R., and Rostagno, C. (1983): L'alterata modulazione vascolare prostaglandinica nella patogenesi della ischemia miocardica. In: *La Cardiopatia Ischemica. Nuovi Aspetti ed Implicazioni*, edited by S. Lenzi, A. Maseri, and G. G. Neri Serneri, pp. 147–185. Edizioni Pozzi, Roma.

58. Neri Serneri, G. G., Masotti, G., Gensini, G. F., Poggesi, L., Abbate, R., and Mannelli, M. (1981): Prostacyclin and thromboxane A₂ formation in response to adrenergic stimulation in human. A mechanism for local control of vascular response to sympathetic activation? *Cardiovasc. Res.*, 15:287–295.

59. Neri Serneri, G. G., Masotti, G., Poggesi, L., Galanti, G., Morettini, A., and Scarti, L. (1982): Reduced prostacyclin production in patients with different manifestation of ischemic heart disease. *Am. J. Cardiol.*, 49:1146–1151.

60. Novak, K. J., Kaijser, L., and Wennmalm, A. (1980): Cardiac synthesis of prostaglandins from arachidonic acid in man. *Prostaglandins Med.*, 4:205–214.

61. Okegawa, T., Jonas, P. E., De Schryver, K., Kawasaki, A., and Needleman, P. (1983): Metabolic and cellular alteration underlying the exaggerated renal prostaglandin and thromboxane synthesis in ureter obstruction in rabbits. Inflammatory response involving fibroblasts and mononuclear cells. *J. Clin. Invest.*, 71:81–90.

62. Patrono, C., Grossi-Belloni, D., Ciabattoni, G., Serra, G. B., Latorre, E., Bombardieri, S., Mancuso, S., and Gorga, C. (1974): Radioimmunoassay measurement of F prostaglandins in the human body fluid. *Horm. Metab. Res.*, 5:190–195.

63. Patrono, C., Pugliese, F., Ciabattoni, G., Maseri, A., and Peskar, B. A. (1982): Evidence for a direct stimulatory effect of prostacyclin on renin release in man. *J. Clin. Invest.*, 69:231–239.

64. Raizner, A. E., and Chahine, R. A. (1979): The treatment of Prinzmetal's variant angina with coronary by-pass surgery. In: *Update II to the Heart*, edited by J. W. Hurst, pp. 85–95. McGraw-Hill, New York.

65. Raz, A., Isakson, P. C., Minkes, M. S., and Needleman, P. (1977): Characterization of a novel metabolic pathway of arachidonate in coronary arteries which generates a potent endogenous coronary vasodilator. *J. Biol. Chem.*, 252:1123–1126.

66. Robertson, R. M., Robertson, D., Friesinger, G. C., Timmons, S., and Hawiger, J. (1980): Platelets aggregates in peripheral and coronary sinus blood in patients with spontaneous coronary artery spasm. *Lancet*, 2:829–831.

67. Robertson, R. M., Robertson, D., Roberts, L. J., Maas, R. L., Fitzgerald, G. A., Friesinger, G. C., and Oates, J. A. (1981): Thromboxane A₂ in vasotonic angina pectoris. Evidence from direct measurements and inhibitor trials. *N. Engl. J. Med.*, 304:998–1003.

68. Sakanashi, M., Arak, H., Furukawa, T., Rokutanda, M., and Yonemura, K. (1981): A study on constrictor response of dog coronary arteries to acetylsalicylic acid. *Arch. Int. Pharmacodyn.*, 252:86–96.

69. Schrör, K., Krebs, R., and Nookhwun, C. K. (1976): Increase in the coronary vascular resistance by indomethacin in the isolated guinea pig heart preparation in the absence of changes in mechanical performance and oxygen consumption. *Eur. J. Pharmacol.*, 39:161–169.

70. Schrör, K., Moncada, S., Ubatuba, F. B., and Vane, J. R. (1978): Transformation of arachidonic acid and prostaglandin endoperoxides by the guinea pig heart. Formation of RCS and prostacyclin. *Eur. J. Pharmacol.*, 47:103–114.

71. Schrör, K., Link, H. B., Rösen, R., Klaus, W., and Rösen, P. (1980): Prostacyclin-induced coronary vasodilatation. Interactions with adenosine, cyclic AMP and energy charge in the rat heart *in vitro*. *Eur. J. Pharmacol.*, 64:341–348.
72. Sivakoff, M., Pure, E., Hsueh, W., and Needleman, P. N. (1979): Prostaglandins and the heart. *Fed. Proc.*, 38:78–82.
73. Sobel, M., Salzman, E. W., Davies, G. C., Haundin, R. I., Sweeney, J., Ploetz, J., and Kurland, G. (1981): Circulating platelet products in unstable angina pectoris. *Circulation*, 63:300–306.
74. Sunahara, F. A., and Talesnik, J. (1979): Myocardial synthesis of prostaglandin-like substances and coronary reactions to cardiostimulation and to hypoxia. *Br. J. Pharmacol.*, 65:71–85.
75. Tada, M., Kuzuya, T., Inoue, M., Kodama, K., Mishima, M., Yamada, M., Inui, M., and Abe, H. (1981): Elevation of thromboxane B_2 levels in patients with classic and variant angina pectoris. *Circulation*, 64:1107–1115.
76. Terashita, Z.I., Fukui, H., and Nishikawa, K. (1978): Coronary vasospastic action of thromboxane A_2 in isolated working guinea pig heart. *Eur. J. Pharmacol.*, 53:49–56.
77. Wennmalm, A. (1975): Hypoxia-induced prostaglandin release from rabbit heart. In: *Recent Advances in Studies on Cardiac Structure and Metabolism, Vol. 10*, edited by P. E. Roy and G. Rona, pp. 379–385. University Park Press, Baltimore.
78. Wennmalm, A. (1979): Prostaglandins and cardiovascular function, some biochemical and physiological aspects. *Scand. J. Clin. Lab. Invest.*, 30:399–405.

*Advances in Prostaglandin, Thromboxane, and
Leukotriene Research, Vol. 13*, edited by G.G. Neri
Serneri, et al. Raven Press, New York © 1985.

Contributory Role of Platelets in Various Manifestations of Ischemic Heart Disease

Jawahar Mehta

*Department of Medicine, Division of Cardiology, University of Florida College of
Medicine, Gainesville, Florida 32610*

Besides hemostasis, platelets play an important role in the evolution of thrombosis in the arterial bed, microvasculature, and on artificial surfaces such as prosthetic cardiac valves and vascular grafts. Platelets also have a role in the genesis of atherosclerosis. The growing information on the contribution of platelets in the evolution of myocardial ischemia has led to platelet-suppressive drug trials in patients with coronary artery disease. The purpose of this chapter is to review the role of platelets in health and in ischemic heart disease.

NORMAL PLATELET FUNCTION

Platelets, small disk-like cells circulating in the blood, have a primary role in hemostasis. On stress to the endothelium and its disruption, platelets adhere to the subendothelial collagen. Other circulating platelets are attracted to the adhering platelets, resulting in platelet aggregation and formation of a platelet thrombus. Red blood cells, leukocytes, and other blood components are incorporated in platelet thrombus with the formation of occlusive clot. Coagulation cascade is also activated at this stage. Platelets on activation release potent hormones, prostaglandins, polypeptides, and other vasoactive substances, some of which promote platelet aggregation, vasoconstriction, and vascular permeability. Following the endothelial reparative process, platelet clumps disaggregate and the vascular lumen becomes recanalized. This, in brief, is a major mechanism by which extravasation of blood following vascular injury is limited. Platelets also play an important role in nurturing vascular endothelium and maintaining its continuity, as is evident from studies showing fenestrations in the endothelial lining in animals with thrombocytopenia or decreased platelet function. Correction of platelet number or the functional defect results in prompt repair of this endothelial injury (18).

PLATELETS, THROMBOSIS, AND ATHEROSCLEROSIS

Arterial thrombosis may be considered an extension of the normal hemostatic mechanism. If the platelets are continuously activated or the endothelial injury is persistent, a thrombotic tendency may ensue. Localized thrombus formation may subsequently result in vasoocclusion and tissue ischemia.

Atherosclerosis

Platelets may also be involved in atherogenesis in regions of blood turbulence or endothelial disruption. Platelet activation may result in release of substances that alter vasomotor tone (thromboxane A_2, serotonin, histamine), increase vascular permeability (β-thromboglobulin), and penetrate the vascular lining (platelet factor 4). In experimental atherosclerosis induced by endothelial injury, platelets release a growth factor responsible for proliferation and migration of smooth muscle cells (14), a key event in atherogenesis. Sequential studies in atherosclerotic pigeons show a persistent increase in platelet factor 4 activity (7). Evidence supporting pathogenic role of platelets also comes from studies demonstrating resistance to the development of atherosclerosis in animals with thrombocytopenia (6) or suppressed platelet function (3,8). However, it should be recognized that atherogenesis is a complex multifactorial process. A variety of plasma proteins, such as pituitary hormones and insulin, are also mitogens. Multiple episodes of injury (9), perhaps coupled with lipid abnormalities, are needed to produce atherosclerosis. Nonetheless, studies briefly mentioned above indicate a link between platelets and atherosclerosis.

PLATELET FUNCTION IN CORONARY "RISK FACTORS"

It has been proposed that so called "risk factors" for atherosclerosis—i.e., hypertension, diabetes mellitus, hyperlipidemia, and smoking—participate in the pathogenesis of atherosclerosis through an abnormal platelet-endothelial interaction (23). Increased platelet activity has been identified in smokers. Patients with hypertension have increased platelet adhesion and increased levels of platelet-released β-thromboglobulin, indicating *in vivo* activation (22). There is evidence for "hyperactive" platelets in diabetic subjects with vascular injury (35). Hyperlipidemia is also associated with increased platelet activity and decreased platelet survival (2). In addition, therapy of hypertension, diabetes mellitus, and hyperlipidemia is associated with reversal of platelet hyperactivity (2,22,35).

PLATELET FUNCTION IN EXPERIMENTAL
MYOCARDIAL ISCHEMIA

Infusion of platelet aggregants, like ADP or epinephrine, results in evidence of focal myocardial infarcts in experimental animals (11,16). Formation of platelet aggregates in the microvasculature causes reduction in blood flow with resultant tissue ischemia, which if sustained can cause tissue death. Platelet aggregates appearing at the site of experimentally-induced vascular injury can lead to vasoocclusion (37). Vik-Mo has observed platelet aggregates in the coronary venous blood obtained from dogs with coronary constriction (39). The contributory role of platelets in myocardial ischemia is also supported by the observations that pretreatment of animals with platelet-suppressive drugs results in decrease in infarct size and improvement in blood flow to the ischemic tissues (1,17).

In dogs with critical coronary narrowing, phasic decrease and increase in blood flow are seen, which relate to spontaneous platelet aggregation and disaggregation, respectively (5). Intracoronary or intravenous administration of platelet aggregants often provokes these phasic changes in coronary blood flow (Fig. 1). These phasic changes in blood flow in animals can be ameliorated with aspirin, prostacyclin, and other platelet-inhibitory agents (5).

PLATELET FUNCTION IN ISCHEMIC HEART DISEASE IN MAN

Studies in patients with ischemic heart disease are fraught with methodologic problems. Platelet function shows diurnal variation and is influenced by the activity status of the individual and a host of drugs. In most studies, platelet function has been measured in the peripheral venous blood, which may not reflect platelet function alterations in the region of interest. Aortic and coronary venous sampling is an attractive approach to evaluate changes in platelet function as blood traverses the atherosclerotic coronary vasculature. However, collection of blood through long indwelling catheters may also influence platelet function. The results obtained from measurement of platelet-specific proteins in plasma have been quite variable because of differences in the methodologies employed. Therefore, only general conclusions relative to platelet function in coronary heart disease in man can be made.

Stable Angina Pectoris

Several years ago, platelet survival was shown to be decreased in patients with stable angina pectoris. Increased platelet sensitivity to aggregating stimuli was described by some investigators (38), but not by others (4,34). Hampton and Gorlin

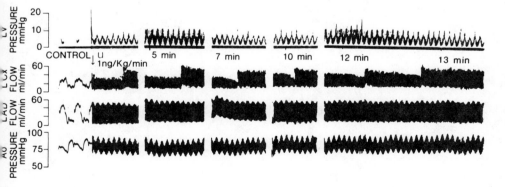

FIG. 1. Cyclical decrease followed by abrupt increase in left circumflex (LCx) coronary artery blood flow in a dog with 60% LCx narrowing following infusion of platelet stimulus U46,619 (U). No changes are seen in left ventricular (LV) and aortic (AO) pressures, and left anterior descending (LAD) coronary artery blood flow.

reported increased platelet electrophoretic mobility in response to ADP not only in patients with coronary artery disease, but also in patients' relatives (12). Neri Serneri et al. (33) found a significant increase in circulating platelet aggregates in all patients with ischemic heart disease, regardless of acuteness of the disease process. The number of megathrombocytes was also increased in all patients, and a close correlation between the number of megathrombocytes and circulating platelet aggregates was observed. However, there was no correlation between the number of circulating platelet aggregates and the severity or extent of coronary artery disease.

We conducted studies on the alteration in platelet function as platelets traverse normal and atherosclerotic vascular beds (25,28,29,31). Blood samples collected from the aorta and coronary sinus (affluent and effluent, respectively) demonstrated no alteration in platelets in subjects with normal coronary arteries. In contrast, platelets seemed to be partially removed in the atherosclerotic vessels, as demonstrated by a significant gradient in platelet counts between aortic and coronary venous blood. Platelet function was also markedly decreased in the effluent, implying passage of biologically less active platelets (Fig. 2).

To determine whether these changes were specific for the coronary vascular bed, we conducted similar studies in another arterial, muscular, and long but isolated vascular bed (30). We demonstrated that the passage through the normal forearm vascular bed did not influence platelet function, size, or shape. To determine the influence of acute regional stress, we paced the heart electrically. During tachycardia stress we found marked activation of platelets exiting in the coronary sinus, but no changes were observed in aortic blood, implying that platelet activation had taken place at the level of the atherosclerotic coronary vascular bed (29). About 15 to 30 min after termination of stress, platelet activation was no longer observed.

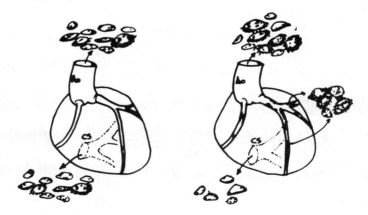

FIG. 2. Schematic representation of effect of passage through the coronary vascular bed at rest on platelets. In normal coronary arteries **(left)**, platelets pass through the vascular bed without any alteration. In contrast, in atherosclerotic vessels **(right)**, platelets are removed in the coronary vessels accounting for fewer platelets in the coronary venous blood compared to the aortic blood.

No similar activation was observed in subjects with normal coronary arteries or in the effluent from the normal forearm during exercise and tissue ischemia.

To examine the concept of platelet sequestration, we studied the effects of platelet-suppressive drugs. With use of aspirin (cyclooxygenase inhibitor) for platelet inhibition, we demonstrated elimination of the gradient in platelet counts and the function across the myocardial vascular bed, although platelet function decreased in both the affluent and the effluent (25). Tachycardia stress also did not evoke coronary venous platelet activation as in the preaspirin state (29). We also examined the effect of dipyridamole (phosphodiesterase inhibitor) and found that the platelet counts increased in coronary venous blood to levels similar to those in arterial blood, while platelet function also became comparable at the two sites (32). Effects of dipyridamole were attributed to the potentiation of prostacyclin and inhibition of platelet adhesion. These studies strongly prove the hypothesis of platelet interaction with atherosclerotic coronary vessels. Platelet activation during tachycardia stress and its inhibition by aspirin also suggest an association of platelet hyperactivity and tissue ischemia.

Studies on measurements of platelet-released products also suggest platelet activation *in vivo* in some patients. Plasma β-thromboglobulin levels increase with exercise in patients with documented coronary artery disease and positive stress test. In contrast, exercise-induced increase in plasma β-thromboglobulin is not observed in patients with negative stress test (24) (Fig. 3). These data are supported by observations of Green et al. (10), who showed plasma platelet factor 4 levels to increase by more than 50% during exercise-induced myocardial ischemia in 11 of 20 patients. The elevated levels returned to baseline within 15 min of termination of exercise. However, other investigators (19) have failed to show similar alterations in release of platelet-specific proteins with exercise. These discrepancies in results reflect methodologic limitations.

Unstable and Vasotonic Angina Pectoris

The role of dynamic factors, such as coronary artery vasospasm and *in vivo* platelet aggregation, as pathogenic factors in spontaneous myocardial ischemia is being increasingly recognized. We have observed spontaneous platelet aggregation in a patient with rest angina (Fig. 4). Robertson et al. (36) have described passage of a large number of platelet aggregates in the coronary venous blood during myocardial ischemia in patients with vasospasm.

Platelets from patients with unstable angina pectoris have been identified to generate large amounts of prostaglandins as well as being "hypersensitive" to thromboxane A_2 and "hyposensitive" to prostacyclin (26). These factors could certainly be pathogenic in the evolution of myocardial ischemia.

It needs to be recognized that these studies were conducted in patients who had spontaneous angina prior to measurement of platelet function. Therefore, it cannot be said with certainty that platelet abnormalities are primary and not secondary to acute myocardial ischemia. Regardless of the primary or secondary nature, these

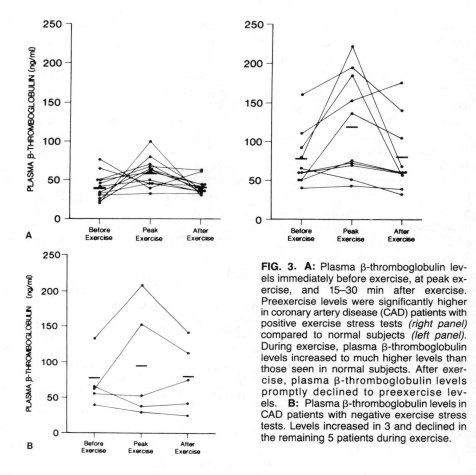

FIG. 3. A: Plasma β-thromboglobulin levels immediately before exercise, at peak exercise, and 15–30 min after exercise. Preexercise levels were significantly higher in coronary artery disease (CAD) patients with positive exercise stress tests *(right panel)* compared to normal subjects *(left panel)*. During exercise, plasma β-thromboglobulin levels increased to much higher levels than those seen in normal subjects. After exercise, plasma β-thromboglobulin levels promptly declined to preexercise levels. **B:** Plasma β-thromboglobulin levels in CAD patients with negative exercise stress tests. Levels increased in 3 and declined in the remaining 5 patients during exercise.

changes in platelet function could be instrumental in the propagation of myocardial ischemia.

Myocardial Infarction

In patients with myocardial infarction, Zahavi and Dreyfuss (40) first showed increased platelet aggregability in response to several stimuli. Others have not observed this phenomenon consistently (4,34). As a more recent study (20) shows, platelet aggregation in response to arachidonic acid may be decreased in the acute stage of myocardial infarction and aggregation response may recover during the recovery state. This "hypoaggregatory" response in the acute state may reflect either "exhausted" platelets or an undefined factor in ischemic plasma that inhibits platelet aggregation.

Circulating platelet aggregates are rather consistently increased in the early stages of acute myocardial infarction, and then decline in the recovery phase (21). In

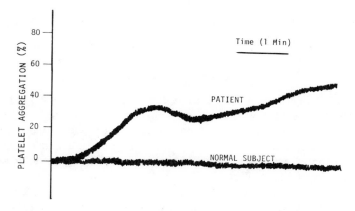

FIG. 4. Spontaneous platelet aggregation in a 51-year-old man hospitalized with unstable angina pectoris. This patient developed anterior wall myocardial infarction a few hours later. Note absence of spontaneous platelet aggregation in the normal subject.

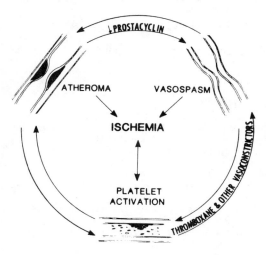

FIG. 5. Proposed relationship between atherosclerosis, platelet activation, vasospasm, and myocardial ischemia. Alterations in prostacyclin and thromboxane may play a key role in the relationship.

patients with extension of myocardial infarction, such decline is not evident. Handin et al. (13) observed marked increases in platelet factor 4 levels in plasma of patients with acute myocardial infarction. Platelet factor 4 levels remained elevated for at least 1 week, and then returned to the normal range. In another study, Heptinstall et al. (15) found no significant differences in platelet release of serotonin in patients with acute myocardial infarction compared to normal subjects. However, 8 of the 26 patients who died within 1 year had significantly more platelet release of serotonin than the 18 survivors. They concluded that the poor prognosis was related to increased platelet release reaction after myocardial infarction.

In 1 patient, we were able to demonstrate marked platelet activation release (coronary venous plasma thromboxane B_2 levels > 2000 pg/ml and β-thromboglobulin

>260 ng/ml) just prior to clinical and laboratory evaluation of acute myocardial infarction (27).

CONCLUSION

In summary, I believe that platelet activation is present in most patients with coronary "risk factors" as well as those with ischemic heart disease. There is evidence for enhanced platelet activation in conjunction with acute myocardial ischemia. If platelet activation were to precede, it could precipitate myocardial ischemia. On the other hand, if platelets are activated secondary to myocardial ischemia, platelet aggregation could cause extension of the ischemic process. A schematic representation of the role of platelets, vasoactive prostaglandins, and atherosclerosis in the genesis of myocardial ischemia is shown in Fig. 5. A contributory role of platelets in ischemic heart disease is also evident from trials of antiplatelet drugs, which have shown beneficial effect when used in proper dosages.

ACKNOWLEDGMENT

The author wishes to thank Kelly Greetham for her assistance in typing the manuscript.

REFERENCES

1. Capurro, N L., Marr, K. C., Aamodt, R., and Goldstein, R. E. (1979): Aspirin-induced increase in collateral flow after acute coronary occlusion in dogs. *Circulation*, 59:744–747.
2. Caravalho, A. C., Colman, R. W., and Lees, R. S. (1974): Platelet function in hyperlipoproteinemia. *N. Engl. J. Med.*, 290:434–438.
3. Cohen, P., and McCombs, H. L. (1968): Platelets and atherogenesis. Part 2. Amelioration of cholesterol atherogenesis in rabbits with reduced platelet counts as a result of ^{32}P administration. *J. Atherosclerosis Res.*, 8:389–393.
4. Enticknap, J. B., Gooding, P. G., Lansley, T. S., and Avis, P. R. D. (1969): Platelet size and function in ischemic heart disease. *J. Atherosclerosis Res.*, 10:41–49.
5. Folts, J. D., Crowell, E. B., and Rowe, G. G. (1976): Platelet aggregation in partially obstructed vessels and its elimination with aspirin. *Circulation*, 54:365–370.
6. Friedman, R. J., Stemerman, M. B., Wenz, B., et al. (1977): The effect of thrombocytopenia on experimental atherosclerotic lesion formation in rabbits. *J. Clin. Invest.*, 60:1191–1201.
7. Fuster, V., Lewis, J. C., Kottke, B. A., Ruiz, C. E., and Bowie, E. J. W. (1977): Platelet factor 4-like activity in the initial stages of atherosclerosis in pigeons. *Thrombosis Res.*, 10:169–172.
8. Fuster, V., Bowie, E. J. W., Fass, D. N., Owen, C. A., and Brown, A. L. (1978): Arteriosclerosis in von Willebrand and normal pigs: Spontaneous and high cholesterol diet-induced. *J. Clin. Invest.*, 61:722–730.
9. Gertz, S. D., Uretsky, G., Wajnbert, R. S., Navot, N., and Gotsman, M. S. (1981): Endothelial cell damage and thrombus formation after partial arterial constriction: Relevance to the role of coronary artery spasm in the pathogenesis of myocardial infarction. *Circulation*, 63:476–486.
10. Green, L. H., Seropplan, E., and Handin, R. I. (1980): Platelet activation during exercise-induced myocardial ischemia. *N. Engl. J. Med.*, 302:193–197.
11. Haft, J. I., and Fani, K. (1973): Intravascular platelet aggregation in the heart induced by stress. *Circulation*, 47:353–358.
12. Hampton, J. R., and Gorlin, R. (1972): Platelet studies in patients with coronary artery disease and in their relatives. *Br. Heart J.*, 34:465–471.

13. Handin, R. I., McDonough, M., and Lesch, M. (1978): Elevation of platelet factor four in acute myocardial infarction: Measurement by radio-immunoassay. *J. Lab. Clin. Med.*, 91:340–349.
14. Harker, L. A., Ross, R., Slichter, S. J., and Scott, C. R. (1976): Homocystine-induced arteriosclerosis: The role of endothelial cell injury and platelet response in its genesis. *J. Clin. Invest.*, 58:731–741.
15. Heptinstall, S., Mulley, G. P., Taylor, P. M., and Mitchell, J. R. A. (1980): Platelet release reaction in myocardial infarction. *Br. Med. J.*, 1:80–81.
16. Jorgenson, L., Rowsell, H. C., Hovig, T., et al. (1967): Adenosinediphosphate-induced platelet aggregation and myocardial infarction in swine. *Lab. Invest.*, 17:616–622.
17. Jugdutt, B. I., Hutchins, G. M., Bulkley, B. H., and Becker, L. C. (1980): Salvage of ischemic myocardium by ibuprofen during infarction in the conscious dog. *Am. J. Cardiol.*, 46:74–82.
18. Kitchens, C. S. (1977): Amelioration of endothelial abnormalities by prednisone in experimental thrombocytopenia in the rabbit. *J. Clin. Invest.*, 60:1129–1134.
19. Mathis, P. C., Wohl, H., Wallach, S. R., and Engler, R. L. (1981): Lack of release of platelet factor four during exercise-induced myocardial ischemia. *N. Engl. J. Med.*, 304:1275–1278.
20. McDaniel, H. G., Maddox, W. T., Poon, M. C., Rogers, W. J., and Rackley, C. E. (1983): Platelet function abnormalities in response to arachidonic acid in the acute phase of myocardial infarction. *Am. J. Cardiol.*, 52:965–970.
21. Mehta, P., and Mehta, J. (1979): Platelet function studies in coronary artery disease. V. Evidence for enhanced platelet micro-thrombus formation activity in acute myocardial infarction. *Am. J. Cardiol.*, 43:757–760.
22. Mehta, J., and Mehta, P. (1981): Platelet function in hypertension and effect of therapy. *Am. J. Cardiol.*, 47:231–234.
23. Mehta, J., and Mehta, P. (1981): Role of blood platelets and prostaglandins in coronary artery disease. *Am. J. Cardiol.*, 48:366–373.
24. Mehta, J., and Mehta, P. (1982): Comparison of platelet function during exercise in normal subjects and coronary artery disease patients: Potential role of platelet activation in myocardial ischemia. *Am. Heart J.*, 103:49–53.
25. Mehta, J., Mehta, P., Burger, C., and Pepine, C. J. (1978): Platelet aggregation studies in coronary artery disease. IV. Effect of aspirin. *Atherosclerosis*, 31:169–175.
26. Mehta, J., Mehta, P., and Conti, C. R. (1980): Platelet function studies in coronary heart disease. IX. Increased platelet prostaglandin generation and abnormal platelet sensitivity to prostacyclin and endoperoxide analog in angina pectoris. *Am. J. Cardiol.*, 46:943–947.
27. Mehta, J., Mehta, P., and Feldman, R. L. (1982): Severe intracoronary thromboxane release preceding acute coronary occlusion. *Prostaglandins, Leukotrienes Med.*, 8:599–605.
28. Mehta, J., Mehta, P., and Pepine, C. J. (1978): Differences in platelet aggregation in coronary sinus and aortic blood in patients with coronary artery disease. II. Effect of propranolol. *Clin. Cardiol.*, 1:96–100.
29. Mehta, J., Mehta, P., and Pepine, C. J. (1978): Platelet aggregation in aortic and coronary venous blood in patients with and without coronary disease. III. Role of tachycardia stress and propranolol. *Circulation*, 58:881–886.
30. Mehta, P., Mehta, J., and Pepine, C. J. (1981): Influence of the normal human forearm vascular bed on platelet aggregation, counts and size. *Microvasc. Res.*, 21:229–233.
31. Mehta, J., Mehta, P., Pepine, C. J., and Conti, C. R. (1980): Platelet function studies in coronary artery disease. VII. Effect of aspirin and tachycardia stress on aortic and coronary venous blood. *Am. J. Cardiol.*, 45:945–951.
32. Mehta, J., Mehta, P., Pepine, C. J., and Conti, C. R. (1981): Platelet function studies in coronary heart disease. X. Effect of dipyridamole. *Am. J. Cardiol.*, 47:1111–1114.
33. Neri Serneri, G. G., Gensini, G. F., Abbate, R., et al. (1981): Increased fibrinopeptide A formation and thromboxane A_2 production in patients with ischemic heart disease: Relationship with coronary pathoanatomy, risk factors and clinical manifestations. *Am. Heart J.*, 101:185–194.
34. O'Brien, J. R., Heywood, J. B., and Heady, J. A. (1969): The quantitation of platelet aggregation induced by four compounds: A study in relation to myocardial infarction. *Thromb. Diath. Haemorrh.*, 16:752–767.
35. Preston, F. E., Ward, J. D., Marcola, B. M., Porter, N. R., Timparkey, W. R., and O'Malley, B. C. (1978): Elevated β-thromboglobulin levels and circulating platelet aggregates in diabetic microangiopathy. *Lancet*, 1:238–240.

36. Robertson, R. M., Robertson, D., Friesinger, G. G., et al. (1980): Platelet aggregates in peripheral and coronary sinus blood in patients with spontaneous coronary artery spasm. *Lancet*, II:829.
37. Rosenblum, W. I., and El-Sabban, F. (1977): Platelet aggregation in the cerebral microcirculation. Effect of aspirin and other agents. *Circ. Res.*, 40:320–328.
38. Steele, P. P., Weily, H. S., Davis, H., and Genton, E. (1973): Platelet function studies in coronary artery disease. *Circulation*, 48:1194–1200.
39. Vik-Mo, H. (1977): Effects of acute myocardial ischemia on platelet aggregation in the coronary sinus and aorta in dogs. *Scand. J. Haematol.*, 19:68–74.
40. Zahavi, J., and Dreyfuss, F. (1969): An abnormal pattern of adenosine diphosphate-induced platelet aggregation in acute myocardial infarction. *Thromb. Diath. Haemorrh.*, 21:76–88.

Advances in Prostaglandin, Thromboxane, and
Leukotriene Research, Vol. 13, edited by G. G. Neri
Serneri, et al. Raven Press, New York © 1985.

Thromboxane in Sudden Death

Adam K. Myers and Peter W. Ramwell

*Department of Physiology and Biophysics, Georgetown University Medical Center,
Washington, D.C. 20007*

Sudden death has been identified as one of the predominant causes of mortality
in human populations (16). Although the final event leading to the sudden death is
considered to be cardiac failure, often associated with ventricular fibrillation, the
etiology of sudden death is obviously more complicated and can involve atherosclerosis, vasospasm, and thromboembolism, as well as cardiac arrhythmias. Indeed, coronary thrombosis and its sequelae may be the precipitating factors in
many sudden death cases (17). In some cases of sudden death, the only significant
finding at autopsy is occlusive pulmonary thrombosis (26). Thus, thrombosis may
have a greater role in sudden death than is commonly thought.

Relatively recent discoveries of the chemistry and biological activities of arachidonic acid metabolites have led to speculation that these agents may be involved
in cardiovascular disease, including sudden death. Of the products of arachidonate,
thromboxane has properties suggesting it may be involved in sudden death, being
a potent platelet aggregating agent, vasoconstrictor, and arrhythmic agent. Thromboxane is the major arachidonate metabolite of platelets and is produced during
release and aggregation.

THROMBOXANE IN ISCHEMIC AND THROMBOTIC
DISEASE STATES

Although cause–effect relationships are difficult to establish, thromboxane has
been found to be elevated in a number of human disease states involving ischemia
and thrombosis. Plasma levels of the thromboxane breakdown product, thromboxane
B_2, are elevated in patients with angina pectoris during pacing-induced ischemia
(15). Likewise, patients with variant angina have elevated plasma levels of thromboxane
B_2 (14). Individuals with unstable angina and recent episodes of pain have elevated
levels of thromboxane B_2 in coronary sinus blood (10). Patients with deep venous
thrombosis display elevated urinary thromboxane B_2 levels (6). Such observations
have led to the suggestion that cyclooxygenase inhibitors may be useful in preventing cardiovascular disease. Overall, clinical trials of cyclooxygenase inhibitors,
usually aspirin, in the prevention of myocardial infarction and stroke show a
moderately protective effect of these agents (8), suggesting the involvement of
thromboxane or other cyclooxygenase products in ischemic and thrombotic disease.

THROMBOXANE IN EXPERIMENTAL SUDDEN DEATH

Several attempts have been made to model sudden death phenomena experimentally. Of these, models involving injection of arachidonic acid or thromboxane mimetics into experimental animals have proved highly useful. The models described below are presently in wide use, particularly in the pharmaceutical industry, for the evaluation of drugs affecting the hemostatic system.

Intravascular Arachidonic Acid Administration

Silver et al. (30) first reported the effects of intravenous arachidonic acid in the rabbit and suggested this model as a method for the study of thrombotic sudden death. Arachidonate injection resulted in respiratory distress, occlusive pulmonary platelet aggregation, and sudden death.

Sudden death induced by arachidonic acid has now been described in several species. Although the dose of arachidonic acid required is species dependent, the effects of i.v. arachidonate are very similar in the various species studied. A survey of the literature suggests that the LD_{50} for arachidonate is approximately 1 mg/kg in the rabbit and 10 mg/kg in the rat (20). In the mouse, the LD_{50} is 33 mg/kg for males and 46 mg/kg for females (19). The sequelae of i.v. arachidonate are presented in Table 1. Based on the work of Kohler et al. (12), we have selected the mouse for our studies due to economic considerations. Its small size also allows conservation of scarce experimental drugs.

The effects of intracarotid and intracoronary arachidonate or thromboxane have also been described. In the rat, intracarotid administration of arachidonate results in cerebrovascular thrombosis and stroke (7). In the rabbit, intracoronary thromboxane injection causes coronary thrombosis and sudden death (29). These techniques are in current use as models of stroke and coronary thrombosis, respectively.

TABLE 1. *Specific manifestations of arachidonate toxicity*

Thrombotic
    Occlusive pulmonary thrombosis (30)
    Thrombocytopenia (2)
    Circulating platelet aggregates (30)
Respiratory
    Respiratory distress (30)
    Apnea (12)
    Cyanosis (12)
Cardiovascular
    Systemic hypotension (2)
    Tachycardia, arrhythmias[a]
    ST segment changes[a]

Numbers in parentheses indicate references for the various pathophysiological effects observed following i.v. administration of arachidonic acid.
[a]A. K. Myers, *unpublished data.*

Thromboxane in Experimental Sudden Death

The protective effect of aspirin against arachidonate-induced sudden death was first reported by Silver et al. (30). DiPasquale and Mellache (5) systematically evaluated the effects of pretreatment with a number of drugs. Cyclooxygenase inhibitors as a class were found to inhibit the lethal effects of arachidonate. These observations suggested that a cyclooxygenase product of arachidonic acid was responsible for the thrombotic sudden death.

Based on its properties, thromboxane A_2 was the most likely mediator of arachidonate-induced sudden death. We therefore tested the effects of a specific thromboxane synthase inhibitor, OKY-1581, on thrombotic death in the mouse (21). OKY-1581, 1 mg/kg, was found to protect against i.v. arachidonate injection, thus supporting our hypothesis. A different thromboxane synthase inhibitor (UK37,248) has been found to enhance survival in rabbits challenged with arachidonate (13). We also tested a specific thromboxane receptor antagonist in the mouse model (19). SQ26,536, a prostaglandin endoperoxide analog that has been described as a thromboxane antagonist (9), provided dose-dependent protection against thrombotic sudden death when administered i.v. 2 min prior to arachidonate. 13-Azaprostanoic acid, another thromboxane receptor antagonist, is protective against arachidonate-induced death in the rabbit (2). Thus, agents that inhibit the production or action of thromboxane A_2 are protective against the pathogenic actions of i.v. arachidonate. The effects of such agents on the experimental sudden death are illustrated in Fig. 1.

We have further tested the hypothesis by studying the effects of i.v. administration of U46619 (19), a thromboxane mimetic (3). U46619 produces sudden death similar in nature to that produced by arachidonate, but is approximately 500-fold more potent. The effects of U46619 cannot be inhibited by indomethacin or OKY-1581, the thromboxane synthase inhibitor, but pretreatment with the thromboxane recep-

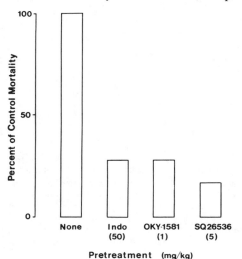

FIG. 1. Effects of cyclooxygenase and thromboxane synthase inhibition and thromboxane receptor antagonism on arachidonate-induced sudden death. Male mice were pretreated with oral indomethacin (Indo), i.v. thromboxane synthase inhibitor OKY-1581, or i.v. thromboxane receptor antagonist SQ26,536, or the appropriate vehicle prior to challenge with arachidonic acid at 50 mg/kg. This dose of arachidonate produces sudden thrombotic death in approximately 60% of untreated mice. All three agents resulted in significantly improved survival compared to the appropriate control groups, suggesting that a cyclooxygenase product of arachidonate, namely thromboxane, mediates the sudden death.

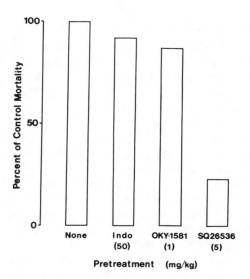

FIG. 2. Effects of cyclooxygenase and thromboxane synthase inhibition and thromboxane receptor antagonism on thromboxane mimetic-induced sudden death. Male mice were pretreated with oral indomethacin (Indo), i.v. thromboxane synthase inhibitor OKY-1581, or i.v. thromboxane receptor antagonist SQ26,536, or the appropriate vehicle prior to challenge with U46619, a thromboxane mimetic, at 0.8 mg/kg. This dose of U46619 produces sudden death in approximately 90% of untreated mice. Of the three agents used as pretreatments, only SQ26,536 significantly improved survival compared to the appropriate control group. These results are in contrast to the arachidonate-induced sudden death model, in which cyclooxygenase and thromboxane synthase inhibitors are also protective (see Fig. 1).

tor antagonist SQ26,536 provides dose-dependent protection (19). For purposes of comparison with arachidonate-induced mortality, the effects of these agents on thromboxane mimetic-induced thrombotic death are illustrated in Fig. 2.

Thus, there is now strong evidence that arachidonate-induced sudden death is mediated by generation of thromboxane from the exogenous arachidonic acid. Furthermore, the fact that thrombotic sudden death can be modeled by either the precursor of thromboxane or by thromboxane agonists supports the suggestion that thromboxane may have a role in the thrombotic aspects of human cardiovascular disease, including sudden death. The proposed mechanism by which arachidonic acid induces sudden death is depicted in Fig. 3.

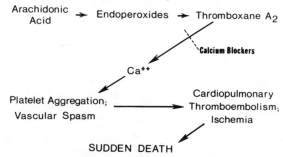

FIG. 3. Proposed mechanism of arachidonic acid-induced sudden death. Intravenous injection of arachidonic acid results in the formation of cyclic endoperoxides and subsequent metabolites, including the major product in platelets, thromboxane A_2. Of the products of arachidonate, thromboxane has characteristics signifying potential importance in cardiovascular disease. Promotion of Ca^{2+} flux into platelets by thromboxane initiates the thrombotic process, while Ca^{2+} induces smooth-muscle contraction in vessels. Cardiopulmonary thromboembolism and ischemia, and hence sudden death, result. The point in this sequence at which calcium-channel blockers are protective against thrombotic sudden death is indicated by the dotted line.

Endocrine Effects on Experimental Sudden Death

Endocrine factors have long been thought to be involved in the gender difference in the incidence of human cardiovascular disease, whereby males are more susceptible than females to nearly all major categories of cardiovascular disease. Because of this marked sex difference, many attempts have been made to investigate the role of gonadal hormones in experimental models of cardiovascular disease.

One of our early observations regarding thrombotic sudden death in mice was that males are more susceptible to the lethal effects of arachidonate than females. Thus, we studied the effects of estrogen, testosterone, and castration on arachidonate-induced thrombotic sudden death (18,25). The adult mouse is relatively refractory to manipulation of the gender difference. Castration of males and females does not alter the sex difference in sudden death. Testosterone pretreatment increases the mortality rate in males but not females; estrogen is protective in castrated males but not in females or intact males (25). Immature mice, on the other hand, are more affected by castration. When mice are castrated prepubertally and challenged several weeks later with arachidonate, the sex difference is no longer in evidence. Furthermore, the sex difference does not develop in intact mice until the approximate time of sexual maturity. Pretreatment of immature mice with estrogen tends to be protective; testosterone has little effect (18). The sum of these observations suggests that the gender difference in experimental sudden death is related to gonadal hormones. However, the mechanism of the hormone action is not known. We have suggested that it may involve differential metabolism of arachidonic acid in males and females. The relevance of these observations to the sex differences in cardiovascular disease remains to be established.

In addition to the gonadal steroids, the glucocorticoids also have an effect on thrombotic sudden death. Because glucocorticoid release is part of the mechanism whereby the organism responds to stress, we tested the effects of adrenalectomy and chronic glucocorticoid treatment on arachidonic acid-induced sudden death (24). Although glucocorticoids are known to inhibit the deacylation of arachidonic acid from membrane phospholipids and thus inhibit production of all products of endogenous arachidonate, they have no well-established effect on the metabolism of exogenously administered arachidonic acid. Not unexpectedly, adrenalectomy significantly exacerbates the response to arachidonic acid. Surprisingly, however, treatment of either adrenalectomized or intact mice with cortisone substantially lowers the mortality rate, compared to intact control animals (24). In addition, glucocorticoids have a beneficial effect against thrombotic sudden death induced by the thromboxane mimetic U46619 (19). Glucocorticoids also have an acute protective action in thrombotic sudden death (27). Intravenous administration of either dexamethasone or hydrocortisone provides protection against arachidonate within a few minutes of administration, lasting for approximately 1 hr. The protective effect of glucocorticoids has been confirmed by others (1), but the mechanism remains to be fully elucidated.

Calcium Blockers in Experimental Sudden Death

Okamatsu et al. (22) have reported that sudden death induced by arachidonate in rabbits is inhibited by pretreatment with the calcium-channel blocking drugs nisoldipine and verapamil. However, statistical analysis of their data reveals that only nisoldipine was significantly beneficial. More recently, a number of groups have reported that calcium blockers have an *in vitro* antiaggregatory effect (11,23,28). This *in vitro* effect appears to be a general property of this class of drugs. This action is not surprising, since Ca^{2+} has several important roles in the hemostatic process. Because of the now widespread use of calcium blockers in cardiovascular disease states and the potential therapeutic importance of any antithrombotic effects of these drugs, we have reinvestigated this phenomenon in three thrombotic sudden death models (A. K. Myers, *in preparation*). For this purpose, arachidonic acid and U46619 were employed as challenges, as well as a combination of epinephrine and collagen, as described recently by DiMinno and Silver (4) as a new thrombosis model.

In all three thrombotic sudden death models, pretreatment with i.v. nifedipine at 0.5 mg/kg enhanced survival of mice following challenge (Fig. 4). Verapamil, on the other hand, had no protective action over a range of doses in any of the models. These results suggest that the antithrombotic action of calcium blockers applies to the *in vivo* situation, since nifedipine enhanced survival of animals challenged with a variety of thrombotic stimuli. Furthermore, although all calcium blockers may have *in vitro* antiaggregatory actions, it is possible that the dihydropyridine agents such as nifedipine and nisoldipine are more efficacious *in vivo* compared to verapamil and related agents. This area is the subject of current investigation in our laboratory. The possible point at which calcium blockers act against experimental sudden death is indicated in Fig. 3.

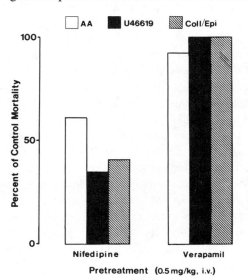

FIG. 4. Differential effects of nifedipine and verapamil on thrombotic sudden death. Groups of 15 male mice were pretreated with i.v. nifedipine, verapamil, or the appropriate vehicle 5 min prior to challenge with 75 mg/kg arachidonate (AA) at 75 mg/kg, U46619 at 0.8 μg/kg, or a combination of collagen (1 mg/kg) and epinephrine (0.12 mg/kg) (Coll/Epi). Pretreatment with nifedipine at 0.5 mg/kg resulted in significant protection against all three thrombotic challenges; verapamil had no protective effect against any of the challenges at the 0.5 mg/kg dose, or at other doses tested.

SUMMARY

Thromboxane has characteristics that signify potential importance in cardiovascular disease states. In models developed for studying thrombotic sudden death, thromboxane appears to be an important mediator. Thus, in arachidonic acid-induced sudden death, agents that either inhibit thromboxane generation or block thromboxane receptor activation prevent the occurrence of thrombotic death. Thromboxane mimetics are also useful in modeling sudden death; when injected i.v., these compounds elicit effects similar to those obtained with arachidonic acid. In this case, however, pretreatment with cyclooxygenase or thromboxane synthetase inhibitors confers no protection, whereas the thromboxane receptor antagonist retains its efficacy.

Other factors that affect susceptibility to experimental sudden death include gender, species, and endocrine status.

Thrombotic sudden death models have now been used to test, *in vivo*, the *in vitro* antiplatelet aggregatory effect of calcium-channel blockers. The data suggest that dihydropyridine agents such as nifedipine and nisoldipine are protective against thrombosis, whereas verapamil may have little such activity. Furthermore, sudden death induced by a variety of thrombotic challenges is prevented by pretreatment with nifedipine.

The thrombotic sudden death models currently employed are useful for the *in vivo* study of the thrombotic process and for the evaluation of agents with potentially thrombotic or antithrombotic properties.

ACKNOWLEDGMENTS

This work was supported in part by National Institutes of Health grants HL18718, HL17516, and HL31498.

REFERENCES

1. Araki, H., Peck, R. C., Lefer, A. M., and Smith, J. B. (1981): Mechanism of protection against arachidonate induced sudden death by glucocorticoid. *Prostaglandins*, 21:387–399.
2. Burke, S. E., Roth, D. M., and Lefer, A. M. (1983): Antagonism of platelet aggregation by 13-azaprostanoic acid in acute myocardial ischemia and sudden death. *Thromb. Res.*, 29:473–488.
3. Coleman, R. A., Humphrey, P. P. A., Kennedy, I., Levy, G. P., and Lumley, P. (1981): Comparison of the actions of U-46619, a prostaglandin H_2-analogue, with those of prostaglandin H_2 and thromboxane A_2 on some isolated smooth muscle preparations. *Br. J. Pharmacol.*, 73:773–778.
4. DiMinno, G., and Silver, M. J. (1983): Mouse antithrombotic assay: A simple method for the evaluation of antithrombotic agents *in vivo*. Potentiation of antithrombotic activity by ethyl alcohol. *J. Pharmacol. Exp. Ther.*, 225:57–60.
5. DiPasquale, G., and Mellace, D. (1977): Inhibition of arachidonic acid induced mortality in rabbits with several non-steroidal anti-inflammatory agents. *Agents Actions*, 7(suppl. 4):481–485.
6. Foegh, M. L., Winchester, J. F., Zmudka, M., Helfrich, G. B., Ramwell, P. W., and Schreiner, G. E. (1982): Aspirin inhibition of thromboxane release in thrombosis and renal transplant rejection. *Lancet*, 1:48–49.
7. Furlow, T. W., and Bass, N. H. (1975): Stroke in rats produced by carotid injection of sodium arachidonate. *Science*, 187:658–660.
8. Harlan, J. M., and Harker, L. A. (1981): Hemostasis, thrombosis, and thromboembolic disorders. The role of arachidonic acid metabolites in platelet-vessel wall interactions. *Med. Clin. North Am.*, 65:855–880.

9. Harris, D. N., Phillips, M. B., Michel, M., Goldenberg, H., Heinkes, J. E., Sprague, P. W., and Antonaccio, M. J. (1981): 9a-Homo-9,11-epoxy-5,13-prostadienoic acid analogues: Specific stable agonist (SQ 26,538) and antagonist (SQ 26,536) of the human platelet thromboxane receptor. *Prostaglandins*, 22:295–308.

10. Hirsh, P. D., Hillis, L. D., Campbell, W. B., Firth, B. G., and Willerson, J. T. (1981): Release of prostaglandins and thromboxane into the coronary circulation in patients with ischemic heart disease. *N. Engl. J. Med.*, 304:685–691.

11. Johnsson, H. (1981): Effects of nifedipine (Aldalat) on platelet function *in vitro* and *in vivo*. *Thromb. Res.*, 21:523–528.

12. Kohler, C., Wooding, W., and Ellenbogen, L. (1976): Intravenous arachidonate in the mouse: A model for the evaluation of antithrombotic drugs. *Thromb. Res.*, 9:67–80.

13. Lefer, A. M., Okamatsu, S., Smith, E. F., and Smith, J. B. (1981): Beneficial effects of a new thromboxane synthetase inhibitor in arachidonate-induced sudden death. *Thromb. Res.*, 23:265–273.

14. Lewy, R. I., Smith, J. B., Silver, M. J., Saia, J., Walinsky, P., and Wiener, L. (1979): Detection of thromboxane B_2 in the peripheral blood of patients with Prinzmetal's angina. *Prostaglandins Med.*, 2:243–248.

15. Lewy, R. I., Wiener, L., Walinsky, P., Lefer, A. M., Silver, M. J., and Smith, J. B. (1980): Thromboxane release during pacing-induced angina pectoris: Possible vasoconstrictor influence on the coronary vasculature. *Circulation*, 61:1165–1171.

16. Lown, B. L. (1979): Sudden cardiac death—1978. *Circulation*, 60:1593–1599.

17. Moore, S. (1976): Platelet aggregation secondary to coronary obstruction. *Circulation*, 53(suppl.I):66–71.

18. Myers, A., Papadopoulos, A., O'Day, D., Ramey, E., Ramwell, P., and Penhos, J. (1982): Sexual differentiation of arachidonate toxicity in mice. *J. Pharmacol. Exp. Ther.*, 222:315–318.

19. Myers, A., Penhos, J., Ramey, E., and Ramwell, P. (1983): Thromboxane agonism and antagonism in a mouse sudden death model. *J. Pharmacol. Exp. Ther.*, 224:369–372.

20. Myers, A., Penhos, J., and Ramwell, P. (1983): Acute arachidonate toxicity. In: *Leukotrienes and Prostacyclin*, edited by F. Berti, G. Folco, and G. P. Velo, pp. 275–284. Plenum Publishing, New York.

21. Myers, A., Rabbani, F., Penhos, J. C., Ramey, E., and Ramwell, P. W. (1981): Protective effects of lidocaine, cyproterone acetate and a thromboxane synthetase inhibitor against arachidonate induced mortality. *Fed. Proc.*, 40:662.

22. Okamatsu, S., Peck, R. C., and Lefer, A. M. (1981): Effects of calcium channel blockers on arachidonate-induced sudden death in rabbits. *Proc. Soc. Exp. Biol. Med.*, 166:551–555.

23. Ono, H., and Kimura, M. (1981): Effects of Ca^{2+}-antagonistic vasodilators, diltiazem, nifedipine, perhexiline and verapamil, on platelet aggregation in vitro. *Arzneim Forsch. Drug Res.*, 31:1131–1134.

24. Penhos, J. C., Montalbert-Smith, M., Rabbani, F., Ramey, E., and Ramwell, P. (1979): Effect of corticosteroids on arachidonate induced mortality in male and female mice. *Prostaglandins*, 18:697–706.

25. Penhos, J. C., Rabbani, F., Myers, A., Ramey, E., and Ramwell, P. (1981): The role of gonadal steroids in arachidonate-induced mortality in mice. *Proc. Soc. Exp. Biol. Med.*, 167:98–100.

26. Pirkle, H., and Carstens, P. (1974): Pulmonary platelet aggregates associated with sudden death in man. *Science*, 185:1062–1064.

27. Rabbani, F., Myers, A., Ramey, E., Ramwell, P., and Penhos, J. C. (1981): Acute protection against arachidonate toxicity by hydrocortisone and dexamethasone in mice. *Prostaglandins*, 21:699–705.

28. Ribeiro, L. G. T., Brandon, T. A., Horak, J. K., Ware, J. A., Miller, R. R., and Solis, R. T. (1982): Inhibition of platelet aggregation by verapamil: Quantification by *in vivo* and *in vitro* techniques. *J. Cardiovasc. Pharmacol.*, 4:170–173.

29. Shimamoto, T. (1978): Stroke and heart attack induced experimentally by thromboxane A_2 in rabbits and effect of EG 626, a thromboxane A_2 antagonist. In: *International Symposium: State of Prevention and Therapy in Human Arteriosclerosis and in Animal Models*, edited by W. H. Hauss, R. W. Wissler, and R. Lehmann, pp. 139–152. Westdeutscher Verlag, Opladen.

30. Silver, M. J., Hoch, W., Kocsis, J. J., Ingerman, C. M., and Smith, J. B. (1974): Arachidonic acid causes sudden death in rabbits. *Science*, 183:1085–1087.

Advances in Prostaglandin, Thromboxane, and Leukotriene Research, Vol. 13, edited by G.G. Neri Serneri, et al. Raven Press, New York © 1985.

Changes in PGE$_2$ Urinary Excretion and Renal Function in Coronary Heart Disease

*P. Bernardi, *L. Bastagli, *F. Ghezzi, *R. Grimaldi, *C. Minelli, *M. A. Mainardi, *A. Bertoldi, *M. Cavazza, **C. Ventura, **C. Clo, and †A. Danieli

*Istituto di Clinica Medica II and **Istituto di Chimica Biologica, University of Bologna; and †Servizio di Fisiopatologia della Riproduzione, Policlinico S. Orsola, 40138 Bologna, Italy*

Our investigation was carried out on 17 patients with uncomplicated acute myocardial infarction (AMI), during a 21-day trial. The functional renal parameters [V_{min}, glomerular filtration rate (GFR), Na$^+$ tubular balance] and prostaglandin (PG) E$_2$ urinary excretion according to Van Orden radioimmunoassay (4) were evaluated every day during the first week from the onset of the illness and then on days 10, 11, 15, 16, 20, and 21.

The usual therapy, nitrates and sedative, was administered when needed. In 5 cases of AMI, indoprophen (i.m.) 200 mg × 2/die was also given during the experimental period.

RESULTS

In the 12 cases not receiving indoprophen, the urinary excretion of PGE$_2$ showed lower than normal values in the first 5 days, reaching normal levels (1) after the fifth day and for the rest of the follow-up period (Fig. 1).

An induced increase in urinary flow and GFR was seen at 1 week from the onset of the disease. The Na$^+$ excretion probably increased with a parallel decreasing Na$^+$ reabsorption percentage on days 5 to 7 (Fig. 2).

In the 5 cases treated with indoprophen, the low levels of urinary PGE$_2$ during the first days did not increase, and no significant changes were observed during the follow-up period. The GFR values were lower than normal, tending toward decreasing levels at the end of the study. The urinary flow and the sodium tubular balance underwent changes that were irregular and not significant.

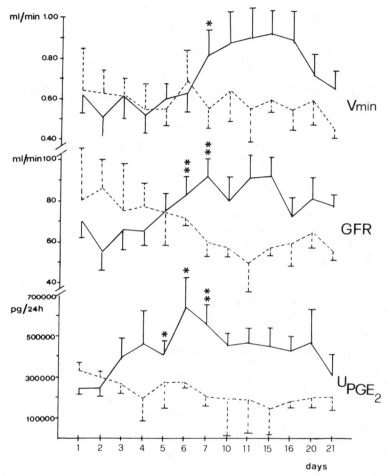

FIG. 1. Changes in V_{min}, GFR, and PGE₂ urinary excretion in 17 subjects with acute myocardial infarction. Solid lines indicate subjects not receiving indoprophen; dashed lines indicate subjects treated with indoprophen (i.m. 200 mg × 2/die). Significant differences between levels in days 5, 6, and 7 and the first day are calculated by Student's t-test ($^*p<0.02$, $^{**}p<0.01$).

CONCLUSIONS

Our findings lead us to hypothesize that an impairment of PG synthesis demonstrated at various levels during coronary heart disease (3) can also involve renal PG synthesis. Therefore the alterations of the renal function during acute myocardial infarction, as observed in this study, could be related to a depression of PGE₂ synthesis.

In our opinion, these observations are confirmed by the results from the indoprophen investigation: the drug was able to prevent the resetting of the renal

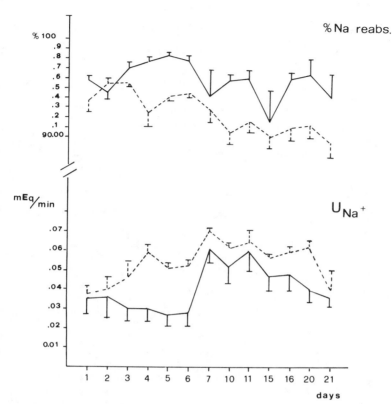

FIG. 2. Changes in Na⁺ tubular balance [Na⁺ excretion (mEq/min) and reabsorption (percentage of Na⁺ filtration rate)].

function, probably by inhibiting PG synthesis (2), as demonstrated by the low urinary excretion of PGE₂ in these cases.

REFERENCES

1. Benzoni, D., Vincent, M., and Sassard, J. (1981): Radioimmunoassay for urinary prostaglandins E and F: Normal values in different age groups. *Clin. Chim. Acta*, 11:9.
2. Dunn, M. J., and Zambraski, E. J. (1980): Renal effects of drugs that inhibit prostaglandin synthesis. *Kidney Int.*, 18:609.
3. Neri Serneri, G. G., Masotti, G., Gensini, G. F., and Abbate, R. (1983): La alterata modulazione vascolare prostaglandinica nella patogenesi della ischemia miocardica. *Soc. It. Med. Int.*, Atti 84th Congresso.
4. Van Orden, D. E., Farley, D. B., and Clancey, C. J. (1977): Radioimmunoassay of PGE and approach to the specific measurement of PGE1. *Prostaglandins*, 13:437.

Advances in Prostaglandin, Thromboxane, and Leukotriene Research, Vol. 13, edited by G. G. Neri Serneri, et al. Raven Press, New York © 1985.

Prostacyclin and Thromboxane Levels During Cardiac Ischemia in Dogs

*M. Prosdocimi, *F. Tessari, *M. Finesso, *A. Gorio,
**E. Dejana, **L. R. Languino, **A. Del Maschio,
and **G. de Gaetano

*Department of Cytopharmacology, Fidia Research Laboratories, Abano Terme, Italy;
and **Mario Negri Institute for Pharmacological Research, Milan, Italy

The relationship between ischemic heart disease and circulating prostanoids is highly debated, because of both the intrinsic complexity of the matter and the methodological difficulties in sampling and measuring blood levels of prostanoids (for review see ref. 4). It has been reported (2) that 6-keto-prostaglandin $F_{1\alpha}$ (6-keto-$PGF_{1\alpha}$) and thromboxane B_2 (TXB_2) are elevated in dog cardiac venous blood after coronary artery ligation and that rabbit isolated perfused hearts *in vitro* release more 6-keto-$PGF_{1\alpha}$ under hypoxic conditions than in control conditions (3).

The aim of our work was to study 6-keto-$PGF_{1\alpha}$ and TXB_2 release in the cardiac venous blood after experimental alterations of coronary circulation in the dog. Male mongrel dogs were anesthetized, artificially ventilated, and instrumented for continuous recording of blood pressure, heart rate, lead II electrocardiogram (ECG), and left ventricular pressure. Left anterior descending coronary artery and left circumflex artery were exposed and coronary blood flow was monitored by electromagnetic flow probes. Blood was obtained from the great cardiac vein, from the aorta, and from a femoral vein, rapidly mixed with sodium citrate containing aspirin, and centrifuged. Plasma levels of 6-keto-$PGF_{1\alpha}$ and TXB_2 were determined in unextracted plasma by radioimmunoassay (RIA) and lactate by enzymatic analysis. Details on the experimental procedure have been described elsewhere (7). Our detection limits were 0.1 pmole/ml for 6-keto-$PGF_{1\alpha}$ and 0.075 pmole/ml for TXB_2. Using unextracted plasma, in control conditions, 6-keto-$PGF_{1\alpha}$ and TXB_2 were below the detection limit in arterial, venous, and cardiac venous blood.

Following left anterior descending coronary artery occlusion, 6-keto-$PGF_{1\alpha}$ rapidly rose in the great cardiac vein and remained elevated for the entire time of observation (60 min). Lactate was also increased, while TXB_2 did not reach detectable values (Table 1). In peripheral circulation no prostanoids were detected, while lactate remained at control levels. Lead II ECG showed signs of ischemia during coronary artery ligation, with frequent episodes of ventricular tachycardia. The second model we used was a critical stenosis of left anterior descending

TABLE 1. Plasmatic levels[a] of 6-keto-PGF$_{1\alpha}$, TXB$_2$, and lactate in the great cardiac vein before and after occlusion of left anterior descending coronary artery

Substance	Minutes from occlusion					
	−12	−2	5	15	30	60
6-Keto-PGF$_{1\alpha}$ (pmoles/ml)	<0.1	<0.1	0.89 ± 0.06	1.02 ± 0.07	1.08 ± 0.13	1.44 ± 0.18
TXB$_2$ (pmoles/ml)	<0.075	<0.075	<0.075	<0.075	<0.075	<0.075
Lactate (μmoles/ml)	0.48 ± 0.03	0.52 ± 0.05	1.06 ± 0.10	1.04 ± 0.16	0.99 ± 0.34	0.79 ± 0.18

[a]Values are the average ± SE of five different experiments.

coronary artery. It has been previously shown (1,5,6) that if a critical stenosis reduces by about 70% the vessel lumen, cyclical declines of blood flow in a coronary artery are induced. These declines are due to platelet thrombi forming in the narrowed vessel. Blood flow is restored either spontaneously or by sliding the plastic cylinder that narrows the vessel. Using this experimental procedure, we examined prostanoids in the great cardiac vein of 11 dogs, before stenotizing the vessel and when cyclical declines in blood flow were evident. In control conditions, 6-keto-PGF$_{1\alpha}$ and TXB$_2$ were undetectable; when blood flow showed cyclical declines, TXB$_2$ was still undetectable but 6-keto-PGF$_{1\alpha}$ increased to detectable levels in the great cardiac vein in 7 of 11 dogs. Lactate was also increased in the great cardiac vein, while in peripheral circulation lactate was unchanged and 6-keto-PGF$_{1\alpha}$ and TXB$_2$ were undetectable. Figure 1 shows a representative experiment. Panel A shows blood flow in the left anterior descending coronary artery in control conditions: 6-keto-PGF$_{1\alpha}$ and TXB$_2$ were undetectable in the great cardiac vein. Panel B shows the cyclical declines in blood flow occurring about 40 min after stenotizing the vessel: while 6-keto-PGF$_{1\alpha}$ was increased, TXB$_2$ was still below detection limit.

In summary, using two different conditions of reduced blood flow in a coronary artery, we observed increased levels of 6-keto-PGF$_{1\alpha}$ in cardiac venous blood, whereas TXB$_2$ was not detectable even when platelet thrombi were continuously forming on a coronary artery. These results support the view that ischemic myocardium releases increased amounts of prostacyclin in acute conditions, possibly as a defense mechanism against cellular damage. On the other hand, the data indicate that it is unlikely that acute focal alterations of coronary blood flow may result in systemic alterations of levels of prostanoids. Further investigations are needed to establish if chronic diffuse alterations of coronary circulation affect plasma prostanoid levels.

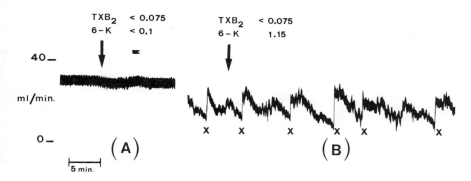

FIG. 1. Blood flow in left anterior descending coronary artery **(A)** before and **(B)** 40 min after stenotizing the vessel. Blood-flow restorations occurred spontaneously and are indicated by *x*. *Arrows* indicate the time when blood was obtained from the great cardiac vein for prostanoid measurement. Levels of 6-keto-PGF$_{1\alpha}$ and TXB$_2$ values are expressed as pmoles/ml.

ACKNOWLEDGMENTS

The excellent technical help of Alberto Zatta is gratefully acknowledged. We thank Patrizia Lentola for typing the manuscript.

REFERENCES

1. Aiken, J. W., Shebushi, R. J., Miller, O. V., and Gorman, R. R. (1981): Endogenous prostacyclin contributes to the efficacy of a thromboxane synthetase inhibitor for preventing coronary artery thrombosis. *J. Pharmacol. Exp. Ther.*, 219:299–308.
2. Coker, S. J., Parrat, J. R., Ledingham, I. McA, and Zeitlin, I. J. (1981): Thromboxane and prostacyclin release from ischemic myocardium in relation to arrhythmias. *Nature (Lond.)*, 291:323–324.
3. Edlund, A., Fredholm, B. B., Patrignani, P., Patrono, C., Wennmalm, A., and Wennmalm, M. (1983): Release of two vasodilators, adenosine and prostacyclin, from isolated rabbit hearts during controlled hypoxia. *J. Physiol.*, 340:487–501.
4. Fitzgerald, G. A., Pedersen, A. K., and Patrono, C. (1983): Analysis of prostacyclin and thromboxane biosynthesis in cardiovascular disease. *Circulation*, 67:1174–1177.
5. Folts, J. D., Crowell, E. B., and Rowe, G. G. (1976): Platelet aggregation in partially obstructed vessels and its elimination with aspirin. *Circulation*, 54:365–379.
6. Folts, J. D., Gallagher, K., and Rowe, G. G. (1982): Blood flow reductions in stenosed canine coronary arteries: Vasospasm or platelet aggregation? *Circulation*, 65:248–255.
7. Prosdocimi, M., Finesso, M., Gorio, A., Languino, L. R., Del Maschio, A., Castagnoli, N. M., de Gaetano, G., and Dejana, E. (1985): Coronary and systemic 6-keto-$PGF_{1\alpha}$ and TXB_2 during myocardial ischemia in the dog. *Am. J. Physiol. (in press)*.

*Advances in Prostaglandin, Thromboxane, and
Leukotriene Research, Vol. 13*, edited by G. G. Neri
Serneri, et al. Raven Press, New York © 1985.

Does Prostacyclin Synthesis Inhibition Significantly Contribute to Nicotine Effects on Coronary Blood Flow?

Lennart Kaijser and Bo Berglund

*Department of Clinical Physiology, Karolinska Hospital,
S-104 01 Stockholm, Sweden*

Nicotine may affect coronary blood flow by multiple, occasionally counteracting mechanisms. Thus, it may alter coronary vascular resistance by a direct smooth-muscle effect of nicotine itself or by stimulated local release of vasoactive substances, e.g., norepinephrine. It may also affect coronary vascular resistance indirectly by producing systemic release of catecholamines, leading to increased cardiac work and thereby metabolically linked coronary vasodilatation (6). Recently nicotine has been shown to inhibit the release of prostacyclin from the heart vasculature (7). Prostacyclin dilates coronary vessels (1), is synthesized in the human coronary vasculature where it is the major arachidonic acid metabolite (5), and under some conditions (e.g., hypoxia) is released from the human heart in substantial amounts (2). The prostaglandin synthesis inhibitor indomethacin has been shown to decrease coronary blood flow, suggesting a role for prostaglandins in coronary flow regulation (3). The present study was undertaken to see if an interference with prostacyclin synthesis explains effects of nicotine on coronary blood flow, fully or in part.

SUBJECTS, PROCEDURES, METHODS

Fourteen healthy male nonsmokers, aged 21 to 55 years, were studied by catheterization of an artery (a) and the coronary sinus (cs). They had not taken aspirin or other nonsteroid antiinflammatory drugs during the week before the study. Blood was sampled for measurement of O_2 saturation in arterial and coronary sinus blood, and in addition the coronary sinus catheter was used for blood flow measurement by thermodilution and atrial pacing (to produce increased cardiac work).

Seven of the patients were studied before and after administration of nicotine, 4 mg orally in a chewing gum (Nicorette®). On each occasion measurements were made at rest, during atrial pacing with stepwise increased heart rate to the highest tolerated rate without atrio–ventricular blocking, and again after pacing. The remaining 7 subjects were studied before drug administration, 60 min after a prostaglandin synthesis inhibitor (ibuprofen 1.2 g orally), and again 30 min after nicotine (4 mg orally). In each situation measurements were made before, during, and after pacing, according to the protocol just given.

RESULTS

Effect of Nicotine

The effect of nicotine is shown in Fig. 1. Nicotine alone increased heart rate by 12 beats/min and arterial mean pressure by 6 mm Hg. Atrial pacing to an average highest heart rate of 120 beats/min increased arterial mean pressure by 3 mm Hg before nicotine but did not alter it significantly after nicotine. Arterial pressure during pacing was essentially the same with as without the drug. At rest, as well as during and after pacing, both coronary blood flow and a–cs O_2 difference were greater with than without nicotine, and so was myocardial O_2 uptake at a given rate × pressure product.

Effect of Ibuprofen

The effect of ibuprofen is shown in Fig. 2. Ibuprofen alone produced an increased arterial mean pressure by 4 mm Hg but did not significantly change heart rate, coronary blood flow, and a–cs O_2 difference. Nicotine after ibuprofen did not increase coronary blood flow but produced changes similar to those without ibuprofen in heart rate, arterial mean pressure, and a–cs O_2 difference, at rest, as well as during and after pacing. Nicotine did not alter the relationship between myocardial O_2 uptake and the rate × pressure product.

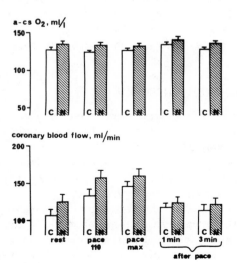

FIG. 1. Coronary blood flow and arterial–coronary sinus O_2 difference at rest, during atrial pacing at heart rate 110 and maximal heart rate without atrio–ventricular blocking, and after pacing, before (C) and after (N) 4 mg nicotine orally. Mean and SE are shown.

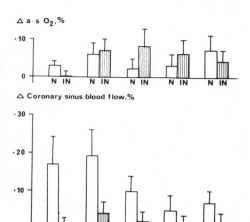

FIG. 2. Changes produced by nicotine at 4 mg orally in coronary blood flow and arterial–coronary sinus O_2 difference before (N) and after (IN) pretreatment by ibuprofen. As in Fig. 1, measurements are taken at rest, pacing at heart rate 110 and maximal heart rate, and 1 and 3 min after pacing. Mean and SE are shown.

DISCUSSION

Nicotine increased coronary blood flow. This was in all probability related to the increased myocardial oxygen consumption produced by increased cardiac work (heart rate × arterial pressure). In addition, nicotine must have had a direct (opposing) vasoconstrictive effect, since the a–cs O_2 difference was increased, indicating that the increase in coronary blood flow did not match the increase in myocardial oxygen consumption.

Ibuprofen did not affect coronary blood flow. It has been observed that indomethacin decreases coronary blood flow (3), and this observation was initially taken to suggest that arachidonic acid metabolites are involved in myocardial blood-flow regulation. However, observations that this effect applies to indomethacin but not to a number of other prostaglandin synthesis inhibitors, including ibuprofen, indicates that the effect is related to pharmacological actions of indomethacin which are not related to prostaglandin synthesis inhibition (4). Yet ibuprofen impeded the coronary blood flow response to nicotine, suggesting that nicotine in the heart releases a cyclooxygenase product that is vasodilating or that increases myocardial contractility.

It is concluded that (a) under both basal conditions and moderately increased cardiac work prostacyclin or other arachidonic acid metabolites have no important blood flow regulation role in the nonischemic human heart; (b) nicotine has a direct coronary vasoconstrictory action in addition to an indirect vasodilatory influence related to the increased cardiac work; and (c) although nicotine inhibits synthesis of the coronary vasodilator prostacyclin in the rabbit heart, pretreatment with a more potent prostaglandin synthesis inhibitor attenuates the coronary flow-increasing effect of nicotine in man.

ACKNOWLEDGMENTS

This study was supported by grants from the Swedish Medical Research Council (4494) and the Swedish Tobacco Company.

REFERENCES

1. Dusting, G. J., Moncada, S., and Vane, J. R. (1977): Prostacyclin (PGX) is the endogenous metabolite of arachidonic acid which relaxes coronary arteries. *Prostaglandins*, 13:3–15.
2. Edlund, A., Bomfim, W., Kaijser, L., Olin, C., Patrono, C., Pinca, E., and Wennmalm, Å. (1982): Cardiac formation of prostacyclin during cardoplegia in man. *Prostaglandins*, 24:5–19.
3. Friedman, P. L., Brown, E. J., Gunther, S., Alexander, R. W., Barry, W. H., Mudge, G. H., and Grossman, W. (1981): Coronary vasoconstrictor effect of indomethacin in patients with coronary-artery disease. *N. Engl. J. Med.*, 305:1171.
4. Kaijser, L. (1982): Release of prostacyclin (PGI$_2$) and adenosine from the heart during angina pectoris. In: *Symposium on Prostaglandins and Cardiovascular Diseases*, edited by M. Winberg, J. E. Olsson, and E. Orinius, pp. 80–83. Boehringer Ingelheim.
5. Nowak, J., Kaijser, L., and Wennmalm, Å. (1980): Cardiac synthesis of prostaglandins from arachidonic acid in man. *Prostaglandins Med.*, 4:205–214.
6. Regan, T. J., Frank, M. J., McGinty, J. F., Zobl, E., Hellems, M. D., and Bing, R. J. (1961): Myocardial response to cigarette smoking in normal subjects and patients with coronary disease. *Circulation*, 23:365–369.
7. Wennmalm, Å. (1978): Nicotine inhibits the release of 6-keto-prostaglandin $F_{1\alpha}$ from the isolated perfused rabbit heart. *Acta Physiol. Scand.*, 103:107–109.

Advances in Prostaglandin, Thromboxane, and Leukotriene Research, Vol. 13, edited by G. G. Neri Serneri, et al. Raven Press, New York © 1985.

Mechanisms of Stroke and Site of Arterial Lesion

Domenico Inzitari, Laura Fratiglioni, and Luigi Amaducci

Department of Neurology, Medical School, University of Florence, 50134 Florence, Italy

There is increasing evidence that different types of strokes and related arterial lesions have different pathogenic mechanisms and risk factors. This concept appears to have gained ground only in the last couple of decades. During a symposium on hypertension in 1972, Sir George Pickering (29) commented on the fact that in the latest World Health Organization (WHO) Report (number 469), intracerebral hemorrhage had been ascribed to atherosclerosis: "Charcot must be turning in his grave, muttering 'How long, oh Lord, how long'" because the role of microaneurysms described by him and Bouchard in 1868 had continued to be ignored. Recently the bulk of physiopathological and clinical work in the field of stroke has, to a large extent, clarified the mechanisms underlying different types of stroke.

However, difficulties in interpreting some epidemiological data, as well as discrepancies in results relating to the role of risk factors, still seem to exist.

Pathological lesions as well as mechanisms and types of stroke are illustrated in Table 1.

Cerebral infarction can be divided into two categories: cortical and deep-seated infarction. Both types may be linked to lesions at different levels of the cerebral

TABLE 1. *Site of cardiovascular lesion and mechanisms of cerebral infarction and hemorrhage*

Site of lesion	Type of lesion	Mechanism of stroke	Site and type of stroke
Heart	Valvulopathy, disrhythmia, parietal diskinesia, etc.	Embolism	Cortical (deep) infarction
Extracranial arteries	Occlusive plaques and thrombosis	Artery-to-artery embolism, hemodynamic	Cortical infarction
Basal and cortical arteries	Occlusive plaques and thrombosis	Hemodynamic	Cortical infarction, deep infarction
Penetrating arteries	Sclero–lipojalinosis, Charcot–Bouchard aneurysms	Lacunar infarction, parenchymal hemorrhage	Deep infarction, intracerebral hemorrhage

101

arterial tree. Cortical infarction appears to be related to occlusive lesions in cervical vessels or to those in larger intracranial arteries, while deep-seated infarctions are generally a consequence of lesions at the ostium or along the course of the smaller penetrating brain arteries. Those lesions in the larger arterial branches, either at the extracranial or intracranial levels, belong to the atherothrombotic type, while those in the small arterial penetrators are of the sclero–lipojaline type. Micro-aneurysms, usually associated with the latter kind of arteriopathy, set the pathologic stage for intracerebral hemorrhage (ICH). Most deep-seated infarctions are so-called lacunar infarctions; as a pathological and clinical entity, these have only recently been reexamined (5,24).

There is strong evidence that the vasal changes associated both with lacunae and with ICH are closely bound, and are both linked to hypertension (32). Cerebral embolism does not appear to be involved in many stroke cases, although more recent studies (25) using more sophisticated diagnosis techniques and more careful pathological criteria have found more embolic cases than had been previously indicated by clinical and epidemiological surveys.

Although many difficulties exist in dealing with the epidemiology of stroke types, a geographical distribution pattern can be identified. In addition, although the pattern of stroke frequency has been known to change over the course of time in different countries, these temporal trends seem to have affected the rates of some clinical varieties of the cardiovascular disease complex more than others (3,7). Moreover, there is strong evidence to suggest that different segments of the cerebral arterial tree tend to be affected in different populations (4,18,28). Finally, it seems that in some countries, the patterns of morbidity and mortality from cerebrovascular and ischemic heart disease (IHD) demonstrate opposite trends, both geographically and temporally, which suggests that cardiovascular risk factors may operate differ-ently in these two pathologies (8).

In 1971, Kuller and Reisler (20) (Table 2) hypothesized that among selected geographic areas and ethnic groups, with elevated blood pressure (BP) and low cholesterol levels, there existed a high risk of cerebrovascular disease (CVD) and a low risk of IHD; the contrary occurred in populations with a high prevalence of hypercholesterolemia and a relatively low prevalence of hypertension. In the first group, according to this theory, there should also be a relatively higher prevalence and incidence of cerebral hemorrhage, and lesions should be predominantly located in the basal arteries and intracerebral penetrating arteries. But in the second group, cerebral infarction should be the most common stroke type, while lesions would be mainly distributed along the large extracranial arteries. Kuller supported his hypothesis with evidence that demonstrated that the stages of pathogenesis of the occlusive lesions in extracranial arteries differ from those in intracranial basal arteries. The etiology of atherosclerotic disease in the extracranial arteries might, according to Kuller's hypothesis, be similar to that found in the coronary arteries and might be related primarily to the levels of blood lipids and secondarily to elevated blood pressure. In the intracranial vessels, however, the atherosclerotic process, according to Baker and Iannone (2), starts with proliferative fibrosis of

TABLE 2. *Risk factor influence on distribution of stroke and coronary heart disease between geographic areas and ethnic groups with associated topography of vascular involvement and proposed model populations*

| | Risk factor | | | Disease | | | |
| | | | | Stroke | | | |
Class	Blood lipid levels	Blood pressure	Incidence	Site of vascular lesion	Coronary heart disease incidence	Model population
1	High	High	High	Both intracranial and extracranial	High	U.S.A. black
2	High	Low	Intermediate	Mainly extracranial	High	U.S.A. white
3	Low	High	High	Mainly intracranial and intracerebral	Low	Japan
4	Low	Low	Low	Few or none	Low	Guatemala

the intima rather than with lipid infiltration. Thus, ranking the risk factors in the pathogenesis of occlusive lesions in the larger intracranial branches, hypertension should have a predominant and earlier role, while blood lipid and glucose levels should play a secondary role, according to Kuller.

In penetrating arteries, the fibrojalinotic changes and microaneurysms should be almost exclusively related to hypertension; blood lipid levels should have little or no effect. The present report adds supporting elements to these hypotheses and is based on data drawn from our own epidemiological and clinical experience, as well as from relevant literature on the subject.

EPIDEMIOLOGICAL OBSERVATIONS

In the larger context of cardiovascular disease, one of the most provocative observations in the last few years has been the fact that trends in CVD and IHD actually seem to be diametrically opposed in some countries over certain time periods.

In Italy, a decline in age-specific death rates for CVD (Fig. 1) and a correspondent decline in the mortality rate from hypertensive disease have been noted since

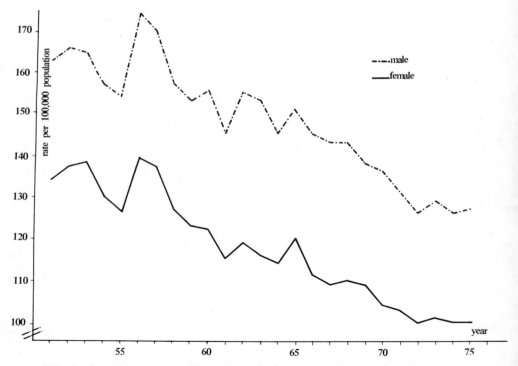

FIG. 1. Annual age-adjusted (to 1960 Italian population) death rates for cerebrovascular disease, Italy 1951–1975.

the 1950s (14). However, mortality from IHD rose until recently; around 1976, a decrease began to be noted. However, in some other countries, the opposite trend continues to be observed (8).

Although various hypotheses may be advanced to explain these phenomena, it may be argued that during this period (from 1950 onward) the prevalence of some of the cardiovascular risk factors such as hypertension (and definitely those more strictly associated with CVD or with particular entities among CVD) has decreased, while the prevalence of other risk factors more strongly associated with IHD (such as hypercholesterolemia) has remained unchanged. The control of hypertension has been claimed to have a major role in the decreasing trend in CVD mortality. Certainly, hypertension is the factor that has undergone the most modification in the years during which CVD mortality fell and IHD mortality rose, but it cannot be said with any certainty that reduced hypertension is the single determining factor in reduced CVD mortality.

The analysis of geographic and temporal trends in the occurrence of specific stroke types adds further elements to this discussion. From the methodological point of view, the validity of epidemiological data in determining the distribution of specific stroke types is questionable. Since it is so difficult to diagnose specific categories of stroke, and hence to register them accurately on death certificates, the validity of type-specific mortality statistics may be compromised. Variations in clinical diagnostic criteria, in the use of certain laboratory diagnostic techniques, and in the frequency of autopsies performed can also help to account for discrepancies in reported incidence of various stroke types. In contrast to mortality studies, incidence studies are not affected by differences in stroke-fatality ratios among stroke subtypes. Therefore, despite the limitations just discussed, incidence rates are more representative of the real distribution of stroke types than are mortality rates.

In Figs. 2, 3, and 4, the percentage frequencies of stroke in different geographic areas, as reflected in the most recent available incidence studies, are shown. The following observations were noted.

Definite clusters of frequency of intracerebral hemorrhage existed. The highest percentages were found in the Scandinavian countries and Japan, and the lowest in the United States, Israel, and other Northern European countries such as Denmark and the Netherlands. Countries such as Nigeria and groups such as Hawaiian men of Japanese extraction and the people of Tartu (Estonia) showed intermediate percentage frequencies.

However, in precisely those countries with the highest percentage of intracerebral hemorrhage rates, the declining rate of CVD has resulted in the last few years in a marked decline of mortality rates from intracerebral hemorrhage. Table 3 shows the percent change in age-adjusted mortality rates from intracerebral hemorrhage in those countries between the periods of 1953–1957 and 1967–1973 (from data elaborated by L. Fratiglioni in collaboration with the neuroepidemiology staff of the National Institute of Neurological and Communicative Disorders and Stroke, Bethesda, Maryland).

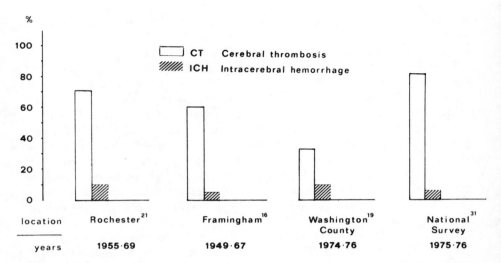

FIG. 2. Percentage frequencies of CT and ICH from selected incidence studies in the United States.

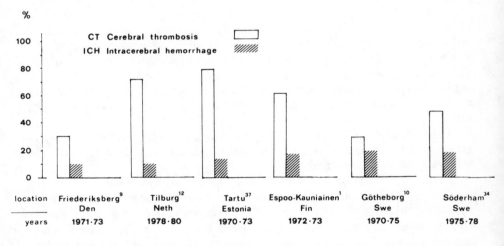

FIG. 3. Percentage frequencies of CT and ICH from selected incidence studies in Scandinavian and other Northern European countries.

As for the distribution pattern of lesions of the cerebral arterial tree in different populations, it has long been recognized that more lesions are found in the basal and cortical intracranial branches of Japanese (4,18) and in African Negroes (24) than in other groups. The Extra/Intracranial Anastomosis Cooperative Study (Fig. 5) confirmed this fact statistically by distributing randomization categories among different geographic areas. As compared with Caucasian subjects, the frequency

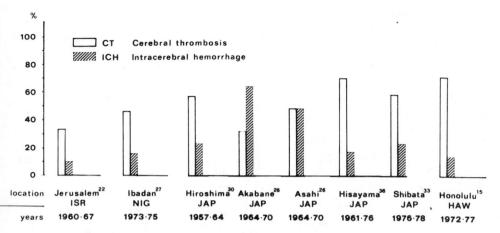

FIG. 4. Percentage frequencies of CT and ICH from selected incidence studies in Israel, Nigeria, and Japan.

TABLE 3. *Percentage changes in average age-adjusted mortality rates for cerebral hemorrhage between 1953 and 1957 and 1967 and 1973 in selected countries*

Country	Cerebral hemorrhage change in rate (%)
United States	−29.8
Finland	−72.2
Sweden	−63.6
Japan	−48.9
Israel	+5.2

of randomizable middle cerebral artery lesions in Japanese was shown to be definitely higher (internal report of EC/IC Bypass Study, 1981).

Regarding the penetrating arteries, recent autopsy studies in Japan (23) have demonstrated that changes in penetrating arteries are more frequent in cases with intracranial occlusion than in cases with extracranial occlusion, confirming the relationship between pathological changes in penetrating arteries and intracranial occlusion. Following these observations, further evidence seems to indicate that in certain defined populations, CVD tends to be distributed predominantly at the intracranial level either in the large basal or in the penetrating arteries. This evidence is pathological, clinical (arteriographic data), and epidemiological (definite clustering of occurrence of intracerebral hemorrhage, which is indicative of severe alterations of the penetrating arteries). At this point, the role of cardiovascular risk factors in relation to these patterns of distribution will be examined.

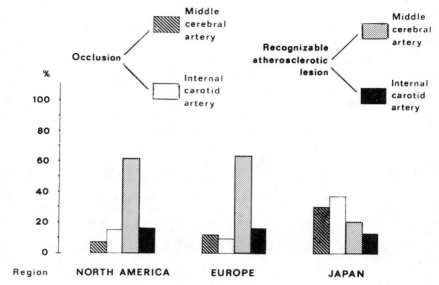

FIG. 5. Extra/Intracranial Bypass Cooperative Study, randomized lesion by region.

ROLE OF CARDIOVASCULAR RISK FACTORS

Hypertension clearly plays a very important role with respect to the occurrence of intracerebral hemorrhage; it also promotes and may maintain pathological changes in the intracranial penetrating arterial branches. However, hypertension is also very important in cases of transient ischemic attack (TIA) in Caucasians, in whom extracranial lesions are predominant.

Many prospective epidemiological surveys have demonstrated that hypertension is a good predictor of the risk of stroke. The Framingham Study (17) has indicated that among the components of BP, systolic BP is the best predictor of atherothrombotic brain infarction. The diastolic component appears to have less importance. Although the specific role of the components of BP in the pathogenesis of intracerebral hemorrhage has not been examined in depth, recent results of a prospective cohort study in Hiroshima and Nagasaki (30) (based on a detailed analysis of the relationship between each of the BP components and cardiovascular risk) have indicated that the incidence of intracerebral hemorrhage was strongly correlated with either recent or remote BP diastolic values. Systolic BP, as already mentioned, was a better predictor of both cerebral infarction and coronary heart disease.

The relative role of BP components in relation to lesion distributions among different segments of the cerebral arterial tree has not often been investigated specifically. The major difficulty is due to the unreliability of antemortem BP registrations. More careful data come from angiographic studies.

In 1975, Harrison and Marshall (11) published an angiographic study on a series of cerebral infarction cases in which there was an inverse relationship between diastolic BP values and the occurrence of carotid artery occlusive disease. This finding may suggest a definite role of diastolic BP levels in relation to the changes in penetrating branches involved in the pathogenesis of cerebral infarction.

Regarding the role of blood lipid levels, evidence indicates an inverse relationship between cholesterol levels and risk of intracerebral hemorrhage. This quite surprising prophylactic effect of hypercholesterolemia on intracerebral hemorrhage has not yet been definitely explained either on pathological or biochemical grounds; however, some evidence exists that intracranial branches may differ from extracranial arteries in the lipid composition of the arterial walls (20). The study of the correlation between blood lipid levels and cerebral infarction, however, has up to now yielded inconsistent results.

In 1970, Heyden and co-workers (13) considered the predisposing factors in a clinical series of ischemic patients, divided into two groups: those who had angiographic evidence of occlusive disease at the intracranial level, and those with similar evidence at the extracranial level. In the first group, with nonembolic occlusion of the middle cerebral artery, there were more hypertensive subjects (defined in relation to the increase of both the BP components); in the second group, with lesions at the carotid bifurcation level, serum cholesterol levels were definitely higher.

More recent clinical studies in patients operated for extracranial stenosis (35) confirm the important role of the blood lipid changes in the extracranial arterial lesion.

In relation to the role of cardiovascular risk factors at different levels of lesion, we are now able to present some preliminary data from the Italian Multicenter Study on reversible cerebral ischemia, in a project supported by the National Research Council of Italy (6). Between 1976 and 1978, 462 patients with reversible cerebral ischemia were enrolled by the eight participating centers in order to undergo an extensive study of risk factors and clinical characteristics. All of the patients underwent angiography. A multivariate analysis of the effect of cardiovascular risk factors on the occurrence and severity of the arterial lesions at different levels was carried out. The discriminant analysis between the two subgroups with and without angiographic signs of atherosclerosis shows a definite role of cholesterol as a discriminating factor of the presence of atherosclerotic lesions at the extracranial level. The severity of atherosclerotic lesion was strongly correlated with systolic BP values in a multiple regression model.

At the same time, smoking and diastolic BP were also significantly involved, although the association appears to be weaker. None of these variables seems to be linked with the presence or severity of intracranial lesions.

The selection criteria adopted and the means of investigation do not allow any evaluation of the state of the penetrating branches; however, these results seem to be generally in line with the quoted literature on the subject, except for the lack of any correlation between the considered risk factors and lesions in the larger intracranial branches.

Finally, the possible role of constitutional factors should not be disregarded, especially in regard to the definite pattern of distribution of the arterial lesions among different racial and ethnic groups.

In concluding this second part of the discussion, the reported evidence indicates that there may be a specific role of cardiovascular risk factors, depending on the site of the arterial lesion. Components of BP may be differentially involved at various levels: systolic hypertension at the extracranial level, and diastolic hypertension at the intracranial one. Cholesterol levels appear to be important only in relation to extracranial lesions.

Certainly, these indications will require further confirmation from either clinical or epidemiological surveys. In addition, an investigation, from the physiopathologic point of view, of the chemical characteristics of the arterial wall would be of interest, as well as an investigation of the role of functional modulators such as prostaglandins at the different levels of the cerebral arterial tree.

ACKNOWLEDGMENT

This work was supported by a grant from the Consiglio Nazionale delle Ricerche (C.N.R.), Rome, number 83.02691.56.

REFERENCES

1. Aho, K., and Fegelholm, R. (1974): Incidence and early prognosis of stroke in Espoo-Kauniainen area, Finland, in 1972. *Stroke*, 5:658–661.
2. Baker, A. B., and Iannone, A. (1958): Cerebrovascular disease I: The large arteries of the circle of Willis. *Neurology*, 9:321–332.
3. Baum, H. M., and Goldstein, M. (1982): Cerebrovascular disease type specific mortality: 1968–1977. *Stroke*, 13:810–817.
4. Brust, R. W. (1975): Patterns of cerebrovascular disease in Japanese and other population groups in Hawaii: An angiographical study. *Stroke*, 6:539–542.
5. Caplan, L. R. (1976): Lacunar infarction: A neglected concept. *Geriatrics*, 31:71–75.
6. Fieschi, C., Mariani, F., Brambilla, G. L., Prencipe, M., Tomasello, F., Argentino, C., Bono, G., Candelise, L., De Zanche, L., Inzitari, D., and Nardini, M. (1983): Italian study of cerebral coversible ischemic attacks: Population characteristics and methodology. *Stroke*, 14:424–430.
7. Furlan, A. J., Whisnant, J. P., and Elveback, L. R. (1979): The decreasing incidence of primary intracerebral hemorrhage: A population study. *Ann. Neurol.*, 5:367–373.
8. Haberman, S., Capildeo, R., and Clifford-Rose, F. (1982): Diverging trends in cerebrovascular disease and ischemic heart disease mortality. *Stroke*, 13:582–589.
9. Hansen, B. S., and Marquardsen, J. (1977): Incidence of stroke in Frederiksberg, Denmark. *Stroke*, 8:663–665.
10. Harmsen, P., Berglund, G., Larsson, O., Tibblin, G., and Wilhelmsen, L. (1979): Stroke registration in Göteborg, Sweden, 1970–1975. Incidence and fatality rates. *Acta Med. Scand.*, 206:337–344.
11. Harrison, M. J. G., and Marshall, J. (1975): The results of carotid angiography in cerebral infarction in normotensive and hypertensive subjects. I. *Neurol. Sci.*, 24:243–250.
12. Herman, B., Leyten, A. C. M., van Luijk, J. H., Frenken, C. W. G. M., Op de Coul, A. A. W., and Schulte, B. P. M. (1982): Epidemiology of stroke in Tilburg, The Netherlands. The population-based stroke incidence register: 2. Incidence, initial clinical picture and medical care, and three week case fatality. *Stroke*, 13:629–634.
13. Heyden, S., Heyman, A., and Goree, J. A. (1970): Nonembolic occlusion of the middle cerebral and carotid arteries—A comparison of predisposing factors. *Stroke*, 1:363–369.
14. Inzitari, D., Fratiglioni, L., Guidi, A., and Amaducci, L. (1981): Epidemiology of cerebrovascular

disease: stroke mortality trends in Italy. In: *Cerebrovascular Disease: New Trends in Surgical and Medical Aspects*, edited by H. Barnett, P. Paoletti, E. Flamm, and G. Brambilla, pp. 169–181. Elsevier/North Holland, Amsterdam.

15. Kagan, A., Popper, J. S., and Rhoads, G. G. (1980): Factors related to stroke incidence in Hawaii Japanese men. The Honolulu heart study. *Stroke*, 11:14–21.
16. Kannel, W. B. (1976): Epidemiology of cerebrovascular disease. In: *Cerebral Arterial Disease*, edited by R. W. Ross Russel, pp. 1–23. Churchill Livingston, Edinburgh.
17. Kannel, W. B., Dawber, T. R., Sorlie, P., and Wolf, P. A. (1976): Components of blood pressure and risk of atherothrombotic brain infarction: the Framingham Study. *Stroke*, 4:327–331.
18. Kikuchi, Y., Yamamoto, H., and Nakamura, M. (1973): Cerebral atherosclerosis in Japanese. 3. Predilection site of atherosclerotic lesions. *Stroke*, 4:768–772.
19. Kramer, S., Diamond, E. L., and Lilienfeld, A. M. (1982): Pattern of incidence and trends in diagnostic classification of cerebrovascular disease in Washington County, Maryland, 1969–1971 to 1974–1976. *Am. J. Epidemiol.*, 115:398–411.
20. Kuller, L., and Reisler, D. M. (1971): An explanation for variations of stroke and arteriosclerotic heart disease among populations and racial groups. *Am. J. Epidemiol.*, 93:1–9.
21. Matsumoto, N., Whisnant, J. P., Kurland, L. T., and Okazaki, H. (1973): Natural history of stroke in Rochester, Minnesota, 1955 through 1969: An extension of a previous study, 1945 through 1954. *Stroke*, 4:20–29.
22. Melamed, E., Cahane, E., Carmon, A., and Lavy, S. (1973): Stroke in Jerusalem district 1960 through 1967: An epidemiological study. *Stroke*, 4:465–471.
23. Mitsuyama, Y., Thompson, L. R., Hayashi, T., Lee, K. K., Keehn, R. J., Resch, J. A., and Steer, A. (1979): Autopsy study of cerebrovascular disease in Japanese men who lived in Hiroshima, Japan, and Honolulu, Hawaii. *Stroke*, 10:389–395.
24. Mohr, J. P. (1982): Lacunes. *Stroke*, 13:3–11.
25. Mohr, J. P., Caplan, L. R., Melski, J. W., Goldstein, R. J., Duncan, G. W., Kislter, J. P., Pessin, M. S., and Howard, L. B. (1978): The Harvard Cooperative stroke registry: A prospective registry. *Neurology*, 28:754–762.
26. Okada, H., Horibe, H., Ohono, Y., Hayakawa, N., and Aoki, N. (1976): A prospective study of cerebrovascular disease in Japanese rural communities, Akabane and Asahi. Part 1: Evaluation of risk factors in the occurrence of cerebral hemorrhage and thrombosis. *Stroke*, 7:599–607.
27. Osuntokun, B. O., Bademosi, O., Akinkugbe, O. O., Oyediran, A. B. O., and Carlisle, R. (1979): Incidence of stroke in an African City: Results from the stroke registry at Ibadan, Nigeria, 1973–1975. *Stroke*, 10:205–207.
28. Osuntokun, B. O. (1977): Stroke in the Africans. *Afr. J. Med. Sci.*, 6:39–53.
29. Pickering, G. (1972): Hypertension. Definition, natural history and consequences. *Am. J. Med.*, 52:570–583.
30. Prentice, L. R., Shinuzu, Y., Lin, C. H., Peterson, A. V., Kato, H., Mason, M. W., and Szatrowski, T. P. (1982): Serial blood pressure measurements and cardiovascular disease in a Japanese cohort. *Am. J. Epidemiol.*, 116:1–27.
31. Robins, M., and Baum, H. T. (1981): The national survey of stroke. Incidence. *Stroke*, 12(suppl. I):45–55.
32. Ross Russel, R. W. (1975): How does blood-pressure cause stroke? *Lancet*, 2:1283–1285.
33. Tanaka, H., Ueda, Y., Date, C., Baba, T., Yamashita, H., Hayashi, M., Shoji, H., Owada, K., Baba, K. I., Shibuya, M., Kon, I., and Detels, R. (1982): Incidence of stroke in Shibata, Japan: 1976–1978. *Stroke*, 12:460–466.
34. Terent, A. (1979): A prospective epidemiological survey of cerebrovascular disease in a Swedish community. *Upsala J. Med. Sci.*, 84:235–246.
35. Terrence, C. F., and Rao, G. R. (1983): Triglycerides as a risk factor in extracranial atherosclerotic cerebrovascular disease. *Angiology*, 34:452–460.
36. Ueda, K., Omae, T., Hirota, Y., Takeshita, M., Katsuki, S., Tanake, K., and Enjoji, M. (1981): Decreasing trend in incidence and mortality from stroke in Hisayama residents, Japan. *Stroke*, 12:154–160.
37. Zupping, R., and Roose, M. (1976): Epidemiology of cerebrovascular disease in Tartu, Estonia, USSR, 1970 through 1973. *Stroke*, 7:187–190.

Advances in Prostaglandin, Thromboxane, and Leukotriene Research, Vol. 13, edited by G.G. Neri Serneri, et al. Raven Press, New York © 1985.

Pathophysiology and Clinical Aspects of Acute Cerebral Ischemia

Cesare Fieschi, Antonio Carolei, Corrado Argentino, and Gian Luigi Lenzi

Department of Neurological Sciences, University of Rome "La Sapienza," 00185 Rome, Italy

GENERAL ISSUES

Cerebral ischemia, although easily recognizable by means of medical history and neurological examination, nevertheless remains an intriguing and fascinating pathophysiological entity. Signs and symptoms of ischemic stroke—transient and incomplete, or prolonged and complete—result from interference with the blood supply to the brain. Cerebral hypoxia, on the other hand, relates to the interference with the oxygen supply to the brain, despite a relatively normal cerebral blood flow and perfusion pressure.

The experimental counterpart of human cerebral ischemia deals with animal models in which the blood supply to the brain is altered by means of selected procedures (4). Regional cerebral ischemia, in stroke, depends on single artery occlusion, while global ischemia depends on failure of the circulation to the entire brain. Cerebral ischemia, when reversible, has time limits and, at present, no definite indicators of selective neuronal damage are available (7). Astrocytes seem to provide a defense against tissue damage but they are potentially vulnerable to high tissue lactate levels.

Neuronal necrosis is always considered irreversible on experimental grounds. At this point in time, protein and neurotransmitter synthesis and mitochondrial enzymatic activities, irreversibly cease. Neurons that are structurally intact but functionally inactive—because of a discrepancy between the threshold for complete electrical and energy failure, and the threshold for release of potassium and Ca^{2+} intracellular uptake—are responsible for the ischemic penumbra (8,9a). When cerebral blood flow in ischemia approaches the level of 10 ml/100 mg·min, cellular potassium efflux causes a massive calcium entry. Raised intracellular calcium activity stimulates breakdown of the phosphatidylinositol pool and phospholipase activity, releasing free fatty acids believed to have further deleterious effects on ischemic cerebral tissue (9). All these experimental data justify a clinical therapeutic approach with calcium entry blockers in the acute phase of stroke.

Luxury perfusion, postischemic hypermetabolism, and ischemic penumbra represent different pathophysiological aspects of regional changes in perfusion after the focal ischemic event. Hypothermia protects the brain in hypoxic hypoxia, shifting the hemoglobin–oxygen dissociation curve towards the left and reducing cellular energy requirements acting on cerebral metabolism (1). When global ischemia lasts 15 min or less, a rapid recovery may occur, without residual neurologic deficits. More protracted ischemia cause severe neuronal multifocal damage in brain areas showing selective vulnerability. A progressive consumptive coagulopathy follows transient global brain ischemia (5).

Microcirculatory flow may be impaired during postischemic reperfusion, because of increased platelet activity and hyperviscosity. On the other hand, symmetrical hyperemia followed by lowered blood flow can occur after short-duration (5 min) oligemia or ischemia, without evidence of the no-reflow phenomenon.

Hyperglycemia worsens brain ischemia, converting an isolated anoxic neuronal damage during normoglycemia into a gross cerebral infarction.

Concepts like delayed postischemic recovery, maturation of neuronal damage, and brain protection represent major advances in the experimental and clinical approach to cerebral ischemia (2a,6,7).

CLINICAL BASIS FOR TREATMENT

Close observation of the acute stroke phase in intensive care units discloses certain similarities with the experimental observations, especially with the concept of progressive establishment of the irreversible damage, in the face of an acute, sudden vascular occlusion (3).

Patients with cerebral ischemia can often display a spontaneous recovery of neurological signs and symptoms after a few minutes or hours. We do not know in advance if recovery will be complete in 24 hr as in a simple transient ischemic attack (TIA) or in more than 24 hr as in a protracted transient ischemic attack (P-TIA), or incomplete, with residual neurological signs, as in a transient ischemic attack with incomplete recovery (TIA-IR), or with both neurological signs and symptoms as a minor stroke.

Epidemiology and natural history of cerebral ischemia have shown that the most part of vertebral basilar and also carotidal episodes—especially if distant in time and single—are low-risk TIAs (9). In these cases, noninvasive tests are mandatory in order to exclude potentially harmful conditions; however, if both clinical and noninvasive data concur to exclude a high risk of repeated TIAs or stroke, these patients only require accurate general medical measures and care of risk factors.

TIAs may repeat themselves within a few hours or days, evolving to a completed stroke after a second and third episode. These are high-risk TIAs, with only two valid alternative therapeutic strategies available: vascular surgery following an urgent angiography, and/or effective anticoagulant treatment.

At the present stage, therefore, a transient ischemic event is only a warning of a situation that must be accurately examined, to select high-risk and low-risk cases, and to introduce them in differential clinical routine and protocols.

As stated before, TIAs clinically prove that focal cerebral ischemia is often reversible. Reversibility is subject to variations, experimentally demonstrated, modifying blood viscosity, blood pressure, or temperature. The brain can also be protected from ischemia with drugs administered in advance. Therefore, preventive brain protection, in high-risk patients or in the acute phase, must be included in the near future in experimental therapeutic protocols (2,3).

Due to the impact of new technologies such as positron emission tomography (PET) and single photon emission tomography (SPECT), cerebral ischemic stroke is now more easily recognizable *in vivo* as an active, dynamic condition, amenable to prevention and treatment by means of assessing cerebral metabolism and the nutrients' regional extraction and utilization (6). The goal of the research in this field is the effort to define the interval of time, after the onset of stroke, in which tissue damage remains potentially reversible (2,7). The concept of brain protection is thus achieving a definite relevance, along with the individuation of the high-risk or excessive-risk TIA patient.

CONCLUSIONS

The decline in mortality from stroke during the last decades has been attributed to effective primary and secondary prevention. In fact, about 10% of patients in the community and 35% of patients in medical centers have TIAs before cerebral infarction (10).

If this is true, more than 60% of stroke-prone subjects have no warnings of their future ischemic stroke.

Nevertheless, the identification of TIA patients helps prevention as well as the identification of high-risk or excessive-risk patients. A further decline of stroke, in the next decades, could be provided by an adequate brain protection, capable of interfering with the theoretically nonreversible maturation of neuronal damage.

REFERENCES

1. Carlsson, C., Hagerdal, M., and Siesjo, B. K. (1976): Protective effect of hypothermia in cerebral oxygen deficiency caused by arterial hypoxia. *Anesthesiology*, 44:27–35.
2. Fieschi, C. (1982): Preventive treatment that might reduce the severity of infarctions in risk patients. *J. Cereb. Blood Flow Metabol.*, 2:582–586.
2a. Carolei, A., Fieschi, C., Prencipe, M., Allori, L., Argentino, C., Brambilla, G. L., Candelise, L., Conforti, P., Ederli, A., Fiorani, P., Frontoni, M., Inzitari, D., Maira, G., Mariani, F., Morocutti, C., Nappi, G., Nardini, M., Pace, A., Paolucci, S., and Servi, M. (1985): Cumulative Italian study on reversible cerebral ischemic attacks (RIAs)—three year follow-up. In: *Proceedings of the World Federation of Neurology 12th Salsburg Conference*. Elsevier, Amsterdam (*in press*).
3. Fieschi, C., Argentino, C., and Carolei, A. (1982): Acute cerebrovascular disorders: An update. In: *International Multidisciplinary Seminar: Cerebral Pathology in Old Age, Neuroradiological and Neurophysiological Correlations*, edited by A. Cecchini, G. Nappi, and A. Arrigo, pp. 245–250. Emiras, Pavia.
4. Hossmann, K-A. (1982): Treatment of experimental cerebral ischemia. *J. Cereb. Blood Flow Metabol.*, 2:275–297.
5. Hossmann, K-A., and Hossmann, V. (1977): Coagulopathy following experimental cerebral ischemia. *Stroke*, 8:77–81.
6. Lenzi, G. L., Frackowiak, R. S. J., and Jones, T. (1982): Cerebral oxygen metabolism and blood flow in human cerebral ischemic infarction. *J. Cereb. Blood Flow Metabol.*, 2:321–335.

7. Plum, F. (1983): What causes infarction in ischemic brain?: The Robert Wartenberg Lecture. *Neurology*, 33:222–233.
8. Siesjo, B. K. (1981): Cell damage in the brain: A speculative synthesis. *J. Cereb. Blood Flow Metabol.*, 1:155–185.
9. Symon, L. (1982): Pathophysiology of brain ischemia: Recent experimental results and early clinical correlations. In: *Advances in Stroke Therapy*, edited by F. C. Rose, pp. 3–10. Raven Press, New York.
9a. Symon, L., Branstou, N. M., Harris, R. J., and Wang, A. (1984): The current status of ischemic thresholds. In: *Cerebral Ischemia*, edited by A. Bes, P. Braquet, R. Paoletti, and B. K. Siesjö, pp. 63–73. Elsevier, Amsterdam.
10. Whisnant, J. P. (1983): The role of the neurologist in the decline of stroke. *Ann. Neurol.*, 14:1–7.

Advances in Prostaglandin, Thromboxane, and Leukotriene Research, Vol. 13, edited by G. G. Neri Serneri, et al. Raven Press, New York © 1985.

Evidence that Hypercapnia-Induced Cerebral Vasodilation in the Conscious Rat Is Not Mediated by Prostaglandins

Ewa Raczka and Antonio Quintana

Departamento de Farmacología, Facultad de Medicina, Universidad del Pais Vasco, Bilbao, Spain

The increase in cerebral blood flow (CBF) induced by hypercapnia has been proposed to require prostaglandin biosynthesis (2,5,6). This assumption is based on the marked reduction in hypercapnia-induced cerebral vasodilation observed after indomethacin administration. Since a similar action with fatty acid–cyclooxygenase inhibitors other than indomethacin has not been reported and indomethacin induces a mesenteric vasoconstriction that is unrelated to the prostaglandin system (3), it cannot be excluded, therefore, that indomethacin affects hypercapnia-induced cerebral vasodilation by other mechanisms not related to cyclooxygenase inhibition.

The aim of the work presented here was to verify whether vascular prostaglandins are required for hypercapnia-induced cerebral vasodilation in the conscious rat.

CBF and cerebral vascular resistances (CVR) were determined using the reference sample radioactive microsphere method, as previously described (1,7). Two injections of microspheres (15 μm in diameter) labeled either with ^{141}Ce or ^{103}Ru (New England Nuclear, specific activity 10 mCi/g) were made on each animal, the first under basal conditions and the second after a period of 5 min in which animals inhaled different concentrations of CO_2 in air. Animals received either i.v. saline (1 ml/kg) or aspirin (50 mg/kg, in the form of its soluble lysine salt) 15 min before the second microsphere injection. The aspirin dose used in this study induces a cerebral vasoconstriction and reduces CBF under normocapnic conditions (7). Arterial blood was sampled immediately before microsphere injections, and PCO_2, PO_2, and pH were measured in an automatic analyzer. Cyclooxygenase inhibition was tested by abolition of the hypotensive effect of arachidonic acid (5 mg/kg).

Figure 1 illustrates that hypercapnia induced a cerebral vasodilation and increased CBF in the conscious rat; however, we did not find a significant correlation between the increase in arterial PCO_2 and either the increase in CBF or the decrease in CVR. Aspirin did not modify the changes in cerebral circulation induced by hypercapnia.

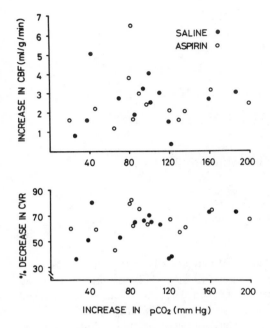

FIG. 1. **Top:** Individual increases in cerebral blood flow (ml/g·min) plotted against increases in arterial blood PCO_2 (mm Hg). **Bottom:** Individual decreases in cerebral-vascular resistance (% of control basal values) plotted against increases in arterial blood PCO_2 (mm Hg).

As shown in Table 1, there were no differences between the pooled data obtained under hypercapnia in rats treated with saline and those obtained in rats treated with aspirin.

The hypotensive effect of i.v. arachidonic acid was always abolished after aspirin, suggesting that cyclooxygenase was inhibited.

Our results are in accordance with recent work of Jackson et al. (4) showing that 1 hr after i.v. administration of indomethacin to anesthetized dogs, prostaglandin synthesis was inhibited but hypercapnia-induced cerebral vasodilation was not modified.

TABLE 1. *Effect of hypercapnia on CBF, CVR, blood gases, and pH in the saline- and aspirin-treated groups[a]*

Parameter	Basal	Saline	Basal	Aspirin
PCO_2	38.4 ± 0.6	135.1 ± 13.2[b]	38.3 ± 0.7	139.6 ± 13.6[b]
PO_2	85.6 ± 1.5	86.0 ± 2.0	85.3 ± 1.8	86.4 ± 2.6
pH	7.40 ± 0.01	7.04 ± 0.04[b]	7.39 ± 0.01	7.02 ± 0.04[b]
CBF (ml/min · g)	1.26 ± 0.08	3.74 ± 0.40[b]	1.19 ± 0.05	3.72 ± 0.38[b]
CVR (mm Hg/ml · min · g)	86.8	33.6[b]	98.5	32.6[b]
	(70.9–106.4)	(25.7–43.9)	(88.0–110.3)	(26.9–39.6)

[a]Values are mean ± SE, except CVR, where mean values and their 95% confidence limits are shown ($n = 13$).
[b]The paired Student's *t*-test has been applied for statistical analysis of the differences between basal and treatment values and shows significance at $p < 0.05$.

Our study demonstrates that, in the conscious rat, hypercapnia-induced cerebral vasodilation is not mediated by vascular prostaglandins and suggests that the reported reduction of the increase in CBF during hypercapnia after indomethacin is not linked to cyclooxygenase inhibition.

REFERENCES

1. Bonaccorsi, A., Dejana, E., and Quintana, A. (1978): Organ blood flow measured with microspheres in the unanaesthetized rat: Effects of three room temperatures. *J. Pharmacol. Methods*, 1:321–328.
2. Dahlgren, N., Nilsson, B., Sakabe, T., and Siesjo, B. K. (1981): The effect of indomethacin on cerebral blood flow and oxygen consumption in the rat at normal and increased carbon dioxide tensions. *Acta Physiol. Scand.*, 111:475–485.
3. Feigen, L. P., King, L. W., Ray, J., Beckett, W., and Kadowitz, P. J. (1981): Differential effects of ibuprofen and indomethacin in the regional circulation of the dog. *J. Pharmacol. Exp. Ther.*, 219:679–684.
4. Jackson, E. K., Gerkens, J. F., Zimmerman, J. B., Uderman, H. D., Oates, J. A., Workman, R. J., and Branch, R. A. (1983): Prostaglandin biosynthesis does not participate in hypercapnia-induced cerebral vasodilatation in the dog. *J. Pharmacol. Exp. Ther.*, 226:486–492.
5. Pickard, J. D., and MacKenzie, E. T. (1973): Inhibition of prostaglandin synthesis and the response of baboon cerebral circulation to carbon dioxide. *Nature [New Biol.]*, 245:187–188.
6. Pickard, J., Tamura, A., Stewart, M., McGeorge, A., and Fitch, W. (1980): Prostacyclin, indomethacin and cerebral circulation. *Brain Res.*, 197:425–431.
7. Quintana, A., Raczka, E., Giralt, M. T., and Quintana, M. A. (1983): Effects of aspirin and indomethacin on cerebral circulation in the conscious rat: Evidence for a physiological role of endogenous prostaglandins. *Prostaglandins*, 25:549–556.

Advances in Prostaglandin, Thromboxane, and
Leukotriene Research, Vol. 13, edited by G. G. Neri
Serneri, et al. Raven Press, New York © 1985.

Arachidonate Metabolism in Renal Injury

James B. Lefkowith and Philip Needleman

*Department of Pharmacology, Washington University Medical School,
St. Louis, Missouri 63110*

ALTERATIONS IN ARACHIDONATE METABOLISM
IN HYDRONEPHROTIC KIDNEYS

The importance of prostaglandin biosynthesis in ureteral obstruction was initially suggested by *in vivo* experiments using cyclooxygenase inhibitors. In a model of acute ureteral obstruction in the cat, it was noted that the vasoconstriction due to adrenergic nerve stimulation or exogenous norepinephrine was blunted and that these effects were abolished by indomethacin (26). These data suggested that a vasodilator prostaglandin was released in response to obstruction. Similarly, experiments in the dog showed that unilateral ligation of the ureter initiated a transient rise in renal blood flow (29) and that pretreatment with indomethacin blocked this response (1).

While the production of vasodilator prostaglandins explains the fall in resistance seen initially with ureteral obstruction (26,29), it does not explain the progressive fall in renal blood flow and glomerular filtration rate (GFR) observed after chronic ureteral obstruction (16). It has been observed that the major cause for the chronic changes is preglomerular vasoconstriction (2). This finding implies that an endogenous vasoconstrictor exists that overrides the effects of vasodilating prostaglandin.

In the rabbit, unilateral ureteral occlusion for 72 hr causes an enhanced basal and hormone (i.e., angiotensin and bradykinin) stimulated prostaglandin biosynthesis. Labeling the perfused hydronephrotic rabbit kidney with [^{14}C]arachidonate and isolating the products from the venous effluent after hormone stimulation showed that the major cyclooxygenase metabolite released was prostaglandin E_2 (22). The role of vasodilating prostaglandins such as prostaglandin E_2 in determining the vascular tone in this model of unilateral hydronephrosis was demonstrated by showing an increase in basal resistance and a potentiation of the vasoconstriction in response to angiotensin II stimulation after indomethacin treatment (22). Since renal vascular resistance is determined mainly by the glomerular arterioles, presumably the prostaglandin released in the hydronephrotic kidney acts at this site.

Subsequently, we found that bradykinin administration to the perfused hydronephrotic rabbit kidney (HNK) released into the venous effluent a substance that contracted a rabbit aorta assay strip and had a rate of disappearance ($t_{1/2} = 30$ sec) identical to that of authentic thromboxane A_2 (17,18). This contractile activity was abolished by indomethacin pretreatment of the kidney and was later confirmed to be thromboxane A_2 by radioimmunoassay of its stable metabolite, thromboxane B_2 (25). In the contralateral unobstructed kidney, even high doses of bradykinin did not release thromboxane into the venous effluent. The importance of thromboxane A_2 in the circulatory adjustments occurring in chronic ureteral obstruction was suggested by the demonstration that the renal vasoconstriction in the postobstructed rat kidney was relieved by pretreatment with imidazole, a thromboxane synthetase inhibitor (31).

The mechanism of the enhanced hormone-stimulated prostaglandin biosynthesis in the hydronephrotic rabbit kidney depends on new protein synthesis (21). Perfusion of a rabbit kidney 72 hr after ureteral obstruction resulted in a progressive time-dependent increase in prostaglandin and thromboxane released into the venous effluent in response to a fixed dose of agonist (e.g., bradykinin or angiotensin). Contralateral or normal kidneys showed no change in prostaglandin release in response to agonists over time. Cycloheximide and actinomycin D, inhibitors of protein synthesis, reversibly blocked this progressive increase in hormone-stimulated prostaglandin release.

This hypothesis is also supported by experiments using aspirin, which covalently acetylates cyclooxygenase. Administration of aspirin to hydronephrotic rabbits inhibited the initial hormone-stimulated prostaglandin biosynthesis in the HNK by 95%. However, within 60 to 90 min of perfusion there was a progressive release of prostaglandin by the aspirin-treated HNK in response to bradykinin that paralleled the prostaglandin release by the nonaspirin-treated HNK control, indicating new cyclooxygenase synthesis. In aspirin-treated contralateral or normal kidneys, hormone-stimulated prostaglandin release was inhibited by 85% and did not recover.

SYNTHESIS AND FUNCTION OF THROMBOXANE IN URETER OBSTRUCTION

By using a selective inhibitor of thromboxane synthetase the role of thromboxane in the pathophysiology of hydronephrosis has been elucidated. Administration of OKY-1581 [sodium-3-(4-3-pyridylmethyl)phenyl-2-methylacrylate] to the isolated perfused rabbit HNK causes a selective inhibition of thromboxane production and does not decrease prostaglandin E_2 or prostacyclin biosynthesis. The selective inhibition of thromboxane production by this agent dramatically alters the vascular response of the rabbit HNK to hormone agonists (10). Bradykinin injected into the perfused HNK during the first few hours of perfusion causes a vasodilation. Prolonged *ex vivo* perfusion of the HNK causes a biphasic vascular response to bradykinin: a brief vasodilation is followed by prolonged vasoconstriction. At this point in time, the administration of OKY-1581 to the HNK abolishes the vasoconstriction and augments the vasodilation seen with bradykinin administration. This effect is reversible with discontinuation of OKY-1581. These data suggest that thromboxane A_2 modulates the effect of bradykinin on the renal vasculature in the

HNK and that this potent vasoconstrictor is capable of overriding the ability of bradykinin to cause vasodilation in this model.

The vascular response to angiotensin II administration is similarly affected by OKY-1581 administration. Angiotensin II causes a monophasic vasoconstriction when injected into the perfused HNK early during perfusion. Later, however, the vascular response is characterized by biphasic vasoconstriction. OKY-1581 inhibits both the second phase of vasoconstriction and the angiotensin II-stimulated thromboxane B_2 release, and unmasks a secondary vasodilation. Indomethacin administration, which inhibits the release of vasodepressor prostaglandins as well as thromboxane, inhibits this secondary vasodilation. Therefore, the vascular tone of the hydronephrotic kidney appears to depend on the interacting influences of hormone agonists, the vasoconstrictor thromboxane A_2, and the vasodilators prostaglandin E_2 and prostacyclin.

These experiments suggest that selective thromboxane synthetase inhibition in the intact kidney is a useful tool to discriminate the participation of thromboxane in various renal pathophysiologic states.

ALTERATION OF CYCLOOXYGENASE AND THROMBOXANE SYNTHETASE IN HYDRONEPHROSIS

Previous studies have established that prostaglandin production by the isolated perfused hydronephrotic kidney increases with the length of perfusion time and that this time-dependent increase is sensitive to inhibitors of protein synthesis (21). Cortical slices display a similar time-dependent increase in prostaglandin production, also inhibited by cycloheximide treatment (4,27). The intact perfused HNK additionally displays an ability to overcome the effect of prior *in vivo* treatment with aspirin. Cortical slices from the hydronephrotic kidneys of animals pretreated with aspirin 3 hr prior to sacrifice initially lack the ability to release prostaglandin E_2; however, after several hours of incubation the slices similarly overcome the effect of aspirin and begin to release prostaglandin E_2 (4). Normal cortical slices cannot overcome the effect of aspirin. Results from hydronephrotic medullary slices do not resemble the isolated perfused hydronephrotic kidney: prostaglandin production in these slices decreases with time of incubation. Thus, these studies indicate that the cortex is responsible for the time-dependent increase in prostaglandin production in the perfused HNK by a mechanism dependent on new protein synthesis.

Microsomal studies also identify the renal cortex as the major site of the metabolic changes in hydronephrosis. Microsomes from the cortex of the hydronephrotic kidney produce predominantly prostaglandin E_2 and thromboxane B_2, whereas microsomes from normal kidney cortex produce much less prostaglandin E2 and no thromboxane B_2 (21,30). Cyclooxygenase and thromboxane synthetase activities are 20- to 40-fold higher in cortical microsomes from the HNK than in those from the contralateral kidney. In the HNK, medullary cyclooxygenase also increases (i.e., prostaglandin E_2, $F_{2\alpha}$, and D_2 synthesis), and thromboxane synthetase activity (blocked by imidazole) becomes apparent (Fig. 1).

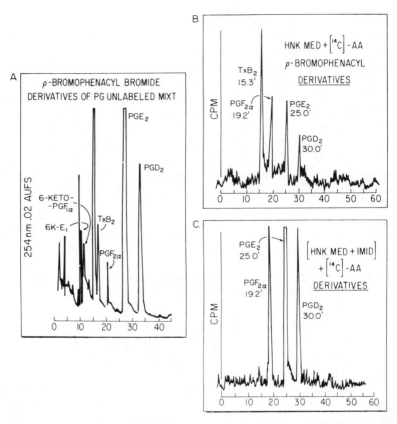

FIG. 1. Hydronephrotic medullary synthesis of cyclooxygenase metabolites analyzed by high-performance liquid chromatography (HPLC). Microsomes from hydronephrotic kidney medulla (HNK MED) were incubated with [^{14}C]arachidonic acid (10 µM) ([^{14}C]-AA) in the absence or presence of imidazole (IMID) (5 mM) for 15 min at 37°C. The reaction mixture was acidified to pH 3.5 with formic acid, extracted with ethyl acetate, and dried under nitrogen. Derivatization was accomplished by adding 0.5 ml p-bromophenacyl bromide (1 mg/ml) in acetonitrile in the presence of diisopropylethylamine for 1 hr at 24°C. HPLC separation was accomplished on an Altex 5 µm octadecasilyl column in an isocratic solvent system of 60% acetonitrile in water.   **A:** Derivatized unlabeled prostaglandin (PG) standards.   **B, C:** Derivatized radioactive cyclooxygenase metabolites produced by the HNK medulla. Imidazole abolished the thromboxane peak (15.3 min retention time on the HPLC) and facilitated the $PGF_{2\alpha}$, PGE_2, and PGD_2 peaks.

The presence of reduced glutathione markedly alters the metabolic capability of renal microsomes from the HNK (30). Cortical and medullary microsomes from hydronephrotic kidneys convert arachidonate into equivalent amounts of prostaglandin E_2 and thromboxane B_2. However, in the presence of reduced glutathione, renal microsomes produce 10-fold more prostaglandin E_2 than thromboxane B_2. This ratio of prostaglandin E_2 to thromboxane B_2 is similar to that seen in the isolated perfused HNK, suggesting that the intact tissue is dominated by the prostaglandin endoperoxide E_2 isomerase and that reduced glutathione may be a key influence on the *in vivo* synthesis of prostaglandin in hydronephrosis.

ROLE OF CORTICAL INFLAMMATORY CELLS IN THE EXAGGERATED ARACHIDONATE METABOLISM AFTER URETERAL OBSTRUCTION

Ureteral obstruction in rabbits results in a diffuse proliferation of fibroblasts and the appearance of mononuclear cells in the renal cortex (19,20). The demonstration of these cell types in the cortex has profound implications in explaining the metabolic changes seen in the renal injury of ureteral obstruction. It has been shown that abolition of circulating blood monocytes by antimacrophage serum and steroids delays the appearance of fibroblasts at sites of injury and suppresses fibroblast proliferation (14). Macrophages also appear to modulate fibroblast prostaglandin biosynthesis. It has been reported that conditioned media obtained from adherent mononuclear cell cultures contain a factor that is mitogenic for fibroblasts (15) and that stimulates prostaglandin E_2 synthesis by fibroblasts (5–7,11).

Consequently we formulated the hypothesis that the invasion of macrophages into the hydronephrotic kidney cortex and the proliferation of fibroblasts in the cortical interstitium might account for the metabolic changes seen in the hydronephrotic kidney. In support of this hypothesis, we were able to grow a monolayer of fibroblasts and monocytes from explants of the HNK cortex, whereas the contralateral kidney cortex yielded only a monolayer of fibroblasts (9). These cultures both released prostaglandin E_2, but the HNK cultures exhibited a threefold to fourfold increase in prostaglandin E_2 in response to endotoxin indicative of the presence of macrophages (9). No response was seen in the contralateral kidney cultures. Bradykinin administration caused a 20-fold stimulation of PGE_2 release from the HNK cultures but only a sevenfold stimulation in contralateral kidney cultures. Using a mild trypsin treatment and passaging the cultures, the phagocytic cells were removed from the HNK cultures. These passaged cultures did not respond to endotoxin, and showed a diminished response to bradykinin and a diminished cyclooxygenase activity when compared to primary cultures. Conditioned media from adherent rabbit peripheral blood mononuclear cells also stimulated prostaglandin E_2 synthesis in HNK and contralateral kidney cultures. These findings suggest that the cortical inflammatory cells are responsible for the changes in arachidonate metabolism seen in the rabbit hydronephrotic kidney.

The role of the cortical inflammatory cells in the metabolic changes of ureteral obstruction was also investigated in the intact hydronephrotic kidney. Macrophages have been shown to produce prostaglandin E_2 and thromboxane in response to endotoxin (8,12). The involvement of macrophages in the increased prostaglandin synthesis of hydronephrosis is demonstrated by the finding that endotoxin stimulates prostaglandin and thromboxane release when injected into the perfused HNK (23,24). Endotoxin has no effect on normal kidneys or on the postobstructed kidney which contains a decreased number of macrophages (24). Hydronephrosis in the cat causes only a modest increase in prostaglandin synthesis and does not induce thromboxane production (24,25). Histologically the hydronephrotic cat kidney contains few macrophages, and when it is perfused it does not respond to endotoxin (24).

The critical role of the macrophage in the metabolic changes of hydronephrosis is demonstrated through the use of endotoxin and nitrogen mustard *in vivo* (13). The *in vivo* administration of endotoxin 1 hr before removal and perfusion of the hydronephrotic kidney markedly enhances the peptide-stimulated arachidonic acid metabolism of the perfused kidney (Fig. 2). Nitrogen mustard renders animals leukopenic and prevents the influx of macrophages into the hydronephrotic kidney. The peptide-stimulated arachidonic acid metabolism of the HNK from the nitrogen mustard-treated animals is suppressed (Fig. 3), and no enhancement is seen when endotoxin is given *in vivo* to these animals. Microsomes from the HNK cortex from nitrogen mustard-treated rabbits show a markedly diminished thromboxane synthetase activity relative to the control HNK cortex implying that the macrophage is the cellular location of the thromboxane synthetase in this model of renal injury. These data suggest that the macrophage is an essential determinant of the enhanced arachidonic acid metabolism seen in experimental hydronephrosis.

An inhibitory effect of prostaglandin E_2 on macrophage function in this model of renal inflammation can also be shown. Prostaglandin E_2 is an *in vitro* inhibitor of macrophage cytolytic function (28). When hydronephrotic animals are given aspirin during the period of ureteral obstruction in order to prevent *in vivo* prostaglandin E_2 production, the peptide-stimulated arachidonic acid metabolism of the

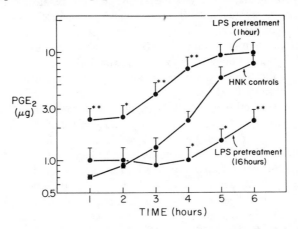

FIG. 2. Prostaglandin (PG) E_2 released into the venous effluent of a perfused HNK (measured by radioimmunoassay) in response to hourly injection of a fixed dose of bradykinin (300 ng). Kidneys from animals receiving endotoxin (LPS) *in vivo* (8 mg/kg) 1 hr before the kidney is removed and perfused show an enhanced release of PGE_2 relative to untreated controls. PGE_2 release is suppressed when endotoxin is given 16 hr before removal of the kidney. Statistical significance: $*p < 0.05$; $**p < 0.01$.

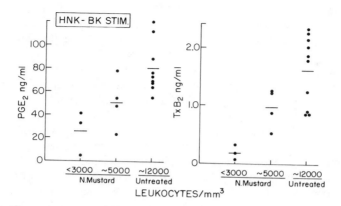

FIG. 3. Prostaglandin E₂ and thromboxane B₂ (TxB₂) released into the venous effluent of a perfused HNK (measured by radioimmunoassay) at hr 9 of perfusion in response to bradykinin (BK) injection (300 ng). Kidneys removed from animals made leukopenic *in vivo* by the administration of nitrogen mustard (N. mustard) show a diminished ability to release these cyclooxygenase metabolites relative to controls.

perfused hydronephrotic kidney, which appears to be a marker of macrophage function in this model, is enhanced (Fig. 4). (13).

SUMMARY

In conclusion, the evidence to date demonstrates that the enhanced arachidonate metabolism seen in hydronephrosis is responsible for the pathophysiological alterations observed in this model of renal injury. The balance between vasodilating prostaglandins and the vasoconstrictor thromboxane A₂ may be critical in determining blood flow to the obstructed kidney. The alterations in arachidonate metabolism in this pathophysiologic state appear to result from the invasion of

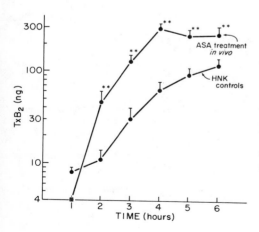

FIG. 4. Thromboxane B₂ (TxB₂) released into the venous effluent of a perfused HNK (measured by radioimmunoassay) in response to hourly injection of a fixed dose of bradykinin (300 ng). Kidneys from animals receiving aspirin (ASA) *in vivo* (50 mg/kg·day) during the period of hydronephrosis show an enhanced release of thromboxane B₂ relative to untreated controls. Statistical significance: $**p < 0.01$.

macrophages and the proliferation of fibroblasts in the cortical interstitium. Additionally, the macrophage appears to be necessary for the expression of the enhanced hormone-stimulated arachidonate metabolism.

We envision the temporal sequence of events in this model to be as follows: ureter obstruction causes a mechanical disruption and/or immunologic stimulus in the cortex, which triggers a regional inflammatory response resulting in the proliferation of interstitial cells and the invasion of mononuclear cells. The macrophages, which are in direct contact with fibroblasts, are capable of releasing a factor that stimulates fibroblast proliferation, cortical microsomal cyclooxygenase activity, and prostaglandin E_2 release (i.e., intrinsic arachidonate metabolism). The enhanced thromboxane synthetase levels and thromboxane A_2 appear to come from the macrophage. The prostaglandin E_2 and thromboxane A_2 released modulate vascular tone. Prostaglandin E_2 may also serve as an inhibitor of macrophage function.

Two other models of renal damage also exhibit marked enhancement of renal prostaglandin synthesis and induction of thromboxane production: renal venous occlusion (32) and glycerol-induced acute renal failure (3). The finding that several models of renal damage have definite quantitative and qualitative alterations in the prostaglandin cascade reflects the importance of this pathway in renal pathophysiology.

ACKNOWLEDGMENTS

This work was supported by National Institutes of Health grants HL-14397, HL-20787, and training grant (to J. Lefkowith) HL-07081.

REFERENCES

1. Allen, J. T., Vaughn, E. D., Jr., and Gillenwater, J. Y. (1978): The effect of indomethacin on renal blood flow and ureteral pressure in unilateral ureteral obstruction in awake dogs. *Invest. Urol.*, 15:324–327.
2. Arendshorst, W. J., Finn, W. R., and Gottschalk, C. W. (1974): Nephron stop flow pressure response to obstruction for 24 hours in the rat kidney. *J. Clin. Invest.*, 53:1497–1500.
3. Benabe, J. E., Klahr, S., Hoffman, M. H., and Morrison, A. R. (1980): Production of thromboxane A_2 by the kidney in glycerol-induced acute renal failure. *Prostaglandins*, 19:333–347.
4. Currie, M. G., Davis, B. B., and Needleman, P. (1981): Localization of exaggerated prostaglandin synthesis associated with renal damage. *Prostaglandins*, 22:933–944.
5. Dayer, J-M., Passwell, J. H., Schneeberger, E. E., and Krane, S. M. (1980): Interactions among rheumatoid synovial cells and monocyte-macrophages: Production of collagenase-stimulating factor by human monocytes exposed to concanavalin A or immunoglobulin Fc fragments. *J. Immunol.*, 124:1712–1720.
6. Dayer, J-M., Robinson, D. R., and Krane, S. M. (1977): Prostaglandin production by rheumatoid synovial cells. Stimulation by a factor from human mononuclear cells. *J. Exp. Med.*, 145:1399–1404.
7. D'Souza, S. M., Englis, D. J., Clark, A., and Russell, R. G. (1981): Stimulation of production of prostaglandin E in gingival cells exposed to products of human blood mononuclear cells. *Biochem. J.*, 198:391–396.
8. Halushka, P. V., Cook, J. A., and Wise, W. C. (1981): Thromboxane A_2 and prostacyclin produc-

tion by lipopolysaccharide-stimulated peritoneal macrophages. *J. Reticuloendothel. Soc.*, 30:445–450.

9. Jonas, P. E., Leahy, K. M., DeSchryver-Kecskemeti, K., and Needleman, P. (1984): Cellular interactions and exaggerated arachidonic acid metabolism in rabbit renal injury. *J. Leukocyte Biol.*, 204:35:55–64.

10. Kawasaki, A., and Needleman, P. (1982): Contribution of thromboxane to renal resistance changes in the isolated perfused hydronephrotic rabbit kidney. *Circ. Res.*, 50:486–490.

11. Korn, J. H., Halushka, P. V., and LeRoy, E. C. (1980): Mononuclear cell modulation of connective tissue function. Suppression of fibroblast growth by stimulation of endogenous prostaglandin production. *J. Clin. Invest.*, 65:543–554.

12. Kurland, J. I., and Bockman, R. (1978): Prostaglandin E production by human blood monocytes and mouse peritoneal macrophages. *J. Exp. Med.*, 147:952–956.

13. Lefkowith, J. B., Okegawa, T., DeSchryver-Kecskemeti, K., and Needleman, P. (1984): Macrophage-dependent arachidonate metabolism in hydronephrosis. *Kidney Int.*, 26:10–17.

14. Leibovich, S. J., and Ross, R. (1975): The role of macrophage in wound repair. A study with hydrocortisone and antimacrophage serum. *Am. J. Pathol.*, 78:71–91.

15. Leibovich, S. J., and Ross, R. (1976): A macrophage-dependent factor that stimulates the proliferation of fibroblasts *in vitro*. *Am. J. Pathol.*, 84:501–513.

16. Moody, T. E., Vaughn, E. D., Jr., and Gillenwater, J. Y. (1975): Relationship between renal blood flow and ureteral pressure during eighteen hours of total unilateral occlusion. Implication for changing sites of renal resistance. *Invest. Urol.*, 13:246–251.

17. Morrison, A. R., Moritz, H., and Needleman, P. (1978): Mechanisms of enhanced renal prostaglandin biosynthesis in ureter obstruction: Role of *de novo* protein synthesis. *J. Biol. Chem.*, 253:8210–8212.

18. Morrison, A. R., Nishikawa, K., and Needleman, P. (1977): Unmasking of thromboxane A_2 synthesis by ureter obstruction in the rabbit kidney. *Nature (Lond.)*, 269:259–260.

19. Nagle, R. B., Bulger, R. E., Cutter, R. E., Jervis, H. R., and Benditt, E. P. (1973): Unilateral obstructive nephropathy in the rabbit. I. Early morphologic, physiologic, and histochemical changes. *Lab. Invest.*, 28:456–467.

20. Nagle, R. B., Johnson, M. E., and Jervis, H. R. (1976): Proliferation of renal interstitial cells following injury induced by ureteral obstruction. *Lab. Invest.*, 35:18–22.

21. Needleman, P., Wyche, A., Bronson, S. D., Holmberg, S., and Morrison, A. R. (1979): Specific regulation of peptide-induced renal prostaglandin synthesis. *J. Biol. Chem.*, 254:9772–9777.

22. Nishikawa, K., Morrison, A. R., and Needleman, P. (1977): Exaggerated prostaglandin biosynthesis and its influence on renal resistance in the isolated hydronephrotic rabbit kidney. *J. Clin. Invest.*, 59:1143–1150.

23. Okegawa, T., DeSchryver-Kecskemeti, K., and Needleman, P. (1983): Endotoxin induces chronic prostaglandin and thromboxane synthesis from ureter-obstructed kidneys: Role of inflammatory cells. *J. Pharmacol. Exp. Ther.*, 225:213–218.

24. Okegawa, T., Jonas, P. E., DeSchryver, K., Kawasaki, A., and Needleman, P. (1983): Metabolic and cellular alterations underlying the exaggerated renal prostaglandins and thromboxane synthesis in ureter obstruction in rabbits. Inflammatory response involving fibroblasts and mononuclear cells. *J. Clin. Invest.*, 71:81–90.

25. Reingold, D. F., Waters, K., Holmberg, S., and Needleman, P. (1981): Differential biosynthesis of prostaglandins by hydronephrotic rabbit and cat kidneys. *J. Pharmacol. Exp. Ther.*, 216:510–515.

26. Schramm, L. P., and Carlson, D. E. (1975): Inhibition of renal vasoconstriction by elevated ureteral pressure. *Am. J. Physiol.*, 228:1126–1133.

27. Schwartzman, M., and Raz, A. (1981): Selective induction of *de novo* prostaglandin biosynthesis in rabbit kidney cortex. *Biochim. Biophys. Acta*, 664:469–474.

28. Taffet, S. M., and Russell, S. W. (1981): Macrophage-mediated tumor cell killing: regulation of expression of cytolytic activity by prostaglandin E. *J. Immunol.*, 126:424–427.

29. Vaughan, E. D., Shenashy, J. H., II, and Gillenwater, J. Y. (1971): Mechanism of acute hemodynamic response to ureteral occlusion. *Invest. Urol.*, 9:109–118.

30. Wu, Y. S., Lysz, T. A., Wyche, A., and Needleman, P. (1983): Kinetic comparison and regulation of the cascade of microsomal enzymes involved in renal arachidonate and endoperoxide metabolism. *J. Biol. Chem.*, 258:2188–2192.

31. Yarger, W. E., Schocken, D. D., and Harris, R. H. (1980): Obstructive nephropathy in the rat. Possible roles for the renin-angiotensin system, prostaglandins, and thromboxanes in postobstructive renal function. *J. Clin. Invest.*, 65:400–412.
32. Zipser, R., Myers, S., and Needleman, P. (1980): Exaggerated prostaglandin and thromboxane synthesis in the rabbit with renal vein constriction. *Circ. Res.*, 47:231–237.

Advances in Prostaglandin, Thromboxane, and Leukotriene Research, Vol. 13, edited by G. G. Neri Serneri, et al. Raven Press, New York © 1985.

Drugs, Prostaglandins, and Renal Function

*C. Patrono, *G. Ciabattoni, *P. Filabozzi, *F. Catella, *L. Forni, *M. Segni, **P. Patrignani, †F. Pugliese, †B. M. Simonetti, and †A. Pierucci

*Department of Pharmacology and **Centro di Studio per la Fisiopatologia dello Shock del C.N.R., Catholic University School of Medicine, 00168 Rome, Italy; and †Division of Nephrology, Department of Medicine, University of Rome La Sapienza, 00100 Rome, Italy*

ORGANIZATION OF THE RENAL PROSTAGLANDIN SYSTEM

Immunofluorescence studies have demonstrated that, in the mammalian kidney, cyclooxygenase [the enzyme converting arachidonic acid into the prostaglandin (PG) cyclic endoperoxides] is localized in the endoplasmic reticulum of three cell types: epithelial collecting tubule cells; medullary interstitial cells, and arterial endothelial cells (26). Further biotransformations of PG cyclic endoperoxides in different cell types, and hence the relative prevalence of individual eicosanoids in discrete segments of the nephron, vary as a function of cellular distribution of specific isomerases converting PGH_2 into PGE_2 (endoperoxide isomerase), $PGF_{2\alpha}$ (endoperoxide reductase), prostacyclin (PGI_2 synthase), and thromboxane (TX) A_2 (TXA_2 synthase).

Medullary and cortical microsomes obtained from human kidneys synthesize PGI_2, $PGF_{2\alpha}$, PGE_2, TXA_2, and PGD_2 (14). The biosynthetic activity is 2- to 24-fold higher in the medulla than in the cortex. PGI_2 is the major cyclooxygenase product of arachidonic acid metabolism in human glomeruli, while in the papilla, PGE_2 is a predominant product (27).

The renal PG system locally modulates cortical and medullary functions, i.e., renal blood flow (RBF), glomerular filtration rate (GFR), renin release, and sodium and water excretion (see ref. 12 for reviews on different aspects of PG action on renal function).

From a merely functional point of view, one can characterize two compartments of the renal PG system: (a) a cortical compartment, whose structures (glomeruli and arterioles) synthesize compounds potentially modulating cortical events, i.e., RBF, renin release and GFR; (b) a medullary compartment, whose structures (interstitial cells, collecting tubules) elaborate PGs capable of modulating medullary events, such as medullary blood flow, collecting-tubule response to vasopressin, and Na and Cl reabsorption in the loop of Henle.

Combined biochemical and functional evidence seems to indicate that, in the human kidney, PGI_2 is primarily involved in the modulation of cortical events, while PGE_2 is largely confined to controlling medullary function.

METHODS FOR THE CLINICAL INVESTIGATION OF THE RENAL PROSTAGLANDIN SYSTEM

In vivo studies on renal PG synthesis, based on the assessment of renal secretory and/or excretory rates of PGE_2 and $PGF_{2\alpha}$, have been reported in several species, including the rat, rabbit, dog, and humans (see ref. 20 for a review). Renal venous PGs are presumably derived from direct venous drainage of cellular sites of synthesis and also from venous removal of readsorbed PGs. Measurement of unmetabolized PGs in renal venous plasma suffers from major limitations, i.e., very low levels, possible platelet contribution, and invasive procedure. As a consequence, measurement of unmetabolized PGs in urine has gained general acceptance following the original report suggesting their renal origin in healthy women (13). Besides having a higher PG concentration, urine has the additional advantage over renal venous plasma of being free of platelet contribution and of providing a continuous and integrated measure of renal PG synthesis. A number of methodologic as well as biologic variables can, however, affect urinary PG measurement in human studies. These include storage and analysis of urine, variable PG excretion rate during the menstrual cycle, and contribution from extrarenal sources (24). The overall validity of estimating renal PG synthesis by urinary PG determinations relies on a crucial assumption, that the lower urogenital tract does not contribute substantial amounts of unmetabolized PGs to urine. On the basis of the available evidence, the validity of such an assumption seems to be limited to women, since trace amounts of seminal fluid may contribute a highly variable fraction of the measured urinary PG in men (21).

It should be pointed out that urinary PGs only represent a fraction of total renal synthesis, which is subtracted to intrarenal metabolism and to secretion into the renal venous blood. Furthermore, renal venous blood as well as urinary unmetabolized PGs probably reflect a heterogeneous origin within the kidney, since no data are available to indicate a preferential secretion or excretion of any particular compartment.

Radioimmunoassay as well as gas chromatography–mass spectrometry (GC-MS) have been employed to assess renal PG production in humans. We have developed radioimmunological techniques to measure urinary PGE_2, $PGF_{2\alpha}$ (6), TXB_2 (the stable hydrolysis product of TXA_2) (23), and 6-keto-$PGF_{1\alpha}$ (the stable hydrolysis product of PGI_2) (22), and we have provided evidence for their identification by means of several independent criteria: (a) characterization of the thin-layer chromatographic pattern of distribution of the extracted PG-like immunoreactivity; (b) use of multiple antisera; (c) comparison with GC-MS determinations.

That urinary 6-keto-$PGF_{1\alpha}$ and TXB_2 excretion may largely reflect the renal synthesis of PGI_2 and TXA_2, respectively, is indicated by several lines of pharmacologic evidence. Thus furosemide, which enhances the intrarenal release of arachidonic acid and hence stimulates renal PG synthesis, also increases the urinary excretion rate of TXB_2 (5) and 6-keto-$PGF_{1\alpha}$ (22) in healthy women. On the other hand, drugs that selectively spare renal cyclooxygenase activity, such as sulindac (7) or low-dose aspirin (17), do not influence the urinary excretion of TXB_2 and 6-keto-$PGF_{1\alpha}$ in health (7,23) and disease (10,23).

More recently, we have been able to demonstrate that, when infused at rates comparable to the endogenous secretion rate, either PGI_2 (24) or TXB_2 *(unpublished data)* failed to influence the urinary excretion of 6-keto-$PGF_{1\alpha}$ or TXB_2, respectively, in healthy subjects.

PHARMACOLOGIC MODULATION OF THE RENAL PROSTAGLANDIN SYSTEM

High-Ceiling Diuretics

The mechanisms by which high-ceiling diuretics induce salt and water loss, lower blood pressure, and increase RBF and renin release are currently considered to be, at least in part, related to activation of the renal PG system. Furosemide induces a prompt and generalized activation of the renal PG system in healthy women, temporally related to the increase of renin release and natriuresis (5,22). The local nature of such activation is further supported by failure of furosemide to raise peripheral plasma levels of 6-keto-$PGF_{1\alpha}$ (22). However, while indomethacin blocks furosemide-induced PG synthesis, it does not affect the natriuretic response (29). On the other hand, PG synthesis inhibition does blunt furosemide-induced vasodilation and renin release (1). Since PGI_2, a potent vasodilator and stimulator of renin release (22), is a major cyclooxygenase product in human glomeruli (27), we have suggested that furosemide-induced renal vasodilation and renin release are mediated by enhanced cortical PGI_2 production (22); similar conclusions were reached by Wilson et al. (30) in the dog.

Angiotensin-Converting Enzyme Inhibitors

Angiotensin-converting enzyme (ACE) inhibitors represent a new class of orally active antihypertensive agents. This enzyme is a COOH-terminal dipeptidyl exopeptidase, with at least two biologically important substrates, angiotensin I and bradykinin. Its action on each is physiologically vasopressor, since (a) it controls the formation of the pressor hormone, angiotensin II, from its inactive precursor, angiotensin I, and (b) it promotes the hydrolytic cleavage of bradykinin, thus inactivating a powerful vasodepressor agent. Therefore, the antihypertensive response to ACE inhibitors, such as captopril or enalapril, might result both from inhibition of angiotensin II formation and from accumulation of bradykinin in the circulation (28). The latter effect might in turn cause an increased release of PGs, especially in the renal vasculature. Since angiotensin II as well as bradykinin are potent releasers of PGI_2 from the lungs and kidney, the stimulatory effects of increased plasma concentrations of bradykinin on PGI_2 release might be offset by decreased levels of angiotensin II, as a consequence of ACE inhibition.

There is conflicting evidence, direct and inferential, that PG release can be increased by ACE inhibitors (16). It is not yet clear whether this release is secondary to changes in kinin degradation or is produced by some other mechanism, i.e., direct stimulation, as suggested by *in vitro* experiments (16). The extent to which such a mechanism contributes to the chronic antihypertensive action of these drugs also remains to be defined.

Nonselective Cyclooxygenase Inhibitors

The vast majority of currently available nonsteroidal antiinflammatory drugs (NSADs) have been reported to inhibit by 50 to 80% renal as well as extrarenal sites of cyclooxygenase activity, in health and disease (7,9,11). The urinary excretion of PGE_2, $PGF_{2\alpha}$, 6-keto-$PGF_{1\alpha}$, and TXB_2 is similarly suppressed by these agents. However, pharmacologic inhibition of the renal PG-system has divergent effects on different cortical events in healthy subjects. Thus, while renin release is substantially reduced, GFR and RBF are largely unaffected. This might imply either that cortical PGI_2 does not participate in the physiologic control of GFR and RBF, or that residual PGI_2 synthesis (approximately 25–35%) is adequate to their maintenance in healthy individuals. In contrast, RBF and GFR become critically dependent on intact renal cyclooxygenase activity under a variety of clinical conditions characterized by ineffective circulatory volume, i.e., volume depletion, congestive heart failure, cirrhosis with ascites, and the nephrotic syndrome (11). A common hallmark of such diverse conditions is represented by an increased renal synthesis of vasodilator PGE_2, currently interpreted as a renal homeostatic response to vasoconstrictor stimuli (11). Besides exaggerated vasoconstrictor stimuli to the kidney, a reduction of local vasodilator influences might create a similar setting. We have recently provided evidence supporting this hypothesis, by showing that the vast majority of female patients with chronic glomerular disease have a significantly lower excretion of 6-keto-$PGF_{1\alpha}$, regardless of the nature of glomerular involvement (10). In these patients, the reduction of RBF and GFR induced by ibuprofen was inversely related to the basal urinary 6-keto-$PGF_{1\alpha}$ excretion in a statistically significant fashion (10). Reduced renal synthesis of PGI_2 might have functional consequences because of (a) lack of direct vasodilatory effect, or (b) enhanced constrictor effects of angiotensin II on glomerular vasculature and glomerular mesangial cells (25).

Increased renal synthesis of vasoconstrictor TXA_2, as detected in patients with systemic lupus erythematosus (SLE) and active renal disease (8), might represent a third mechanism underlying the cyclooxygenase-dependence of renal function, because of important effects on glomerular contraction, thereby reducing the glomerular ultrafiltration coefficient (K_f) (25).

Although the role played by advanced age and concomitant diuretic therapy in NSAD-induced renal insufficiency has been emphasized in recent case reports (2), the relation of a number of pathophysiologic variables to the cyclooxygenase dependence of renal function remains to be determined.

Selective Cyclooxygenase Inhibitors

A number of mechanisms have been proposed to explain the differential inhibition by some drugs of PG synthesis in different human tissues. These are listed in Table 1.

Selective sparing of renal cyclooxygenase activity has been demonstrated with sulindac (7), low-dose aspirin (17), and sulfinpyrazone (3).

In contrast to other NSADs, sulindac does not affect renal PG synthesis in healthy subjects (7), in patients with Bartter's syndrome (7), and in patients with chronic glomerular disease (10), i.e., under conditions of normal, enhanced, or reduced glomerular PGI_2 production. In the latter, sulindac treatment was not associated with any statistically significant change of renal function, in contrast to the consistent reduction of GFR (Fig. 1) and RBF detected in patients treated with ibuprofen (10). These findings establish, for the first time, a cause–effect relation between changes in glomerular PGI_2 synthesis and renal function. Although the precise mechanism for this selectivity remains to be elucidated, it appears likely to be related to the redox pro-drug nature of sulindac affecting its intrarenal distribution and metabolism. Thus, oxidative enzymes of renal cortical structures may oxidize the active sulfide metabolite back to the inactive sulfoxide (i.e., sulindac itself), thereby protecting the physiologically relevant site(s) of cyclooxygenase activity from inhibition. Experimental data consistent with this hypothesis have been reported by Miller et al. (15). Further support to this interpretation is provided by our recent finding that renal PG synthesis is not inhibited by sulfinpyrazone (3), a drug sharing with sulindac a reversible reduction to a more potent sulfide metabolite. Consistently with this biochemical observation, Choudhury et al. (4) found no evidence that sulfinpyrazone reduced GFR in patients with uncomplicated acute myocardial infarction.

Another example of selective sparing of renal PGI_2 production is provided by low-dose aspirin (Fig. 2). The mechanism underlying this selectivity is probably related to a different rate of recovery of cyclooxygenase activity in glomeruli versus platelets, following irreversible inactivation of the enzyme, and possibly to a different aspirin sensitivity of glomerular cyclooxygenase (17). The finding of a normal

TABLE 1. *Mechanisms underlying differential inhibition of prostaglandin synthesis in human tissues*

Different "sensitivity" of cyclooxygenase of different cell types
Different rate of recovery of enzyme activity following
  irreversible inactivation
Different drug affinity for the binding site versus the catalytic site
  of the enzyme
Different tissue distribution of the drug
Tissue-selective inactivation of active metabolites of the drug

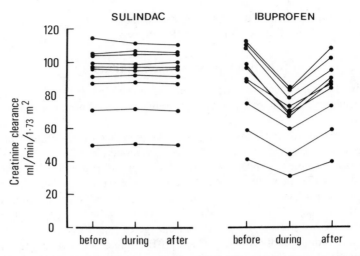

FIG. 1. Changes in creatinine clearance in 20 patients with chronic glomerular disease during sulindac (400 mg/day for 7 days) or ibuprofen (1,200 mg/day for 7 days) treatment. Individual values for all patients are shown. Each point represents the mean of three separate measurements performed in the same patients in each phase of the study. (For details see ref. 10.)

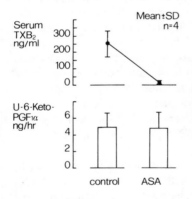

FIG. 2. Selective sparing of renal PGI_2 production by low-dose aspirin (ASA, 0.45 mg/kg·day for 7 days). Serum TXB_2 concentrations and urinary 6-keto-$PGF_{1\alpha}$ excretion were measured in 4 healthy subjects under control conditions and after daily dosing with aspirin (0.45 mg/kg·day) for 7 days.

pattern of furosemide-induced increase of renin release and urinary 6-keto-$PGF_{1\alpha}$ excretion after 3 to 4 weeks of low-dose aspirin treatment (17) indicates that renal PGI_2-producing cells are readily activatable at a time of virtually complete suppression of platelet cyclooxygenase activity. Thus, low-dose aspirin might have an additional advantage over high-dose aspirin in patients chronically treated with both drugs.

Selective Thromboxane Synthase Inhibitors

Besides being explored as potential antithrombotic agents, TX synthase inhibitors are currently being explored as pharmacologic tools to investigate the role of glomerular TXA_2 production in renal pathophysiology and may provide a novel therapeutic strategy in TXA$_2$-dependent deterioration of renal function (25). We have recently examined the effects of three orally active TX-synthase inhibitors, i.e., dazoxiben (19), OKY-046 (18), and UK-38,485 *(unpublished data)* on renal PG endoperoxide metabolism in healthy subjects. Despite variable biological half-life of platelet TX-synthase inhibition (4 to >8 hr), the three drugs only caused a marginal reduction of urinary TXB$_2$ excretion by approximately 30% at doses maximally inhibiting platelet TXB$_2$ production (Figs. 3 and 4; effect of OKY-046 not shown). Redirection of PG endoperoxide metabolism could be demonstrated in platelets but not in the kidney, either *in vivo* or *in vitro*, possibly because of widely different relative abundance of TXA$_2$ (18,19). Oral dosing with OKY-046 (200 mg t.i.d. for 3 days) was not associated with any statistically significant change of GFR or RBF *(unpublished observations)*. Similarly, Zipser et al. (31) recently reported a partial reduction in urinary TXB$_2$ by dazoxiben in the hepatorenal syndrome, a clinical condition characterized by increased TXB$_2$ excretion. No consistent improvement of renal function was associated in these patients with a 54% reduction of urinary TXB$_2$ excretion (31). Thus, definition of the pathophysiologic role of glomerular TXA$_2$ production in human disease states has to wait the development of tissue-selective TX synthase inhibitors or perhaps TXA$_2$ receptor antagonists.

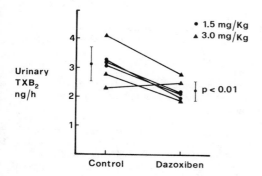

FIG. 3. Effect of dazoxiben on renal TXA$_2$ production. The 8-hr urinary TXB$_2$ excretion was measured before and after the oral administration of dazoxiben, 1.5 or 3.0 mg/kg, to 6 healthy volunteers. Individual and mean ($\pm$ SD) values are plotted.

FIG. 4. Effect of UK-38,485 (50 mg p.o. at *arrow*) on platelet and renal TXA$_2$ production. Serum TXB$_2$ concentrations and 8-hr urinary TXB$_2$ excretion were measured before and after the oral administration of UK-38,485, 50 mg, to 3 healthy subjects. Each subject was studied on 3 consecutive days. The different symbols used in the lower panel of the figure denote different subjects. Mean ($\pm$ SD) values are also plotted.

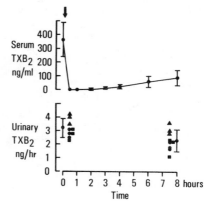

ACKNOWLEDGMENTS

The authors wish to thank Angelamaria Zampini for expert editorial assistance; Dr. J. E. Pike (Upjohn Company, Kalamazoo, Michigan) for several generous gifts of PGs and TXB_2; Dr. H. M. Tyler (Pfizer Central Research, Sandwich, Kent, England) for a gift of dazoxiben and UK-38,485; and M. Tsuboshima (Ono Pharmaceutical Company, Osaka, Japan) for a gift of OKY-046.

These studies were supported by grants from Consiglio Nazionale delle Ricerche (82.00389.96 and 83.02535.04) and Ministero della Pubblica Istruzione (60/82, 60/83).

REFERENCES

1. Attallah, A. (1979): Interactions of prostaglandins with diuretics. *Prostaglandins*, 18:369–375.
2. Blackshear, J. L., Davidman, M., and Stillman, M. T. (1983): Identification of risk for renal insufficiency from nonsteroidal antiinflammatory drugs. *Arch. Intern. Med.*, 143:1130–1134.
3. Catella, F., Pugliese, F., Patrignani, P., Filabozzi, P., Ciabattoni, G., and Patrono, C. (1984): Differential platelet and renal effects of sulfinpyrazone in man. *Clin. Res. (Abstr.)*, 32:239A.
4. Choudhury, S. L., Taylor, S. H., Wieringa, G., Swaminathan, R., and Morgan, D. B. (1983): Sulphinpyrazone and renal function following myocardial infarction. *Eur. J. Clin. Pharmacol.*, 24:747–750.
5. Ciabattoni, G., Pugliese, F., Cinotti, G. A., Stirati, G., Ronci, R., Castrucci, G., Pierucci, A., and Patrono, C. (1979): Characterization of furosemide-induced activation of the renal prostaglandin system. *Eur. J. Pharmacol.*, 60:181–187.
6. Ciabattoni, G., Pugliese, F., Spaldi, M., Cinotti, G. A., and Patrono, C. (1979): Radioimmunoassay measurement of prostaglandin E_2 and $F_{2\alpha}$ in human urine. *J. Endocrinol. Invest.*, 2:173–182.
7. Ciabattoni, G., Pugliese, F., Cinotti, G. A., and Patrono, C. (1980): Renal effects of antiinflammatory drugs. *Eur. J. Rheumatol.*, 3:210–221.
8. Ciabattoni, G., Patrignani, P., Filabozzi, P., Pierucci, A., Simonetti, B. M., Cinotti, G. A., Pinca, E., Gotti, E., Remuzzi, G., and Patrono, C. (1982): Increased renal thromboxane production in systemic lupus erythematosus. *Clin. Res.*, 30:445A.
9. Ciabattoni, G., Bianchi Porro G., Caruso, I., Fumagalli, M., Pugliese, F., and Patrono, C. (1984): Differential inhibition of prostaglandin and thromboxane synthesis in human tissues by nonsteroidal antiinflammatory drugs. *Clin. Res. (Abstr.)*, 32:462A.
10. Ciabattoni, G., Cinotti, G. A., Pierucci, A., Simonetti, B. M., Manzi, M., Pugliese, F., Barsotti, P., Pecci, G., Taggi, F., and Patrono, C. (1984): Effects of Sulindac and Ibuprofen in patients with chronic glomerular disease. *N. Engl. J. Med.*, 310:279–283.
11. Dunn, M. J., and Zambraski, E. J. (1980): Renal effects of drugs that inhibit prostaglandin synthesis. *Kidney Int.*, 18:609–622.
12. Dunn, M. J., Patrono, C., and Cinotti, G. A., editors (1983): *Prostaglandins and the Kidney. Biochemistry, Physiology, Pharmacology, and Clinical Applications*. Plenum Press, New York.
13. Frölich, J. C., Wilson, T. W., Sweetman, B. J., Smigel, M., Nies, A. S., Carr, K., Watson, J. T., and Oates, J. A. (1975): Urinary prostaglandins. Identification and origin. *J. Clin. Invest.*, 55:763–770.
14. Hassid, A., and Dunn, M. J. (1980): Microsomal prostaglandin biosynthesis of human kidney. *J. Biol. Chem.*, 255:2472–2475.
15. Miller, M. J. S., Bednar, M. M., and McGiff, J. C. (1983): Renal metabolism of sulindac, a novel nonsteroidal antiinflammatory agent. In: *Advances in Prostaglandin, Thromboxane and Leukotriene Research, vol. 11*, edited by B. Samuelsson, R. Paoletti, and P. Ramwell, pp. 487–491. Raven Press, New York.
16. Mullane, K., Moncada, S., and Vane, J. R. (1983): Does prostaglandin release contribute to the hypotension induced by inhibitors of angiotensin converting enzyme? In: *Prostaglandins and the Kidney. Biochemistry, Physiology, Pharmacology, and Clinical Applications*, edited by M. J. Dunn, C. Patrono, and G. A. Cinotti, pp. 213–233. Plenum Press, New York.

17. Patrignani, P., Filabozzi, P., and Patrono, C. (1982): Selective cumulative inhibition of platelet thromboxane production by low-dose aspirin in healthy subjects. *J. Clin. Invest.*, 69:1366–1372.
18. Patrignani, P., Catella, F., Filabozzi, P., Pugliese, F., Pierucci, A., Simonetti, B. M., Forni, L., Segni, M., and Patrono, C. (1984): Differential effects of OKY-046, a selective thromboxane-synthase inhibitor, on platelet and renal prostaglandin endoperoxide metabolism. *Clin. Res.* (Abstr.), 32:246A.
19. Patrignani, P., Filabozzi, P., Catella, F., Pugliese, F., and Patrono, C. (1984): Differential effects of dazoxiben, a selective thromboxane-synthase inhibitor, on platelet and renal prostaglandin-endoperoxide metabolism. *J. Pharmacol. Exp. Ther.*, 288:472–477.
20. Patrono, C., and Pugliese, F. (1980): The involvement of arachidonic acid metabolism in the control of renin release. *J. Endocrinol. Invest.*, 3:193–201.
21. Patrono, C., Wennmalm, Å., Ciabattoni, G., Nowak, J., Pugliese, F., and Cinotti, G. A. (1979): Evidence for an extra-renal origin of urinary prostaglandin E$_2$ in healthy men. *Prostaglandins*, 18:623–629.
22. Patrono, C., Pugliese, F., Ciabattoni, G., Patrignani, P., Maseri, A., Chierchia, S., Peskar, B. A., Cinotti, G. A., Simonetti, B. M., and Pierucci, A. (1982): Evidence for a direct stimulatory effect of prostacyclin on renin release in man. *J. Clin. Invest.*, 69:231–239.
23. Patrono, C., Ciabattoni, G., Patrignani, P., Filabozzi, P., Pinca, E., Satta, M. A., Van Dorne, D., Cinotti, G. A., Pugliese, F., Pierucci, A., and Simonetti, B. M. (1983): Evidence for a renal origin of urinary thromboxane B$_2$ in health and disease. In: *Advances in Prostaglandin, Thromboxane and Leukotriene Research*, edited by B. Samuelsson, R. Paoletti, and P. Ramwell, pp. 493–498. Raven Press, New York.
24. Pugliese, F., and Ciabattoni, G. (1983): Investigations of renal arachidonic acid metabolites by radioimmunoassay. In: *Prostaglandins and the Kidney. Biochemistry, Physiology, Pharmacology and Clinical Applications*, edited by M. J. Dunn, C. Patrono, and G. A. Cinotti, pp. 83–98. Plenum Press, New York.
25. Scharschmidt, L. A., Lianos, E., and Dunn, M. J. (1983): Arachidonate metabolites and the control of glomerular function. *Fed. Proc.*, 42:3058–3063.
26. Smith, W. L., and Bell, T. G. (1978): Immunohistochemical localization of the prostaglandin-forming cyclooxygenase in renal cortex. *Am. J. Physiol.*, 235:F451–F457.
27. Sraer, J., Ardaillou, N., Sraer, J.-D., and Ardaillou, R. (1982): *In vitro* prostaglandin synthesis by human glomeruli and papillae. *Prostaglandins*, 23:855–864.
28. Swartz, S. L., Williams, G. H., Hollenberg, N. K., Crantz, F. R., Moore, T. J., Levine, L., Sasahara, A. A., and Dluhy, R. G. (1980): Endocrine profile in the long-term phase of converting-enzyme inhibition. *Clin. Pharmacol. Ther.*, 28:499–508.
29. Weber, P. C., Scherer, B., and Larsson, C. (1977): Increase of free arachidonic acid by furosemide in man as the cause of prostaglandin and renin release. *Eur. J. Pharmacol.*, 41:329–332.
30. Wilson, T. W., Loadholt, C. B., Privitera, P. J., and Halushka, P. V. (1982): Furosemide increases urine 6-keto-prostaglandin F$_{1\alpha}$. Relation to natriuresis, vasodilation and renin release. *Hypertension*, 4:634–641.
31. Zipser, R., Kronborg, I., Rector, W., and Reynolds, T. (1984): Therapeutical trial of the thromboxane synthase inhibitor, dazoxiben, in the hepatorenal syndrome. *Clin. Res.* (Abstr.), 32:288A.

Advances in Prostaglandin, Thromboxane, and Leukotriene Research, Vol. 13, edited by G. G. Neri Serneri, et al. Raven Press, New York © 1985.

Effects of Indomethacin and Polyunsaturated Phosphatidylcholine on Short-Term Control of Renal Water Excretion

G. C. Agnoli, P. Andreone, M. Cacciari, C. Garutti, and E. Ikonomu

Cattedra di Fisiopatologia Medica, University of Bologna, 40138 Bologna, Italy

The biological action of prostaglandins (PG) on renal function *in vivo* has been studied by evaluating the functional effects of increment or decrement of PG production. However, precise deductions regarding mechanism of actions must be approached with caution (9).

In the present study we have estimated the effects of indomethacin or/and phosphatidylcholine (rich in linoleic acid) on the short-term control of diuresis.

The renal function has been investigated during steady hypotonic polyuria and during antidiuresis induced by *in bolo* injection of lysine-8-vasopressin (LVP). Urine PGE has been measured as index of renal medullary PG synthesis (3).

METHODS

Five voluntary healthy females (ranging in age from 20–40 years) have been studied in four different experimental conditions: (a) absence of treatment (TA); (b) after treatment with indomethacin (Merck Sharp & Dohme) (I), 2.5 mg/kg·day *per os* for the 2 days preceding study plus 100 mg i.m. 60 min prior to experiment; (c) after treatment with polyunsaturated phosphatidylcholine (EPL, Nattermann, containing 80% linoleic acid of total polyunsaturated fatty acids) (E), 13 mg/kg·day *per os* for the 2 days preceding study plus 300 mg 60 min prior to experiment; and (d) after treatment with both drugs (E + I) at the same doses previously mentioned.

In each experimental condition, hypotonic polyuria was induced by oral water load (20 mg/kg in 60 min) and was maintained by a 5% dextrose infusion. After a period of equilibration, three 30-min clearances (C, LVP_1, LVP_2) were carried out; LVP was injected *in bolo* (1.5 mU/kg) at the end of the C period. Urine and serum were analyzed for sodium and potassium concentrations (flame photometer), for endogenous creatinine concentration (7), and for total solutes concentration (Fiske osmometer). Urine flow rate was measured by bladder catheter. Clearances of endogenous creatinine, sodium, potassium, total solutes, and urine/plasma

(U/P) osmotic ratio were estimated by usual methods. Mean arterial pressure (MAP) has been evaluated by sphygmomanometer. Urine PGE was assayed by radioimmunoassay (RIA) using antiserum anti-PGE_2-1-BTG, which is indifferent to PGE_1 and PGE_2 (1); recovery of labeled PGE was about 65 to 70%.

RESULTS AND DISCUSSION

Hypotonic polyuria is shown in Fig. 1. As compared to TA condition, I treatment significantly decreases urinary PGE excretion, while E treatment fails to produce a significant increase. As compared to E condition, I treatment results in a greater number of differences in the renal functional parameters: (a) glomerular filtration rate (GFR), solutes, and sodium excretions tend to decline, and potassium excretion increases, although the differences do not attain statistical significance; and (b) urine flow rate decreases, and urine osmolarity and MAP increase. These effects are significantly different as compared to E condition. It is possible that these

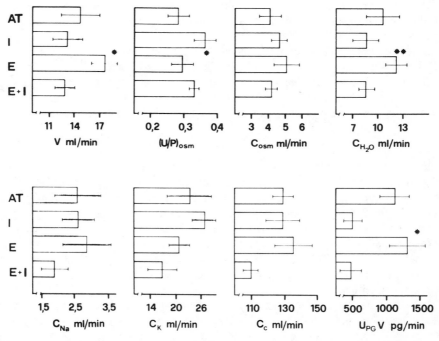

FIG. 1. Hypotonic polyuria in different experimental conditions: TA, absence of treatment; I, treatment with indomethacin; E, treatment with polyunsaturated phosphatidylcholine; E + I, treatment with both drugs. Values are mean ± SEM for each experimental condition. V, urinary flow rate; (U/P)$_{osm}$, urine/plasma osmotic ratio; C_{osm}, osmolar clearance; C_{H_2O}, free-water clearance; C_{Na}, sodium clearance; C_K, potassium clearance; C_c, endogenous creatinine clearance; $U_{PG}V$, urinary PGE excretion. The significant differences of E versus I values (paired t-test) are marked: $^*p < 0.05$; $^{**}p < 0.01$.

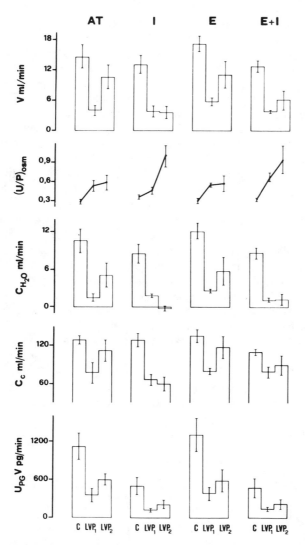

FIG. 2. Renal effects of lysine-vasopressin on hypotonic polyuria induced in different experimental conditions: AT, absence of treatment; I, treatment with indomethacin; E, treatment with polyunsaturated phosphatidylcholine; E + I, treatment with both drugs. See Fig. 1 for other abbreviations.

opposite functional patterns depend on a different availability of PGE at glomerular and medullary level.

In I condition, water reabsorption is improved: a possible explanation for this finding is that inhibition of PG synthesis by indomethacin enhances the effects of residual circulating vasopressin on the collecting tubule and increases NaCl reabsorption by the medullary thick ascending limb of Henle's loop with consequent increment of medullary solutes content (5,8).

Antidiuresis is shown in Fig. 2. In all our experimental conditions, LVP fails to increase PGE urinary excretion. PGE urinary concentration is directly related to urine flow rate; thus it is unlikely that LVP effects regression depends on enhanced PGE production induced by hormone. In all experimental conditions, LVP increases MAP while it reduces GFR and excretions of solutes, sodium, and potassium. (a) In TA, the lack of increment of the U/P ratio is probably attributable to medullary washout induced by maximal water diuresis (6), and by rapid degradation of hormone (*in bolo* infusion). The increment of MAP is not significant. The regress of LVP effects occurs during the interval of 30 to 60 min. (b) Indomethacin pretreatment (I) prolongs and intensifies the effects of LVP. In LVP_2 the decrease of GFR and the increment of water reabsorption are unchanged or further accentuated. The U/P ratio is greater than that observed in TA. It is conceivable that persistent action of hormone unmasks its effects on medullary interstitial osmolarity (2) in addition to those on water permeability of collecting tubule (9). The MAP is significantly higher. Because an increment of PGE production stimulated by LVP cannot be demonstrated, it seems possible that indomethacin prolongs its effects by enhancing, through a mechanism not dependent on PG, the intracellular events following the hormone–receptor binding (phosphodiesterase blocking?) (4). (c) In $E + I$, phosphatidylcholine is shown to depress the enhancement of LVP renal effects elicited by indomethacin. In LVP_1 the increment of MAP is not significant, and the decreases of GFR and of solutes and sodium excretions are attenuated. In LVP_2 a greater degree of recovery of GFR and a slight trend to prolong water saving occur; nevertheless the increment of the U/P ratio is not significantly different in these two experimental conditions. Since urinary PGE excretion does not significantly differ in $E + I$ compared to I, the hypothesis that prostaglandins mediate the effects of phosphatidylcholine cannot be supported.

REFERENCES

1. Andreone, P., Bolelli, G., Cacciari, M., Celani, M. F., Franceschetti, F., Garutti, C., and Salvini, M. (1981): Prostaglandine urinarie del gruppo E: Relazione tra la loro escrezione e flusso urinario rispettivamente in diuresi da carico idrico e in antidiuresi. *Bull. Sci. Med. (Bologna)*, CLIII(3/4):1–17.
2. Atherton, J. C., Green, R., and Thomas, S. (1971): Influence of lysine-vasopressin dosage on the course of changes in renal tissue and urinary composition in the conscious rat. *J. Physiol. (Lond.)*, 213:291–309.
3. Dunn, M. J., and Hood, V. L. (1977): Prostaglandins and the kidney. *Am. J. Physiol.*, 2:F169–F184.
4. Dunn, M. J., and Zambraski, E. J. (1980): Renal effects of drugs that inhibit prostaglandin synthesis. *Kidney Int.*, 18:609–622.
5. Kaojarern, S., Chennavasin, P., Anderson, S., and Brater, D. C. (1983): Nephron site of effect of nonsteroidal anti-inflammatory drugs on solute excretion in humans. *Am. J. Physiol.*, 244:F134–F139.
6. Levitin, H., Goodman, A., Pigeon, G., and Epstein, F. H. (1962): Composition of the renal medulla during water diuresis. *J. Clin. Invest.*, 41:1145–1151.
7. Steinitz, K., and Thürkand, H. (1940): The determination of the glomerular filtration rate by the endogenous creatinine clearance. *J. Clin. Invest.*, 19:285–298.

8. Stokes, J. B. (1979): Effect of prostaglandin E_2 on chloride transport across the rabbit thick ascending limb of Henle. Selective inhibition of the medullary portion. *J. Clin. Invest.*, 64:495–502.

9. Stokes, J. B. (1981): Integrated actions of renal medullary prostaglandins in the control of water excretion. *Am. J. Physiol.*, 240:F471–F480.

Advances in Prostaglandin, Thromboxane, and
Leukotriene Research, Vol. 13, edited by G. G. Neri
Serneri, et al. Raven Press, New York © 1985.

The Influence of Selective and Nonselective Prostaglandin Inhibition on Renin

R. Pedrinelli, A. Magagna, B. Abdel-Haq, and A. Salvetti

Clinica Medica I, University of Pisa, Pisa, Italy

The finding that sulindac, in contrast to indomethacin, does not inhibit renal prostaglandins (PGs) can offer the means to study the role of systemic and/or renal PGs in the control of renin. Therefore we studied, using a randomized cross-over design, the influence of treatment with sulindac and indomethacin on plasma renin activity (PRA) of essential hypertensive patients, which was measured either after standing or after chronic captopril and chlorthalidone administration.

In the captopril-treated group, serum thromboxane B_2 (TXB_2) and urinary 6-keto-$PGF_{1\alpha}$ were significantly reduced by indomethacin, while sulindac reduced only serum TXB_2. PRA was significantly reduced by indomethacin in the three groups and by sulindac only in standing and captopril-treated patients. These findings suggest that systemic PGs are mainly involved in the control of renin during standing and angiotensin-converting enzyme (ACE) inhibition, while mainly renal PGs play a role in the control of renin during chronic thiazide-like diuretic administration.

INTRODUCTION

It is now established that prostaglandins can stimulate renin release (6,7), and it is assumed that this role is mainly played by renal PGs. Recently it has been shown that sulindac is able to inhibit systemic, but not renal, PG synthesis, while indomethacin inhibits both (1,9). This finding can offer a way to study the role that systemic and/or renal prostaglandins can play in the control of renin secretion. On these bases we performed the following three studies.

MATERIAL AND METHODS

The first study was done on 6 hospitalized patients (2 males, 4 females, age range 32–56 years) with mild moderate uncomplicated essential hypertension who were on a diet of constant sodium (60–100 mmole/day) and potassium (60–80 mmole/day) content for all the period of the study. At the attainment of the equilibrium state the patients received both indomethacin (50 mg twice daily) for 1 day and sulindac (200 mg twice daily) for 7 days. The sequence of the treatment was randomized and 48 hr were allowed to pass between the two treatments. Blood pressure, heart rate, PRA, and plasma potassium (PlK$^+$) were measured before and at the end of each treatment with the patients in upright position for 1 hr, while urinary sodium excretion was measured daily.

In the second study, 11 out-patients (7 males, 4 females, age range 33–62 years) with mild moderate uncomplicated essential hypertension while on continued treatment (3–12 months) with captopril (50 mg twice daily) were randomly asked to take sulindac (200 mg twice daily) or indomethacin (50 mg twice daily) alone for 1 week and the reverse treatment after 2 weeks. Blood pressure, heart rate, body weight, plasma potassium, PRA, creatinine clearance, serum TXB$_2$, and urinary 6-keto-PGF$_{1\alpha}$ were measured the day before giving indomethacin and sulindac and at day 7 of treatment with these two drugs.

The third study was done in 10 out-patients (8 males, 2 females, age range 20–55 years) with mild moderate uncomplicated essential hypertension chronically (2–6 months) treated with chlorthalidone (25 mg/day), who followed the same protocol as that described for captopril. PRA (11), serum TXB$_2$ (5), and urinary 6-keto-PGF$_{1\alpha}$ (1) were measured by radioimmunoassay. Blood pressure was measured by mercury sphygmomanometer and heart rate by palpatory method for 30 sec after 15 min of recumbency, each value of these variables representing the mean of six determinations. Means and SEM were calculated according to standard methods, and the difference between mean values was obtained by paired Student's t-test.

RESULTS

In the first study, sulindac (SUL) and indomethacin (IND) did not significantly change mean blood pressure (mmHg) (B: 113.9 ± 4.7, SUL: 113 ± 4.3, IND: 115.1 ± 7.1), plasma potassium (mEq/l) (B: 4.2 ± 0.1, SUL: 4.1 ± 0.2, IND: 4.1 ± 0.2), and body weight (kg) (B: 68.7 ± 6, SUL: 68.7 ± 6, IND: 69.6 ± 7.2). Both drugs tended to reduce creatinine clearance (ml/min) (B: 115.2 ± 15.8, SUL: 108.8 ± 13.1, IND: 96.6 ± 11.6), although not to a significant extent, and sulindac reduced urinary sodium excretion in the first 2 to 3 days so that it caused a slight positive ($+ 25.1 \pm 32.8$ mEq/7 days) sodium balance. PRA (Fig. 1) was significantly reduced by both drugs.

In the second study (Table 1), while indomethacin significantly increased blood pressure, reduced creatinine clearance, and tended to increase plasma potassium, sulindac did not change these variables. Both drugs significantly reduced PRA and to the same extent PRA (Fig. 1). In 5 out of 11 patients, serum TXB$_2$ (ng/ml) (B: 269.5 ± 49.3, SUL: 13.6 ± 2.5, IND: 5.09 ± 1.24) was significantly ($p<0.001$) reduced and to the same extent (SUL: -95%, IND: -98.1%) by both drugs, while only indomethacin significantly ($p<0.001$) reduced urinary 6-keto-PGF$_{1\alpha}$ (ng/h) (B: 6.91 ± 3.2, SUL: 6.64 ± 1.26, IND: 3.21 ± 0.84; SUL: -3.7%, IND: 53.2%).

In the third study, blood pressure, creatinine clearance, plasma potassium, and body weight did not show any significant change, although indomethacin tended to

TABLE 1. *Behavior of mean blood pressure (MBP), creatinine clearance (CrCl), plasma potassium (PIK⁺), and body weight (BW) before (B) and after sulindac (SUL) and indomethacin (IND) administration in patients treated with captopril and chlorthalidone*[a]

Treatment	Time observed	MBP (mm Hg)	CrCl (ml/min)	PIK⁺ (mEq/l)	BW (kg)
Second study (captopril)	B	105.0 ± 2.5	129.1 ± 7.2	4.0 ± 0.1	76.0 ± 3.0
	SUL	107.9 ± 4.2	125.9 ± 9.4	4.0 ± 0.1	76.6 ± 2.9
	IND	$113.5 \pm 4.1^*$	$103.9 \pm 9.4^{**}$	4.2 ± 0.1	76.6 ± 2.9
Third study (chlorthalidone)	B	100.2 ± 2.2	106.2 ± 8.7	3.4 ± 0.1	75.6 ± 2.9
	SUL	102.1 ± 2.9	100.8 ± 9.3	3.6 ± 0.1	76.0 ± 2.9
	IND	105.7 ± 3.6	111.8 ± 12.9	3.9 ± 0.1	76.0 ± 2.9

[a]Mean and SEM are reported. The asterisks indicate the significance in comparison to basal values: $^*p < 0.02$; $^{**}p < 0.01$.

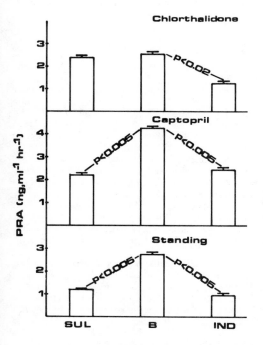

FIG. 1. Behavior of plasma renin activity (PRA) before (B) and after sulindac (SUL) and indomethacin (IND) administration in the three protocols.

increase blood pressure and plasma potassium (Table 1). PRA was significantly reduced only by indomethacin (Fig. 1).

DISCUSSION

In the present study we have indirectly evaluated the role of systemic and/or renal PGs in the control of renin, assuming that sulindac can inhibit only systemic but not renal PG synthesis while indomethacin inhibits both (1,9). Our findings in captopril-treated patients seem to confirm this hypothesis. We gave indomethacin and sulindac to patients whose renin had been stimulated by sympathetic nervous system (SNS) activation induced by standing and by chronic treatment with captopril and chlorthalidone, that is, in conditions in which PG synthesis seems to be activated (3,4,10). Thus, as expected (8), indomethacin was able to reduce PRA in the three groups of patients, but sulindac exerted the same effect in standing and in captopril-treated patients. We can reasonably assume that sulindac did not influence renin by acting on mechanisms unrelated to PG synthesis inhibition, since it did not cause any evident sodium retention, nor did it increase blood pressure and plasma potassium, well-known mechanisms through which renin can be reduced (2). To the extent that we can assume that sulindac is a selective inhibitor of PGs synthesis, we can hypothesize that systemic PGs are mainly involved in the control of renin release during SNS activation and ACE inhibition, while mainly renal PGs play a role in the control of renin during chronic thiazide-like diuretic administration.

REFERENCES

1. Ciabattoni, G., Pugliese, F., Cinotti, G. A., and Patrono, C. (1980): Renal effects of anti-inflammatory drugs. *Eur. J. Rheumatology*, 3:210–221.
2. Davis, J. O., and Freeman, A. H. (1976): Mechanisms regulating renin release. *Physiol. Rev.*, 56:1–56.
3. Lopez-Ovejero, J. A., Weber, M. A., Drayer, J. L. M., Sealey, J. E., and Laragh, J. H. (1978): Effects of indomethacin alone and during diuretic or β-adrenoreceptor-blockade therapy on blood pressure and the renin system in essential hypertension. *Clin. Sci. Mol. Med.*, 55:203s–205s.
4. Nadler, J., Zipser, R. D., and Horton, R. (1983): The effect of adrenergic stimulation on urinary prostaglandin E_2 and 6-keto-PGF_1 in man. *Prostaglandins*, 26(4):519–530.
5. Patrono, C. (1980): Radioimmunoassay of serum thromboxane B_2: A simple method to assess pharmacological effects on platelet function. *Adv. Prostaglandin Thromboxane Res.*, 6:187–195.
6. Patrono, C., Pugliese, F., Ciabattoni, G., Patrignani, P., Maseri, A., Chierchia, S., Peskar, B. A., Cinotti, G. A., Simonetti, B. M., and Pierucci, A. (1982): Evidence for a direct stimulatory effect of prostacyclin on renin release in man. *J. Clin. Invest.*, 69:231–239.
7. Salvetti, A., Pedrinelli, R., Sassano, P., Arzilli, F., and Turini, F. (1982): Effects of prostaglandins inhibition on changes in active and inactive renin induced by antihypertensive drugs. *Clin. Exp. Hypertension Theory Pract.*, A4:2435–2448.
8. Salvetti, A., and Pedrinelli, R. (1982): Pharmacological evaluation of prostaglandins and their interaction with renin secretion in human hypertension. In: *Endocrinology of Hypertension*, edited by F. Mantero, F. G. Biglieri, and C. R. W. Edwards, pp. 243–256. Academic Press, London.
9. Salvetti, A., Pedrinelli, R., Magagna, A., and Ugenti, P. (1982): Differential effects of selective and nonselective prostaglandin-synthesis inhibition on the pharmacological responses to captopril in patients with essential hypertension. *Clin. Sci.*, 63:261s–263s.
10. Swartz, S. L., William, G. H., Hollemberg, H. K., Cranz, F. R., Levine, L., Moore, T. J., and Dluhy, R. G. (1980): Increase in prostaglandins during converting enzyme inhibition. *Clin. Sci.*, 59(suppl. 6):133s–135s.
11. Zucchelli, G. C., Malvano, R., and Salvetti, A. (1973): Control of the enzyme system in plasma renin activity measurement by angiotensin 1 radioimmunoassay. *J. Nucl. Biol. Med.*, 17:187–195.

Advances in Prostaglandin, Thromboxane, and
Leukotriene Research, Vol. 13, edited by G. G. Neri
Serneri, et al. Raven Press, New York © 1985.

Mechanisms of Arterial Hypertension: Role of Neural Control of Renal Functions

Alberto Zanchetti, Andrea Stella, and Raffaello Golin

*Istituto di Clinica Medica IV, University of Milan, and Centro di Fisiologia Clinica e
Ipertensione, Ospedale Maggiore, Milan, Italy*

The role of any mechanism that may be involved in a complex disease of regulation such as arterial hypertension has long been the subject of discussion and controversy. It would be impossible to summarize all the aspects of the various controversies in this short review. Attention has been concentrated mostly on the role of the sympathetic nervous system and of neural mechanisms in the pathogenesis and maintenance of high blood pressure. There is also a large body of evidence that neural and renal influences can interact, and it is to these interactions and especially to neural influences on renal function that this review is addressed.

There is evidence that the three main sets of renal functions are under sympathetic control: the vasomotor function; the secretion of renin; and tubular reabsorption of sodium and water.

NEURAL CONTROL OF RENAL CIRCULATION

That the renal vasculature, and particularly preglomerular resistance vessels, can be constricted by sympathetic fibers has long been known, but more recently important evidence has been added that marked alterations in renal circulation accompany spontaneous behavioral changes in conscious animals (15,16,26). During a brief emotional confrontation, vasoconstriction is observed in an innervated kidney only, whereas on more prolonged or intense fighting a delayed vasoconstriction, probably mediated through circulating catecholamines, also occurs in the contralateral denervated kidney (16). On the other hand, approximately the same degree of vasodilatation occurs in an innervated and a denervated kidney during sleep, probably as the expression of a transient decrease in vasomotor activity on the innervated side and as the expression of vasodilator autoregulation to the fall in blood pressure in the denervated side (16).

Sympathetic influences on renal circulation have been shown to be controlled by reflex by both sinoaortic and vagal receptors. The vagally innervated receptors in the low-pressure area in the heart and lungs responsive to changes in blood volume are those exerting the most important reflex influence on the kidney vasculature, whereas other vascular beds, e.g., that in skeletal muscles, are under a predominant control from the sino–aortic areas (19).

NEURAL CONTROL OF RENIN RELEASE

In the last few years evidence has accumulated that renal secretion of renin is also under a sympathetic excitatory influence directly exerted on juxtaglomerular cells and mediated through beta-adrenoreceptors (30,31). Figure 1 summarizes some work of our group (22). Electrical stimulation of the vasomotor center in the pons and medulla produces a sharp increase in renin release and a fall in renal blood flow to the innervated kidney, whereas no change in renin release and a slight passive increase in blood flow occur in the contralateral denervated kidney. Dissociation of vasomotor and renin-releasing effects of brainstem stimulation was obtained either by intrarenal artery infusion of the alpha-adrenergic blocker, phenoxybenzamine (which abolished vasoconstriction but left renin release intact), or by intravenous propranolol (which abolished the renin releasing effect but left the vasoconstrictive response intact).

Further evidence for a direct sympathetic action on juxtaglomerular cells independent of vascular and macula densa receptors comes from experiments in non-filtering and papaverine-treated kidneys (5) and by low-frequency stimulation of renal nerves (25). This beta-receptor-mediated stimulation of renin release appears to be largely independent of renal prostaglandins (13).

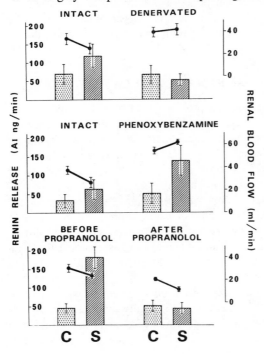

FIG. 1. Effect of electrical stimulation of the vasomotor center in the brainstem. Mean values ± SEM are shown for renin release *(histograms and bars, left ordinates)* and for renal blood flow *(filled circles, right ordinates)*. C, control; S, after a 5-min stimulation period. AI, angiotensin I. (From Richardson et al., ref. 22.)

Sympathetic control of renin release has also been shown to be under a powerful reflex control, mostly from low-pressure cardiopulmonary receptor afferents running in the vagi. This conclusion has been drawn from experiments we have performed in the anesthetized cat, using tilting head-up as an experimental model. Tilting head-up seems to release renin solely through reflex sympathetic activation, as increased secretion occurs only from the innervated kidney, whereas on the denervated side there is no releasing effect (23). Section of cardiopulmonary afferents by vagotomy does not disturb pressure homeostasis but prevents reflex activation of juxtaglomerular cells: after vagotomy, innervated and denervated kidneys both have a similarly mild increase in renin during tilting (4). On the other hand, after sino–aortic denervation, cardiovascular adjustment to tilting is conspicuously impaired and blood pressure markedly falls in the upright posture. In this condition, the increment of renin release from the innervated kidney is not impaired, but is rather augmented. The response, however, does not appear to be mediated through the vagi, as it is maintained after combined sino–aortic denervation and vagotomy. It is likely to be due to stimulation of intrarenal mechanisms by the conspicuous fall in renal perfusion pressure. The observation that only the innervated kidney responds with an increment in renin release, even when tilting is associated with a large hypotension, confirms that only innervated juxtaglomerular cells can promptly and markedly respond to reduction in perfusion pressure (4).

We have also evidence in humans about the possible role of various reflex mechanisms in modulating renin release. Both stimulation and deactivation of carotid sinus reflexes by means of a variable pressure neck chamber caused only minor decreases and increases in renin release (17). On the other hand, recent experiments by our group (11) showed that stimulation or deactivation of low-pressure cardiopulmonary receptors by leg raising or lower body suction could clearly affect renin release.

NEURAL CONTROL OF RENAL TUBULAR REABSORPTION

A sympathetic influence facilitating tubular reabsorption of sodium and water has also been identified (10). Denervation of one kidney results in the well-known phenomenon of denervation diuresis and natriuresis, a phenomenon that, in micropuncture experiments, has been shown not to be accompanied by changes in single nephron glomerular filtration rate and to be due to removal of an influence exerted on proximal tubule reabsorption. Di Bona's group has induced a reduction in natriuresis by low-voltage, low-frequency stimulation of renal nerves, and has also shown that this antinatriuretic action of renal sympathetic innervation is independent of angiotensin and prostaglandins (7).

Little is known of a possible reflex control of the sympathetic influence on tubular reabsorption of sodium and water. It is reasonable to expect that this sympathetic renal influence is also regulated by cardiopulmonary low-pressure receptors, but it is particularly difficult to unravel the effects that low-pressure receptors may directly exert on tubular reabsorption from indirect effects exerted through control of vasomotor phenomena and renin release. Recent evidence, however, suggests that a direct neural facilitation of tubular reabsorption may be reflexly released during the first few minutes of tilting (8).

RENO–RENAL REFLEXES

For all renal functions, but particularly for tubular reabsorption, the existence has been suggested of reno–renal reflexes, i.e., of mechanisms by which renal functions are self-controlled or one kidney controls the other one (3,6). These might be particularly useful mechanisms in the fine regulation of the kidney, but although reno–renal reflexes have been suggested for some time, crucial proof of their existence has been obtained only recently.

There is evidence of the existence of both mechanoreceptors and chemoreceptors in the kidney. Mechanoreceptors can be excited mostly by increasing pressure in the renal vein or ureter. My colleague Recordati and his group have recently produced evidence of other renal receptors that can be considered to convey information on chemical rather than mechanical, intrarenal events. Two groups of renal chemoreceptors were identified and termed R1 and R2 chemoreceptors (21). Furthermore, their stimulation by backflow or by renal ischemia was shown to increase electrical activity in ipsilateral and contralateral efferent renal nerve fibers (20), thus substantiating the existence of reno–renal reflexes.

Electrophysiological techniques have a well-known limitation, however: they cannot indicate the renal functions on which the reflex influence is exerted. We have therefore resorted to stimulation and denervation experiments. The stimulation experiments have failed to give evidence of either excitatory or inhibitory reno–renal reflexes (2,23a), whereas the denervation approach has been remarkably successful.

To obtain more definite information on the existence and the significance of reno–renal reflexes, we have developed a model of reversible and hence repeatable renal denervation, under which renal functions are monitored separately from the two kidneys of an anesthetized cat while conduction in one renal nerve is temporarily blocked by cooling through a local thermode (9). Renal nerve cooling did not cause any change in arterial pressure. A slight increase in blood flow, no change in glomerular filtration rate, and a large increase in water and sodium excretion occurred in the ipsilateral kidney; simultaneously, no change in blood flow, a slight and transient decrease in glomerular filtration rate, and a significant decrease in diuresis and natriuresis were observed in the contralateral kidney. Ipsilateral and contralateral renal changes were equally evident in the early (min 0–8) and late (min 8–16) phases of the cooling period. Finally, when renal nerve cooling was repeated after surgical denervation of the contralateral kidney, all contralateral effects were abolished (9).

In a more recent series of investigations, we have sought to obtain further and more direct evidence of these reno–renal reflexes by selective interruption of the afferent fibers responsible for the reflex. Afferent fibers present in the renal nerves are spinal afferents, which are known to enter the spinal cord through the dorsal roots T9 to L4, and can be interrupted by cutting these dorsal roots. In these recent experiments (24), separate renal functions were measured during transient cooling of the left renal nerve in cats in which central connections of the left renal nerve had been left intact (sham operated) and in cats in which they had been interrupted by cutting dorsal roots T9 to L4. Left renal nerve cooling induced the usual decrease in sodium and water excretion from the contralateral (right) kidney in animals with intact dorsal roots; the contralateral response was still present and substantially unchanged in animals in which the ipsilateral (left) dorsal roots T9 to L4 had been cut, but the response was entirely abolished when dorsal roots were sectioned bilaterally. This suggests that afferent renal nerve fibers project bilaterally, rather than unilaterally, to the spinal cord.

By showing that the integrity of afferent renal nerve fibers is necessary, our data provide the missing evidence that a reno–renal reflex mediates the effects of renal denervation on the contralateral kidney. Furthermore, as contralateral changes in glomerular filtration rate and blood flow, and changes in arterial pressure are negligible when cooling of one renal nerve induces contralateral antidiuresis, it is likely that the sympathetic activity involved in these reno–renal reflexes is that controlling proximal tubular reabsorption of sodium and water.

In conclusion, reno–renal reflexes seem definitely to exist. The one we have described consists of a tonic inhibition of contralateral sympathetic activity controlling tubular reabsorption of sodium and water, and renin release. This tonic inhibition does not involve blood pressure, renal blood flow, and glomerular filtration rate. However, we do not know the receptors from which this inhibitory input originates, and the nature and the role of this reno–renal reflex still remain to be elucidated. We also have electrophysiological evidence of an opposite, excitatory, reno–renal reflex, originating from Recordati's chemoreceptors (20), but we ignore the renal functions on which it is exerted. We also ignore the possible interactions between these two types of reflexes.

DOES NEURAL CONTROL OF THE KIDNEY PLAY A ROLE IN HYPERTENSION?

There are several lines of evidence suggesting that the various mechanisms by which the sympathetic nervous system influences various renal functions may play a role in hypertension, either in participating in the processes leading to high blood pressure or in maintaining abnormally elevated blood pressure.

Figure 2 summarizes the numerous levels at which angiotensin II can stimulate the sympathetic nervous system (29). As sympathetic activity can release renin and consequently increment angiotensin II generation, the interactions between the sympathetic and the renin–angiotensin systems have the characteristics of a positive feedback system, i.e., of a mechanism suitable to cause and to maintain a rise in blood pressure. That the role of these interactions may be really important is suggested by the recent clinical experience with angiotensin-converting-enzyme

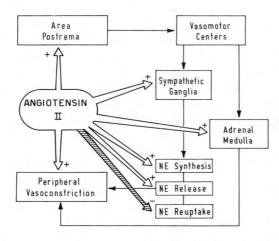

FIG. 2. Summary of the actions of angiotensin II on the sympathetic nervous system. NE, norepinephrine. (From Zanchetti and Bartorelli, ref. 29.)

inhibitors, the blood-pressure lowering effect of which is not limited to hypertensive patients with high renin. Recent observations of ours (18) have shown that captopril alters the carotid sinus baroreflex in human hypertension in such a way as to emphasize the pressor and tachycardic response to baroreceptor deactivation. This suggests that captopril might remove a tonic inhibitory influence exerted by physiological levels of angiotensin II on the baroreflex.

In support of a role of renal innervation in hypertension, there are also a number of observations showing that several experimental models of hypertension are delayed in onset or moderated in severity by previous renal denervation (14,27).

This conception of neural and renal interactions in the pathogenesis of arterial hypertension must be considered in face of the classical hypothesis elaborated by Guyton and co-workers (12) that hypertension can only result from a primary alteration of the kidney's ability to excrete sodium, that is, of the so-called pressure–natriuresis curve. This physiological relationship is normally so steep that even a small increase in arterial pressure causes a very great increase in sodium excretion, and this promptly and entirely corrects the rise in pressure. This is the reason why Guyton defines the kidney as a pressure-regulating mechanism with infinite gain and claims that any nonrenal factor, neural factors included, can increase blood pressure only transiently, as pressure natriuresis would promptly nullify the initial rise in pressure. On the other hand, an alteration of the function of the kidney would cause sodium retention and lead to a permanent increase in pressure through a chain of events including as a primary hemodynamic change an increase in extracellular fluid volume, in plasma volume, and in cardiac output.

There are very important points in Guyton's conception of the key role of pressure natriuresis in hypertension, but the main limitation is represented by the fact that extracellular fluid volume and plasma volume, which are regularly increased in primary aldosteronism, are generally found to be slightly decreased, rather than increased, in essential hypertension (1).

We think that, without disputing the possibility that the pressure-natriuresis curve has indeed a key role in hypertension, this key role can be interpreted in two different ways. In Fig. 3 (left), the curve is shifted to the right and/or its slope depressed by a primary disturbance of renal sodium excretion or by some agent acting only on renal sodium excretion; as a consequence, there will be a transient phase of sodium retention and volume expansion, lasting until the consequent blood pressure increase will bring sodium excretion back to equilibrium. This is the mechanism that can easily explain hypertension in renal insufficiency and in primary aldosteronism.

In Fig. 3 (right), a primary pressor agent may both increase arterial pressure by means of diffuse vasoconstriction and simultaneously shift to the right and/or depress the renal excretion curve, thus preventing the primary blood pressure increase from being corrected by a large pressure natriuresis. This interpretation does not imply any phase—even a transient one—in which hypertension is accompanied by volume increase; the readjustment of renal function is only instrumental in preventing too great a reduction in plasma and extracellular fluid volume. This is what seems to occur in pheochromocytoma with continuous hypertension, in which volume contraction is a well known characteristic; it may also be what occurs in essential hypertension, in which volumes are also decreased, although to a much smaller extent.

Figure 4 summarizes a hypothetical sequence of physiological events leading to raised blood pressure (28). It is conceivable that sympathetic activity may be primarily increased either centrally or by reflex, through a primary resetting of negative feedback reflexes as sino-aortic baroreflexes. Sympathetic activity by augmenting cardiac output and arteriolar resistance can reproduce the hemodynamic pattern characterizing essential hypertension, either borderline or established hypertension. Maintenance of sympathetic activity in spite of the increased blood pressure will be assured by further resetting of depressor reflexes, while pressure natriuresis will be reduced through the various mechanisms of sympathetic control

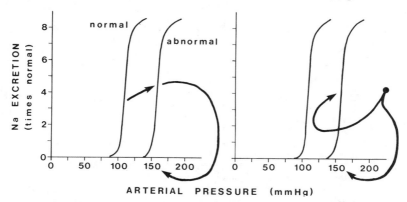

FIG. 3. Resetting of pressure–natriuresis curve. **Left:** By a primary intrinsic renal abnormality. **Right:** By a primary extrarenal pressor system.

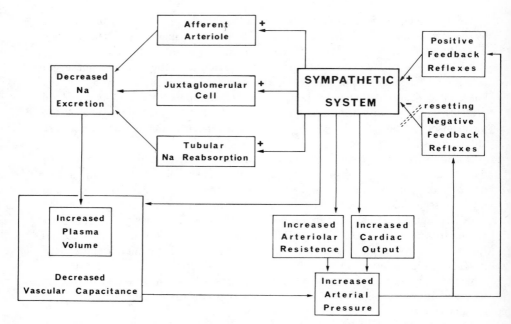

FIG. 4. Role of sympathetic system, cardiovascular reflexes, and sympathetic control of renal function in hypertension. (From Zanchetti, ref. 29.)

of renal function. Eventually, as vascular hypertrophy develops, the participation of sympathetic activity in sustaining the hypertension might become less necessary.

This is, of course, just one of the many possible sequences of events that could lead to elevated blood pressure, and involve central and reflex sympathetic activity, the kidney, the heart, and the vascular smooth muscle. Genetic factors play an important role in determining arterial pressure levels, but we still must learn at which level these factors intervene; if inheritance of blood pressure is polygenic, several functions may well be involved simultaneously or differently in different individuals. It remains to be more firmly established whether sympathetic activity and its reflex influences on the cardiovascular system are inherited and to what degree.

REFERENCES

1. Beretta-Piccoli, C., Davies, D. L., Boddy, K., Brown, J. J., Cumming, A. M. M., East, B. W., Fraser, R., Lever, A. F., Padfield, P. L., Semple, P. F., Robertson, J. I. S., Weidmann, P., and Williams, E. D. (1982): Relation of arterial pressure with body sodium, body potassium and plasma potassium in essential hypertension. *Clin. Sci.*, 63:257–270.
2. Calaresu, F. R., Stella, A., and Zanchetti, A. (1976): Hemodynamic responses and renin release during stimulation of afferent renal nerves in the cat. *J. Physiol. (Lond.)*, 255:687–700.
3. Colindres, R. E., Spielman, W. S., Moss, N. G., Harrington, W. W., and Gottschalk, C. W. (1980): Functional evidence for reno-renal reflexes in the rat. *Am. J. Physiol.*, 239:F265–F270.
4. Dampney, R. A. L., Stella, A., Golin, R., and Zanchetti, A. (1979): Vagal and sinoaortic reflexes in postural control of circulation and renin release. *Am. J. Physiol.*, 237:H146–H152.

5. Davis, J. O., and Freeman, R. H. (1976): Mechanisms regulating renin release. *Physiol. Rev.*, 56:1–56.
6. Di Bona, G. F., and Rios, L. L. (1980): Renal nerves in compensatory renal response to contralateral renal denervation. *Am. J. Physiol.*, 238:F26–F30.
7. Di Bona, G. F., Zambraski, E. J., Aguilera, A. J., and Kalayanides, G. J. (1977): Neurogenic control of renal tubular reabsorption in the dog. *Circ. Res.*, 40(suppl. I):I-127–I-130.
8. Golin, R., Stella, A., Genovesi, S., and Zanchetti, A. (1983): Role of renal nerves in mediating the renal response to tilting. *J. Hypertension*, 1(suppl. II):210–211.
9. Golin, R., Stella, A., and Zanchetti, A. (1982): Reversible renal nerve denervation in the cat: Effects on hemodynamic and excretory functions of the ipsilateral and contralateral kidneys. *Clin. Sci.*, 63:215s–217s.
10. Gottschalk, C. W. (1979): Renal nerves and sodium excretion. *Ann. Rev. Physiol.*, 41:229–240.
11. Grassi, G., Gavazzi, C., Ramirez, A., Sabadini, E., Turolo, L., and Mancia, G. (1984): Role of cardiopulmonary receptors in reflex control of renin release in man. *Abstr. 10th Annual Meeting Int. Soc. Hypertension*, Interlaken.
12. Guyton, A. C., Coleman, T. G., Cowley, A. W., Manning, R. D., Norman, R. A., and Ferguson, J. D. (1974): A systems analysis approach to understanding long-range arterial blood pressure control and hypertension. *Circ. Res.*, 35:159–176.
13. Henrich, W. L. (1981): Role of prostaglandins in renin secretion. *Kidney Int.*, 19:822–830.
14. Katholi, R. E., Whitlow, P. L., Winternitz, S. R., and Oparil, S. (1982): Importance of the renal nerves in established two-kidney, one clip Goldblatt hypertension. *Hypertension*, 4(suppl. II):II-166–II-174.
15. Kirchheim, H. (1969): Effect of common carotid occlusion on arterial blood pressure and on kidney blood flow in unanesthetized dogs. *Arch. Gesamte Physiol.*, 306:119–134.
16. Mancia, G., Baccelli, G., and Zanchetti, A. (1974): Regulation of renal circulation during behavior in the cat. *Am. J. Physiol.*, 227:536–542.
17. Mancia, G., Leonetti, G., Terzoli, L., and Zanchetti, A. (1978): Reflex control of renin release in essential hypertension. *Clin. Sci.*, 54:217–222.
18. Mancia, G., Parati, G., Pomidossi, G., Grassi, G., Bertinieri, G., Buccino, N., Ferrari, A., Gregorini, L., Rupoli, L., and Zanchetti, A. (1982): Modification of arterial baroreflexes by captopril in essential hypertension. *Am. J. Cardiol.*, 49:1415–1419.
19. Mancia, G., Shepherd, J. T., and Donald, D. E. (1975): Role of cardiac, pulmonary and carotid mechanoreceptors in the control of hindlimb and renal circulation in the dog. *Circ. Res.*, 37:200–208.
20. Recordati, G., Genovesi, S., and Cerati, D. (1982): Renorenal reflexes in the rat elicited upon stimulation of renal chemoreceptors. *J. Autonomous Nerv. Syst.*, 6:127–142.
21. Recordati, G., Moss, N. G., Genovesi, S., and Rogenes, P. (1981): Renal chemoreceptors. *J. Autonomous Nerv. Syst.*, 3:237–251.
22. Richardson, D., Stella, A., Leonetti, G., Bartorelli, A., and Zanchetti, A. (1974): Mechanisms of renal release of renin by electrical stimulation of the brainstem in the cat. *Circ. Res.*, 34:425–434.
23. Stella, A., and Zanchetti, A. (1977): Effects of renal denervation on renin release in response to tilting and furosemide. *Am. J. Physiol.*, 232:H500–H507.
23a. Stella, A., Golin, R., Busnardo, I., and Zanchetti, A. (1984): Effects of afferent renal nerve stimulation on renal hemodynamic and excretory function. *Am. J. Physiol.*, 247:H576–H583.
24. Stella, A., Golin, R., Genovesi, S., and Zanchetti, A. (1983): Do renal afferent fibres modulate the function of the contralateral kidney? *J. Hypertension*, 1(suppl. II):66–67.
25. Taher, M. S., McLain, L. G., McDonald, K. M., and Schrier, R. W. (1976): Effect of beta-adrenergic blockade on renin response to renal nerve stimulation. *J. Clin. Invest.*, 57:459–465.
26. Vatner, S. F. (1978): Effect of exercise and excitement on mesenteric and renal dynamics in conscious, unrestrained baboons. *Am. J. Physiol.*, 234:H210–H214.
27. Winternitz, S. R., Katholi, R. E., and Oparil, S. (1980): Role of the renal sympathetic nerves in the development and maintenance of hypertension in the spontaneous hypertensive rat. *J. Clin. Invest.*, 66:971–978.
28. Zanchetti, A. (1979): Overview of cardiovascular reflexes in hypertension. *Am. J. Cardiol.*, 44:912–918.
29. Zanchetti, A., and Bartorelli, C. (1977): Central nervous mechanisms in arterial hypertension:

experimental and clinical evidence. In: *Hypertension*, edited by J. Genest, E. Koiw, and O. Kuchel, pp. 59–76. McGraw-Hill, New York.

30. Zanchetti, A., and Stella, A. (1975): Neural control of renin release. *Clin. Sci. Mol. Med.*, 48:215s–233s.

31. Zanchetti, A., Stella, A., Leonetti, G., Morganti, A., and Terzoli, L. (1980): Control of renin release: Experimental evidence and clinical implications. In: *Topics in Hypertension*, edited by J. H. Laragh, pp. 122–158. Yorke Medical Books, New York.

Advances in Prostaglandin, Thromboxane, and
Leukotriene Research, Vol. 13, edited by G.G. Neri
Serneri, et al. Raven Press, New York © 1985.

Renal Prostaglandins and Hypertension

*John C. McGiff, *Michal Schwartzman, and
**Nicholas R. Ferreri

*Department of Pharmacology, New York Medical College, Valhalla, New York 10595; and
**Department of Molecular Immunology, Scripps Clinic & Research Foundation,
La Jolla, California 92037

Renal prostaglandin (PG)-dependent mechanisms participate in the regulation of blood pressure by: (a) modulating the action of vasoactive agents including ADH, angiotensin II, neurotransmitters and kinins; (b) regulating tubular function at critical sites in the nephron involved in the control of extracellular fluid volume, such as the thick ascending limb of the loop of Henle (TALH) and the collecting ducts; and (c) contributing to the control of renin and kallikrein release.

PROSTAGLANDINS MODULATE THE VASCULAR ACTIONS OF PEPTIDES AND ADRENERGIC NERVOUS ACTIVITY

Prostacyclin (PGI_2), having been discovered in blood vessels, has been assumed to be the principal product of enzymatic transformation of the cyclic endoperoxides PGG_2 and PGH_2 in all vascular elements (16). Prostaglandin-dependent mechanisms within blood vessels are usually considered to be mediated by prostacyclin (3); other prostaglandins identified in vascular tissues are thought to be less important. However, several findings preclude the unqualified acceptance of prostacyclin as the only important vascular prostaglandin.

1. In some blood vessels there is evidence that prostacyclin is not the principal product of enzymatic transformation of the cyclic endoperoxides (24). Further, in the microcirculation of the heart (7) and brain (6), the principal products of cyclooxygenase have been reported to be PGE_2 and PGD_2, respectively.

2. PGE_2, which is also synthesized in the vascular wall (22), may be the principal modulator prostaglandin affecting the vascular actions of peptides and neurotransmitters. For example, PGI_2, unlike PGE_2, did not inhibit the effects of angiotensin II on the microcirculation, rather potentiation occurred (15). This finding challenges the proposed modulator role for PGI_2 in the vasculature.

3. Prostacyclin may be transformed by some tissues to a more stable product, 6-keto-PGE_1, having similar biological activity (14,27). In addition, rapid termination of the action of prostacyclin can occur as it can be rapidly metabolized by

15-hydroxyprostaglandin dehydrogenase (28), an enzyme having high activity in blood vessels.

In 1969, Weiner and Kaley (26) advanced the hypothesis that prostaglandins are local regulators of the circulation through their direct vasodilator effects and their ability to antagonize the vascular actions of pressor hormones. Prostaglandins of the E series were shown to dilate the rat mesenteric vasculature and to inhibit the vasoconstrictor effects of diverse stimuli, peptides as well as catecholamines. Further, this capacity to antagonize pressor hormone-induced vasoconstriction was independent of the vasodilator effect of the prostaglandin, as the antagonism lasted well beyond the waning of the direct vascular action. PGE_2 has been shown to attenuate the vasoconstrictor response to adrenergic nerve stimulation in the rabbit isolated kidney at a concentration 200-fold less than the concentration that dilates this vascular bed (12). This concentration of PGE_2, 20 pg/ml, is likely to be realized intrarenally, as levels of PGE_2 in renal venous blood and urine, which reflect tissue levels intrarenally, are usually well above this concentration. Indeed, as much as a 100-fold increase in PGE_2 levels in renal venous blood occurred in response to infusion of norepinephrine into the renal artery of the dog (13). These peak levels occurred coincidentally with recovery of depressed renal blood flow despite continued infusion of norepinephrine. $PGF_{2\alpha}$ concentrations measured simultaneously in renal venous blood were unaffected. The importance of renal prostaglandin release to attenuation of the vasoconstriction of pressor hormones was evident after inhibition of cyclooxygenase (1). After indomethacin administration, potentiation of the renal vasoconstrictor action of the pressor agent occurred as prostaglandin release was inhibited.

When prostaglandins were called forth by an appropriate stimulus such as norepinephrine, prostaglandins were released within seconds—peak levels occurred within 60 to 90 sec, representing increases of as much as several hundredfold (4) (Fig. 1). The decline from peak values was equally rapid, falling to control levels within several minutes after bolus injections of norepinephrine. Renal perfusion pressure and prostaglandin release showed a dose-dependent response to norepinephrine. It is of interest to note that in the isolated kidney of the rat, the principal prostaglandin released was PGE_2, which exceeded the levels of $PGF_{2\alpha}$ and PGI_2, the latter measured as the hydrolysis product, 6-keto-$PGF_{1\alpha}$, by a factor of five- to tenfold.

Compartmentalization of prostaglandins within the kidney became evident when the efflux of prostaglandins into the separate urinary and venous effluents was measured during infusion of a vasoactive agent into the renal artery (4). Thus, infusion of bradykinin into the rabbit isolated kidney caused a surge of PGE_2 into the urinary effluent, whereas 6-keto-$PGF_{1\alpha}$ was the principal product exiting in the venous effluent. Selective release of a prostaglandin should not be surprising, as structures within the kidney differ greatly in their capacity to generate prostaglandins as well as differing in the profile of arachidonic acid products that they synthesize. Variations in the profile of prostaglandins among renal structures is

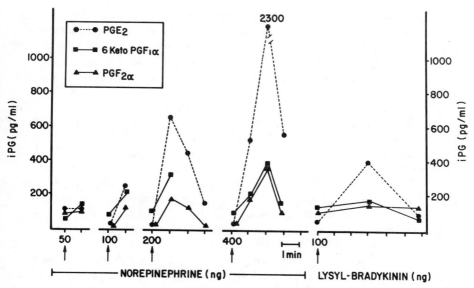

FIG. 1. Release of immunoreactive prostaglandins (iPG) from the rat isolated kidney induced by norepinephrine and lysyl-bradykinin. (From Samuelsson et al., ref. 18.)

evident when comparing the prostaglandin-synthesizing capacity of the renal tubules with both large and small renal arterial elements (23). The principal product of all of the arterial elements both large and small, at least up to the interlobular arteries, is PGI_2, although significant amounts of PGE_2 and $PGF_{2\alpha}$ are also formed. Convoluted tubules, on the other hand, have a low capacity to generate prostaglandins, and even this is suspect as it may result from contamination of the tubules with adherent small blood vessels. These data should not lead one to conclude that the renal microcirculation and veins demonstrate the same capacity to generate PGI_2 as arterial elements. For example, the coronary microcirculation exhibits a different profile of prostaglandins than those of the larger arteries of the same vascular bed (7).

It is also possible to distinguish regional variations in prostaglandin synthesis using slices of renal cortex and medulla. Medullary slices demonstrate a greater capacity to transform added arachidonic acid to prostaglandins, chiefly PGE_2 and $PGF_{2\alpha}$, whereas cortical slices show a much lesser capacity and produce primarily PGI_2 (23).

ARACHIDONIC ACID METABOLISM IN THE NEPHRON

In addition to differences in the profile of eicosanoids generated by zones and structures within the kidney, prostaglandin-synthesizing capacity varies longitudinally within the nephron (19). Thus, as noted, the convoluted tubules demonstrated a low capacity in contrast to the collecting ducts, which had a high density of cyclooxygenase. This study was based on immunohistofluorescence techniques for detecting cyclooxygenase. Of particular note was the reduced cyclooxygenase antigenicity in the TALH, suggesting low prostaglandin-forming capacity in this portion of the nephron. This region has been identified, at least in the medulla, as a principal site of the inhibitory action of PGE_2 on sodium chloride absorption (21).

Because of the importance of prostaglandin-dependent mechanisms to renal function and the heterogeneous nature of the nephron with respect to ion transport and hormonal responsiveness, we deemed it important to associate the pattern of arachidonic acid metabolism with specific cells within the nephron (5). The thick ascending limb was of particular concern because of its importance to the regulation of extracellular fluid volume, as well as containing the principal target cells for the most potent diuretics, the loop diuretics: furosemide, ethacrynic acid, and bumetanide (10). We studied arachidonic acid metabolism in a cell suspension containing principally cells of the TALH, obtained from the excised inner stripe of the outer medulla of the rabbit kidney. Based on comparison of specific activities of enzymes before and after separation—alkaline phosphatase, Na^+,K^+-ATPase, as well as Tamm–Horsfall glycoprotein and electron microscopic appearance—80% of these cells were estimated to be TALH in origin. We also found that TALH cells had low cyclooxygenase activity. However, TALH cells selectively converted exogenous arachidonic acid to oxygenated metabolites by cytochrome P-450-related mechanisms. Arachidonic acid metabolites were produced in large quantities, representing 30 to 40% conversion of [^{14}C]arachidonic acid, that is, 1 to 5 μg/mg protein·hr, and were increased fivefold after separation of TALH cells from a suspension of outer medullary cells (5). Preliminary gas chromatographic–mass spectroscopic analysis indicated that one of the metabolites was an epoxide of arachidonic acid with three unconjugated double bonds.

What has this to do with the regulation of blood pressure? Jacobson et al. (9) have recently reported that the same or a similar compound, also an epoxide, when injected into perfused rabbit cortical collecting tubules was able to inhibit sodium transport. The potential significance of our study is that one or more of the arachidonic acid metabolites arising from the cytochrome P-450 dependent-pathway in the TALH plays a vital role in the regulation of salt and water transport and, thereby, extracellular fluid volume. Moreover, preliminary observations indicate that one or more of the oxygenated arachidonic acid metabolites recovered from TALH cells was capable of inhibiting Na^+,K^+-ATPase activity and might be the link that relates changes in Na^+,K^+-ATPase activity to increased vascular reactivity.

6-KETO-PGE$_1$: A POTENT RENIN SECRETAGOGUE

Prostaglandin-dependent mechanisms have also been shown to contribute to the regulation of renin release (25) (Fig. 2). PGI_2 has been proposed to be the eicosanoid mediating renin release. However, 6-keto-PGE_1, which is thought to arise from PGI_2, is a more potent renin secretagogue than prostacyclin (8,14). The

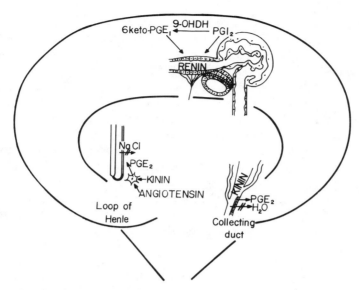

FIG. 2. Prostaglandin (PG) interactions with the kallikrein–kinin and renin–angiotensin systems intrarenally. Three major sites have been identified: on the *left*, within the interstitium of the medulla and adjacent loop of Henle; in the *center*, the juxtaglomerular apparatus; on the *right*, kinin–prostaglandin interactions in the distal nephron and collecting ducts. PGI_2 = prostacyclin. (From McGiff, ref. 14a.)

capacity of 6-keto-PGE_1 to release renin from rabbit renal cortical slices into the incubating medium was compared to that of PGI_2. The threshold dose of 6-keto-PGE_1, which released renin, was tenfold lower than the dose of PGI_2. A dose–response relationship was noted, and the effects of 6-keto-PGE_1 on renin release from cortical slices persisted through the second 20-min period of incubation, whereas the effects of PGI_2 on renin release were restricted to the initial 20-min period. An unexpected effect was registered by 6-keto-$PGF_{1\alpha}$, which resulted in renin release only after a latent period of 20 min. We interpreted this finding to signify delayed metabolic transformation of 6-keto-$PGF_{1\alpha}$ to either 6-keto-PGE_1 or a similar substance. Pretreatment of the rabbit with indomethacin caused potentiation of 6-keto-PGE_1-induced renin release into the incubating medium and had the expected effect of reducing renin release from renal cortical slices before addition of the prostaglandin (20). The enzyme responsible for transformation of PGI_2 to 6-keto-PGE_1, 9-hydroxy prostaglandin dehydrogenase, showed a similar zonal distribution within the kidney, as did renin, having highest activity in the cortex and negligible activity in the papilla (14).

RENAL KALLIKREIN–KININ–PROSTAGLANDIN INTERACTIONS

Close coupling of the renal kallikrein–kinin and prostaglandin systems was demonstrated in the conscious rat during administration of mineralocorticoids given to elevate the activity of each vasodilator–diuretic system (Fig. 3). At the end of 1 week of deoxycorticosterone administration, a severalfold increase in urinary kallikrein occurred together with a threefold increase in excretion of PGE_2 and lesser increases in $PGF_{2\alpha}$ excretion (17). On day 11, the serine protease inhibitor aprotinin was given for an additional 4 days and caused the expected decline in urinary kallikrein activity associated with a *pari passu* decline in PGE_2 excretion, despite continued administration of either deoxycorticosterone or aldosterone. Reduced activity of the renal kallikrein–kinin–prostaglandin system induced by aprotinin was associated with an antidiuresis lasting for 3 days and an antinatriuresis for 2 days. Despite diminished activity of the renal kallikrein–kinin and prostaglandin systems, as reflected in urinary kallikrein activity and PGE_2 excretion, sodium and water excretion returned to preaprotinin levels by day 4 of aprotinin treatment. These results suggest that the concerted activity of the kallikrein–kinin–prostaglandin systems intrarenally is involved in the short- and intermediate-term regulation

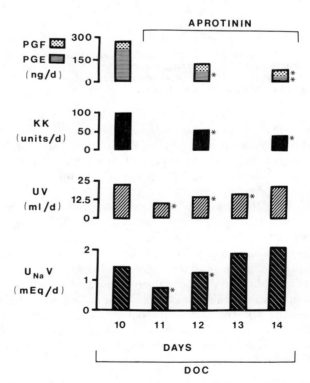

FIG. 3. Rats were treated with deoxycorticosterone (DOC) 5 mg/day subcutaneously for 14 days. On days 11 to 14, aprotinin (100,000 kIU/day) was administered also subcutaneously. Daily excretion of prostaglandins (PG) E_2, $F_{2\alpha}$, and kallikrein (KK), as well as urinary volume (UV) and sodium excretion ($U_{Na}V$), were measured in six rats. Significant differences are indicated by $^*p < 0.05$; $^{**}p < 0.01$, when compared to day 10.

of extracellular fluid volume and that mineralocorticoid "escape" is dependent on heightened intrarenal activities of these hormonal systems.

CONCLUSION

If one assumes tonic activity of the opposing blood-pressure-regulating systems, a deficiency of the vasodepressor system may lead to hypertension without an increase in the basal activity of the blood-pressure-elevating system. Within the kidney, and probably within extrarenal blood vessels as well, prostaglandins interact with the principal blood-pressure-regulating systems, the kallikrein–kinin and the adrenergic nervous–renin–angiotensin, reinforcing the former and buffering the latter.

If a deficiency in prostaglandin production initiates or exaggerates hypertension, chronic administration of a cyclooxygenase inhibitor should result in hypertension. In the anesthetized dog, the immediate hemodynamic effects of indomethacin resembled those of uncomplicated essential hypertension: elevated blood pressure, unchanged cardiac output, marked increase in the vascular resistance of the kidneys, and a smaller increase in that of the limbs (11). However, most attempts to produce chronic hypertension with nonsteroidal antiinflammatory agents have failed, probably because the dose was too small and the reserve capacity for prostaglandin generation is so great. In a recent study, daily administration of indomethacin to the rabbit—the dose is critical and is highly toxic to most animals—resulted in sustained elevation in blood pressure (2); it was several days before the full effect was obtained (Fig. 4). For elevation of blood pressure to occur during inhibition of prostaglandin synthesis, renal cyclooxygenase activity must be decreased by more than 80% as reflected in diminished excretion of PGE_2. The demonstration that inhibition of prostaglandin synthesis by nonsteroidal antiinflammatory drugs can result in hypertension urges consideration of the contribution of deficiencies in vasodepressor systems to hypertensive disease in humans.

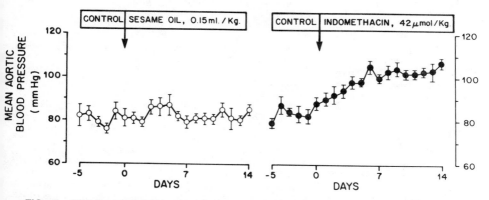

FIG. 4. Effects on arterial blood pressure of the cyclooxygenase inhibitor indomethacin in conscious rabbits. Animals were injected subcutaneously each day with indomethacin (15 mg/kg) ($n = 7$) or vehicle ($n = 6$). (From Colina-Chourio et al., ref. 2.)

ACKNOWLEDGMENTS

This work was supported by the National Institutes of Health grants (HL25406-NHLBI and HL25394-NHLBI), and by the Fogarty International Center of the National Institutes of Health grant of M. Schwartzman (FO5TW03100). The authors thank Shirley Klein, Sallie McGiff, and Pat Scholl for their assistance in preparing the manuscript.

REFERENCES

1. Aiken, J. W., and Vane, J. R. (1973): Intrarenal prostaglandin release attenuates the renal vaso-constrictor activity of angiotensin. *J. Pharmacol. Exp. Ther.*, 184:678–687.
2. Colina-Chourio, J., McGiff, J. C., and Nasjletti, A. (1979): Effect of indomethacin on blood pressure in the normotensive unanesthetized rabbit: Possible relation to prostaglandin synthesis inhibition. *Clin. Sci.*, 57:359–365.
3. Dusting, G. J., Moncada, S., and Vane, J. R. (1979): Prostaglandins, their intermediates and precursors: Cardiovascular actions and regulatory roles in normal and abnormal circulatory systems. *Prog. Cardiovasc. Dis.*, 21:405–430.
4. Ferreri, N. R., McGiff, J. C., Miller, M. J. S., Schwartzman, M., Spokas, E. G., and Wong, P. Y-K. (1983): The kidney and arachidonic acid. In: *Advances in Prostaglandin, Thromboxane, and Leukotriene Research, Vol. 11*, edited by B. Samuelsson, R. Paoletti, and P. Ramwell, pp. 481–485. Raven Press, New York.
5. Ferreri, N. R., Schwartzman, M., Ibraham, N., Chander, P. N., and McGiff, J. C. (1984): Arachidonic acid metabolism in a cell suspension isolated from rabbit renal outer medulla. *J. Pharmacol. Exp. Ther.*, 231:441–448.
6. Gerritsen, M. E., and Printz, M. P. (1981): Prostaglandin D synthase in microvessels from the rat cerebral cortex. *Prostaglandins*, 22:553–566.
7. Gerritsen, M. E., and Printz, M. P. (1981): Sites of prostaglandin synthesis in the bovine heart and isolated bovine coronary microvessels. *Circ. Res.*, 49:1152–1163.
8. Jackson, E. K., Herzer, W. A., Zimmerman, J. B., Branch, R. A., Oates, J. A., and Gerkins, J. F. (1981): 6-Keto-prostaglandin E_1 is more potent than prostaglandin I_2 as a renal vasodilator and renin secretagogue. *J. Pharmacol. Exp. Ther.*, 216:24–27.
9. Jacobson, H. R., Corona, S., Capdevila, J., Chacos, N., Manna, S., Womack, A., and Falck, J. R. (1983): Effects of epoxyicosatrienoic acids on ion transport in the rabbit cortical collecting tubule. Nato Advanced Research Workshop on Icosanoids and Ion Transport. Paris, November 17–18. (Abstract) p. 9.
10. Jørgensen, P. L. (1980): Sodium and potassium ion pump in kidney tubules. *Physiol. Rev.*, 60:864–917.
11. Lonigro, A. J., Itskovitz, H. D., Crowshaw, K., and McGiff, J. C. (1973): Dependency of renal blood flow on prostaglandin synthesis in the dog. *Circ. Res.*, 32:712–717.
12. Malik, K. U., and McGiff, J. C. (1975): Modulation by prostaglandins of adrenergic transmission in the isolated perfused rabbit and rat kidney. *Circ. Res.*, 36:599–609.
13. McGiff, J. C., Crowshaw, K., Terragno, N. A., Malik, K. U., and Lonigro, A. J. (1971): Differential effect of noradrenaline and renal nerve stimulation on vascular resistance in the dog kidney and the release of a prostaglandin E-like substance. *Clin. Sci.*, 42:223–233.
14. McGiff, J. C., Spokas, E. G., and Wong, P. Y.-K. (1982): Stimulation of renin release by 6-oxo-prostaglandin E_1 and prostacyclin. *Br. J. Pharmacol.*, 75:137–144.
14a. McGiff, J. C. (1981): Prostaglandins, prostacyclin, and thromboxanes. *Ann. Rev. Pharmacol. Toxicol.*, 21:479–509.
15. Messina, E. J., and Kaley, G. (1980): Microcirculatory responses to prostacyclin and PGE_2 in the rat cremaster muscle. In: *Advances in Prostaglandin and Thromboxane Research, Vol. 7*, edited by B. Samuelsson, P. W. Ramwell, and R. Paoletti, pp. 719–722. Raven Press, New York.
16. Moncada, S., Gryglewski, R. J., Bunting, S., and Vane, J. R. (1976): A lipid peroxide inhibits the enzyme in blood vessel microsomes that generates from prostaglandin endoperoxides the substance (prostaglandin X) which prevents platelet aggregation. *Prostaglandins*, 12:715–737.
17. Nasjletti, A., McGiff, J. C., and Colina-Chourio, J. (1978): Interrelations of the renal kallikrein-kinin system and renal prostaglandins in the conscious rat. *Circ. Res.*, 43:799–807.

18. Samuelsson, B., Paoletti, R., and Ramwell, P., editors (1983): *Advances in Prostaglandin, Thromboxane and Leukotriene Research*. Raven Press, New York.
19. Smith, W. L., and Wilkin, G. P. (1977): Immunochemistry of prostaglandin endoperoxide-forming cyclooxygenases: The detection of the cyclooxygenases in rat, rabbit, and guinea pig kidneys by immunofluorescence. *Prostaglandins*, 13:873–892.
20. Spokas, E. G., Wong, P. Y.-K., and McGiff, J. C. (1982): Prostaglandin-related renin release from rabbit renal cortical slices. *Hypertension*, 4(suppl. 2):96–100.
21. Stokes, J. B. (1979): Effect of prostaglandin E_2 on chloride transport across the rabbit thick ascending limb of Henle. *J. Clin. Invest.*, 64:495–502.
22. Terragno, D. A., Crowshaw, K., Terragno, N. A., and McGiff, J. C. (1975): Prostaglandin synthesis by bovine mesenteric arteries and veins. *Circ. Res.*, 36&37(suppl. 1):76–80.
23. Terragno, N. A., McGiff, J. C., and Terragno, D. A. (1979): Synthesis of prostaglandins by vascular and nonvascular renal tissues and the presence of an endogenous prostaglandin synthesis inhibitor in the cortex. In: *Advances in Pharmacology and Therapeutics, Vol. 4, Prostaglandins-Immunopharmacology*, edited by B. B. Vargaftig, pp. 39–46. Pergamon Press, Oxford.
24. Terragno, N. A., Terragno, A., McGiff, J. C., and Rodriguez, D. J. (1977): Synthesis of prostaglandins by the ductus arteriosus of the bovine fetus. *Prostaglandins*, 14:721–726.
25. Weber, P. C., Larsson, C., Änggård, E., Hamberg, M., Corey, E. J., Nicolaou, K. C., and Samuelsson, B. (1976): Stimulation of renin release from rabbit renal cortex by arachidonic acid and prostaglandin endoperoxides. *Circ. Res.*, 39:868–874.
26. Weiner, R., and Kaley, G. (1969): Influence of prostaglandin E_1 on the terminal vascular bed. *Am. J. Physiol.*, 217:563–566.
27. Wong, P. Y.-K., Malik, K. U., Desiderio, D. M., McGiff, J. C., and Sun, F. F. (1980): Hepatic metabolism of prostacyclin (PGI_2) in the rabbit: Formation of a potent novel inhibitor of platelet aggregation. *Biochem. Biophys. Res. Commun.*, 93:486–494.
28. Wong, P. Y.-K., Sun, F. F., and McGiff, J. C. (1978): Metabolism of prostacyclin in blood vessels. *J. Biol. Chem.*, 253:5555–5557.

Advances in Prostaglandin, Thromboxane, and Leukotriene Research, Vol. 13, edited by G. G. Neri Serneri, et al. Raven Press, New York © 1985.

Prostaglandins, Renin–Angiotensin System, and Hypertension

Alberto Nasjletti and Philip G. Baer

Department of Pharmacology, University of Tennessee Center for the Health Sciences, Memphis, Tennessee 38163

The level of arterial blood pressure is a function of cardiac output and vascular resistance. In turn, cardiac output and vascular resistance are determined by many factors working in an interrelated manner. Axiomatically, hypertension develops when the balance between factors that increase and factors that decrease blood pressure is disrupted. Such an imbalance may result (a) from primary increases in the activity of pressor systems such as the sympathetic nervous system, the renin–angiotensin system, vasopressin, or aldosterone, which elevate vascular resistance and promote conservation of salt and water, or (b) from reduction in the levels of vasodilatory prostaglandins (PG), kinins, and antihypertensive renal lipids, which promote diuresis and natriuresis and/or decrease vascular resistance. The concept that an interplay between prostaglandins and the renin–angiotensin system contributes to blood pressure control was first advanced in 1970 by McGiff et al. (13), who reported release of a prostaglandin-like substance into renal venous blood in response to renal artery constriction or angiotensin II infusion. Subsequently, this notion gained strength with reports that the vascular effects of angiotensin II are augmented by prostaglandin synthesis inhibitors (1) and attenuated by both PGE_2 and prostacyclin (PGI_2) (29) and that, in conditions featuring activation of the renin–angiotensin system, inhibition of prostaglandin synthesis causes renal vasoconstriction and compromises renal excretory functions (2,22). This chapter considers the relationship between angiotensin II and prostaglandins and discusses the significance of that relationship to the regulation of vascular tone and blood pressure.

PROSTAGLANDIN SYSTEM DURING ANGIOTENSIN II-INDUCED HYPERTENSION

It is now well established that angiotensin II increases the synthesis of prostaglandins in a variety of organs, including kidneys, lungs, heart, and blood vessels, an action related to stimulation of phospholipid deacylation resulting in elevation of free arachidonic acid available to cyclooxygenase for metabolism to prostaglandins (11,17). As a result of promotion of prostaglandin synthesis, short-term exposure to angiotensin II increases the release of PGE_2 from most tissues and the release of PGI_2 from the kidney, heart, lung, and arterial blood vessels (8,10,11,17). Also, there are reports that the pressor peptide induces release of $PGF_{2\alpha}$ from the dog kidney, and of thromboxane A_2 from the hydronephrotic kidney and the kidney of spontaneously hypertensive rats (8,15,25).

These observations demonstrating stimulation of prostaglandin synthesis and release during the course of *in vitro* or acute *in vivo* experiments are complemented by our recent report (7) on the consequences of prolonged elevation of angiotensin II levels on the plasma concentration, urinary excretion, and the *in vitro* tissue release of PGE_2 and 6-keto-$PGF_{1\alpha}$, a PGI_2 metabolite. Intraperitoneal angiotensin II infusion at 125 to 200 ng/min for 12 days in conscious rats increased systolic blood pressure progressively (Fig. 1) and elevated fluid intake and urine volume. Urinary 6-keto-$PGF_{1\alpha}$ increased from 38 ± 6 to 55 ± 5 and 51 ± 7 ng/day on days 8 and 11, respectively, of angiotensin infusion at 200 ng/min (Fig. 2), but urinary PGE_2 excretion did not change. Rats made hypertensive by angiotensin II infusion also exhibited increased plasma arterial concentration of 6-keto-$PGF_{1\alpha}$ (Fig. 3) and of 13,14-dihydro-15-keto-PGE_2, and augmented net release of 6-keto-$PGF_{1\alpha}$ from aortic rings and renal medulla slices during incubation in Krebs solution.

It is intriguing that under *in vitro* conditions that did not preserve a critical feature of the *in vivo* environment—i.e., high angiotensin II levels—rings of aorta and renal medullary tissue obtained from rats infused with angiotensin II for 12 days still released more 6-keto-$PGF_{1\alpha}$ than did corresponding tissues from vehicle-infused rats. In this regard, one must consider the possibility that in rats with angiotensin II-induced hypertension the enhancement of 6-keto-$PGF_{1\alpha}$ release from aortic rings and renal medulla slices relates to one or more slowly developing and persistent alterations in function and/or tissue structure rather than to a direct, immediate, and rapidly reversible action of angiotensin II on the phospholipid–

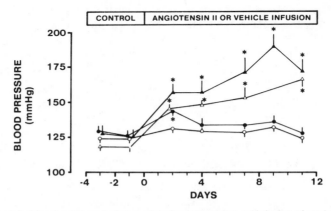

FIG. 1. Systolic blood pressure before and during intraperitoneal infusion of angiotensin II (AII) in rats. Results are expressed as means ± SE. * = $p < 0.05$ relative to corresponding values in vehicle-infused rats; ○ = Vehicle; ● = AII,75 ng/min; △ = AII,125 ng/min; ▲ = AII, 200 ng/min. (From Diz et al., ref. 7.)

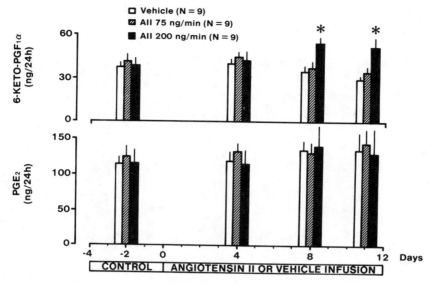

FIG. 2. Urinary excretion of immunoreactive 6-keto-PGF$_{1\alpha}$ and PGE$_2$ before and during intra-peritoneal infusion of angiotensin II (AII) in rats. Results are expressed as means ± SE. * = $p < 0.05$ relative to values in vehicle-infused rats. (From Diz et al., ref. 7.)

arachidonate system. Relative to this view, several investigators have suggested a causal association between high blood pressure and increased vascular prostaglandin synthesis (7). Regardless of the mechanism involved, our study suggests that augmentation of vascular production and plasma levels of PGI$_2$ is a feature of the response to angiotensin II-induced hypertension in the conscious rat.

MODIFICATION BY PROSTAGLANDINS OF ANGIOTENSIN II VASCULAR EFFECTS

Angiotensin II-induced vasoconstriction in the renal, coronary, and mesenteric vasculature is associated with augmentation of prostaglandin synthesis, as evidenced by increased blood levels of PGE$_2$ and/or PGI$_2$. These two prostaglandins produce vasodilation and counteract the vasoconstrictor action of angiotensin II in the kidney (29) and probably in other vasculatures as well. That induction of prostaglandin synthesis by angiotensin II influences the vascular actions of the peptide is evidenced by observations that such actions are magnified by the administration of inhibitors of prostaglandin synthesis. For example, when generation of prostaglandins is prevented by inhibition of cyclooxygenase with indomethacin or like-acting drugs, the vasoconstrictor effect of angiotensin II in the kidney and heart is substantially enhanced (1,10). Collectively, these observations suggest that one or more endogenous prostaglandins serve to attenuate the constrictor action of angiotensin II on resistance blood vessels and, consequently, may weaken its pressor effect.

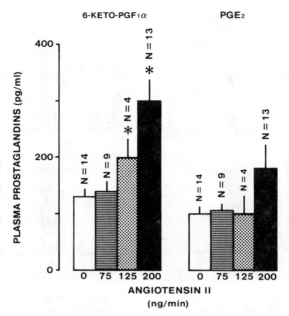

FIG. 3. Immunoreactive 6-keto-PGF$_{1\alpha}$ and PGE$_2$ concentrations in arterial plasma on day 12 of angiotensin II intraperitoneal infusion. Results are expressed as means ± SE. * = $p < 0.05$ relative to values in vehicle-infused rats. (From Diz et al., ref. 7.)

Several studies comparing the pressor effect of angiotensin II before and during cyclooxygenase inhibition suggest that prostaglandins attenuate the pressor action of the peptide. For example, the administration of prostaglandin synthesis inhibitors increases the duration of the angiotensin II pressor effect in the rabbit (23). Inhibitors of prostaglandin synthesis also were reported to augment the rise in blood pressure caused by angiotensin II in normal subjects, subjects on a low-sodium diet, and patients with Bartter's syndrome (17,18,27). As a whole, these observations suggest that prostaglandins are a feature of mechanisms that curtail the pressor effect of angiotensin II. In agreement with this view, the duration of the pressor effect of angiotensin II in the rabbit correlates inversely with the plasma level of 6-keto-PGF$_{1\alpha}$ (23).

INTERACTION OF PROSTAGLANDINS AND ANGIOTENSIN II

A growing body of experimental and clinical observations suggests that during activation of the renin–angiotensin system the renal circulation becomes critically dependent on an interplay between prostaglandins and vasoconstrictor mechanisms implemented by angiotensin II. The interaction between prostaglandins and vaso-constrictor systems plays a prominent role in maintenance of renal hemodynamics in experimental animals during renal ischemia, surgical stress, hypovolemia, or sodium depletion (2,17,22,24). Most of these conditions have three features in common. First, the activity of the renin–angiotensin system is elevated. Second, the production of renal prostaglandins is increased, probably as a response to stimulation by angiotensin II. Third, in contrast with the lack of effects on renal hemodynamics in animals and subjects having "normal" renin–angiotensin system activity, in all four states the administration of an inhibitor of prostaglandin synthesis brings about lowering of renal blood flow and/or glomerular filtration, indicative of renal vasoconstriction (2,17,22,24). In this regard, the reduction in renal blood flow and glomerular filtration rate that follows the administration of a cyclooxygenase inhibitor, such as indomethacin, may be an expression of diminished synthesis of a vasodilator prostaglandin, resulting in augmentation of the renal vasoconstriction elicited by angiotensin II. Involvement of angiotensin II in the renal vasoconstriction produced by cyclooxygenase inhibition is supported by reports that the degree of vasoconstriction (a) correlates positively with the prevailing plasma renin activity in the sodium deficient dog (2) and (b) is blunted by blockade of angiotensin II vascular receptors in the dog during partial renal artery occlusion (24) or sodium depletion (2). It would appear, then, that in states characterized by augmented activity in the renin–angiotensin system, the kidney produces one or more vasodilator prostaglandins that are instrumental in counteracting the vasoconstrictor actions of angiotensin II and thereby contribute to maintenance of the renal circulation.

Information on whether an interplay between prostaglandins and angiotensin II affects vascular tone in organs other than the kidney is scant. During pregnancy in the dog, a condition characterized by marked activation of the renin–angiotensin system, the administration of indomethacin produces a striking reduction of uterine blood flow, suggesting that a prostaglandin mechanism contributes to support the uterine circulation in the face of elevated angiotensin II levels. Augmented prostaglandin synthesis may account for reduction in the pressor responsiveness of angiotensin II and norepinephrine in patients with Bartter's syndrome, a feature of the condition that is blunted by treatment with cyclooxygenase inhibitors (26).

Thus in humans and in animals prostaglandins appear to support blood flow to the kidney and probably to other organs in the face of activation of the renin–angiotensin system.

CONTRIBUTION OF PROSTAGLANDINS TO THE REGULATION OF BLOOD PRESSURE

That angiotensin II induces synthesis of one or more prostaglandins that counteract its vasoconstrictor effect fits well with the concept that an interplay between prostaglandins and pressor mechanisms implemented by angiotensin II contributes to set the level of arterial blood pressure. Implied in this concept is that a disturbance in such an interplay because of impaired prostaglandin production could, if uncompensated, cause blood pressure to rise, thereby initiating hypertension or aggravating preexisting hypertension. There have been numerous attempts to produce by administration of cyclooxygenase inhibitors an imbalance between prostaglandins and pressor mechanisms. Colina-Chourio et al. (4) reported that daily administration of indomethacin at 15 mg/kg subcutaneously in the rabbit elevates mean arterial blood pressure without altering plasma volume or increasing sodium retention. Also, in normal and in sodium-depleted (28) subjects, and in patients with idiopathic orthostatic hypotension (5) or with heart failure (9), the administration of indomethacin was reported to produce modest but significant elevations in blood pressure. However, these observations are at variance with reports that indomethacin does not alter blood pressure in normotensive animals or humans (16,18,22). Studies of the effects of inhibitors of cyclooxygenase on blood pressure in hypertensive states also have yielded conflicting results. Reports that indomethacin or like-acting drugs aggravate hypertension in humans (19) and in rats with spontaneous hypertension (3), deoxycorticosterone acetate–salt hypertension (21), and Goldblatt hypertension (20) contrast with reports that they do not (14,30). Indeed, in one study the administration of indomethacin to two siblings with renin-dependent hypertension and aldosteronism resulted in lowering of blood pressure associated with reduction of plasma renin activity and serum aldosterone (6). Similarly, the administration of indomethacin caused reduction of blood pressure and plasma renin in rats made hypertensive by ligation of the aorta between the renal arteries (12). Seminal to the disagreement noted in reports regarding the effect of cyclooxygenase inhibitors on blood pressure is the effect of such drugs in reducing renin secretion and, consequently, plasma renin activity (22). Thus, the antihypertensive effect of lowering plasma renin activity during treatment with indomethacin or like-acting drugs may offset any tendency of blood pressure to rise because of reduced synthesis of antihypertensive prostaglandins. This view is in accord with the results of Romero and Strong (22), who studied the effect of indomethacin in two subgroups of rabbits with one-clip, two-kidney Goldblatt hypertension of 5 weeks duration. Hypertensive animals in one subgroup had normal renal blood flow and plasma renin activity, and in those animals administration of indomethacin did not increase blood pressure further or produce sustained alterations in renal blood flow, but it did produce a profound and sustained reduction of plasma renin. Rabbits in the second subgroup had lower renal blood flow and higher blood pressure and plasma renin activity; administration of indomethacin in these animals resulted in further augmentation of blood pressure associated with marked reduction of renal blood flow. It is most important that plasma renin activity, which initially was reduced by indomethacin, returned on subsequent days to the pretreatment level *pari passu* with the increase of blood pressure. Thus, when indomethacin did not cause sustained reduction of plasma renin activity, it did aggrevate hypertension, an outcome consistent with the proposed role of prostaglandins in counteracting pressor mechanisms implemented by angiotensin II.

ACKNOWLEDGMENTS

This study was supported by U.S. Public Health Service grants HL-18579 and HL-23548. Dr. Philip Baer is the recipient of National Institutes of Health Career Research Development Award 1 KO4 HL-00806.

REFERENCES

1. Aiken, J. W., and Vane, J. R. (1973): Intrarenal prostaglandin release attenuates the renal vaso-constrictor activity of angiotensin. *J. Pharmacol. Exp. Ther.*, 184:678–687.
2. Blasingham, M. C., and Nasjletti, A. (1980): Differential renal effects of cyclooxygenase inhibition in sodium-replete and sodium-deprived dog. *Am. J. Physiol.*, 239:F360–F365.
3. Chrysant, S. G., Townsent, S. M., and Morgan, P. R. (1978): The effects of salt and meclofenamate administration on the hypertension of spontaneously hypertensive rats. *Clin. Exp. Hypertension*, 1:381–391.
4. Colina-Chourio, J., McGiff, J. C., and Nasjletti, A. (1974): Effect of indomethacin on blood pressure in the normotensive unanesthetized rabbit: Possible relation to prostaglandin synthesis inhibition. *Clin. Sci.*, 57:359–365.
5. Davies, I. B., Bannister, R., Hensby, C., and Sever, P. S. (1980): The pressor actions of noradren-aline and angiotensin II in chronic autonomic failure treated with indomethacin. *Br. J. Clin. Pharmacol.*, 10:223–229.
6. DeJong, P. E., Donker, A. J. M., Van der Wall, E., Erkelens, D. W., Van der Hem, G. K., and Doorenbos, H. (1980): Effect of indomethacin in two siblings with a renin-dependent hypertension, hyperaldosteronism and hypokalemia. *Nephron*, 25:47–52.
7. Diz, D. I., Baer, P. G., and Nasjletti, A. (1983): Angiotensin II-induced hypertension in the rat. Effects on the plasma concentration, renal excretion, and tissue release of prostaglandins. *J. Clin. Invest.*, 72:466–477.
8. Dunn, J. J., Liard, J. F., and Dray, F. (1978): Basal and stimulated rates of renal secretion and excretion of prostaglandins E_2, $F_{2\alpha}$, and 13,14-dihydro-15-keto F_α in the dog. *Kidney Int.*, 13:136–143.
9. Dzau, V. J., Lilly, L., Swartz, S., and Packer, M. (1983): Role of endogenous prostaglandins in circulatory homeostasis in human heart failure. *Circulation (Abstr.)*, 68:129.
10. Gunther, S., and Cannon, P. J. (1980): Modulation of angiotensin II coronary vasoconstriction by cardiac prostaglandin synthesis. *Am. J. Physiol.*, 238:895–901.
11. Isakson, P. C., Raz, A., Denny, S. E., Wyche, A., and Needleman, P. (1977): Hormonal stimulation of arachidonate release from isolated perfused organs. Relationship to prostaglandin biosynthesis. *Prostaglandins*, 14:853–871.
12. Jackson, E. K., Oates, J. A., and Branch, R. A. (1981): Indomethacin decreases arterial blood pressure and plasma renin activity in rats with aorta ligation. *Circ. Res.*, 49:180–185.
13. McGiff, J. C., Crowshaw, K., Terragno, N. A., and Lonigro, A. J. (1970): Release of a prosta-glandin-like substance into renal venous blood in response to angiotensin II. *Circ. Res.*, 26–27(suppl. 1):I-121–I-130.
14. McQueen, D., and Bell, K. (1976): The effects of prostaglandin E_1 and sodium meclofenamate on blood pressure in renal hypertensive rats. *Eur. J. Pharmacol.*, 37:223–235.
15. Morrison, A. R., Mishikawa, K., and Needleman, P. (1978): Thromboxane A_2 biosynthesis in the ureter obstructed isolated perfused kidney of the rabbit. *J. Pharmacol. Exp. Ther.*, 205:1–8.
16. Muirhead, E. E., Brooks, B., and Brosius, W. L. (1976): Indomethacin and blood pressure control. *J. Lab. Clin. Med.*, 88:578–583.
17. Nasjletti, A., and Malik, K. U. (1982): Interrelations between prostaglandins and vasoconstrictor hormones: Contribution to blood pressure regulation. *Fed. Proc.*, 41:2394–2399.
18. Negus, P., Tannen, R. L., and Dunn, M. J. (1976): Indomethacin potentiates the vasoconstrictor actions of angiotensin II in normal man. *Prostaglandins*, 12:175–180.
19. Patak, R. B., Mookerjee, C., Bentzel, P., Hysert, P., Babe, M., and Lee, J. (1975): Antagonism of the effects of furosemide by indomethacin in normal and hypertensive man. *Prostaglandins*, 10:649–659.
20. Pugsley, D. J., Beilin, L. J., and Petro, R. P. (1975): Renal prostaglandin synthesis in the Goldblatt hypertensive rat. *Circ. Res.*, 36(suppl. 1):81–88.
21. Pugsley, D. J., Mullins, R., and Beilin, L. J. (1976): Renal prostaglandin synthesis in hypertension induced by deoxycorticosterone and sodium chloride in the rat. *Clin. Sci. Mol. Med.*, 51(suppl. 3):253s–256s.
22. Romero, J. D., and Strong, J. C. (1977): The effect of indomethacin blockade of prostaglandin synthesis on blood pressure of normal rabbits and rabbits with renovascular hypertension. *Circ. Res.*, 40:35–41.

23. Rowe, B. P., and Nasjletti, A. (1983): Biphasic blood pressure response to angiotensin II in the conscious rabbit: Relation to prostaglandins. *J. Pharmacol. Exp. Ther.*, 225:559–563.

24. Satoh, S., and Zimmerman, B. G. (1975): Influence of the renin-angiotensin system on the effect of prostaglandin synthesis inhibitors in the renal vasculature. *Circ. Res.*, 36–37(suppl. I):189–195.

25. Shibouta, Y., Inada, Y., Terashita, Z.; Nishikawa, K., Kikuchi, S., and Shimamoto, K. (1979): Angiotensin II-stimulated release of thromboxane A_2 and prostacyclin (PGI_2) in isolated, perfused kidneys of spontaneously hypertensive rats. *Biochem. Pharmacol.*, 28:3601–3609.

26. Silverberg, A. B., Mennes, P. A., and Cryer, P. E. (1978): Resistance to endogenous norepinephrine in Bartter's syndrome. Reversion during indomethacin administration. *Am. J. Med.*, 64:231–235.

27. Speckart, P., Zia, P., Zipser, R., and Horton, R. (1977): The effect of sodium restriction and prostaglandin inhibition on the renin-angiotensin system in man. *Clin. Endocrinol. Metab.*, 44:832–837.

28. Staessen, J., Eagard, R., Lijnen, P., and Amery, A. (1983): Effect of prostaglandin synthesis inhibition on blood pressure and humoral factors in normal, sodium-deplete man at exercise. *Circulation*, 68:150 (abstract).

29. Susic, H., Nasjletti, A., and Malik, K. U. (1981): Inhibition by bradykinin of the vascular actions of angiotensin II in the dog kidney: Relationship to prostaglandins. *J. Pharmacol. Exp. Ther.*, 218:103–107.

30. Yun, J., Kelly, G., and Bartter, F. C. (1979): Effect of indomethacin on renal function and plasma renin activity in dogs with chronic renovascular hypertension. *Nephron*, 24:278–282.

Advances in Prostaglandin, Thromboxane, and
Leukotriene Research, Vol. 13, edited by G.G. Neri
Serneri, et al. Raven Press, New York © 1985.

The Relevance of Prostaglandins in Human Hypertension

Michael J. Dunn and *Hermann-Josef Gröne

*Department of Medicine, Case Western Reserve University, and *Division of Nephrology,
University Hospitals of Cleveland, Cleveland, Ohio 44106*

This chapter summarizes the data for and against the hypothesis that vascular and renal prostaglandins (PG) are important in the control of blood pressure in both normotensive and hypertensive humans. Although there is extensive literature on the interaction of prostaglandins with the renin–angiotensin and kallikrein–kinin systems in experimental animals, this discussion will be restricted to human experimentation. Primary emphasis is placed on studies that have assessed prostaglandin synthesis in human hypertension, the effects of cyclooxygenase-inhibitory drugs on blood pressure control in normotensive and hypertensive subjects, and the possible beneficial effects of dietary supplements of polyunsaturated fatty acids on blood-pressure control.

MECHANISM OF PROSTAGLANDIN ACTION ON BLOOD PRESSURE CONTROL

The actions of prostaglandins to alter blood pressure can be summarized under five major headings. Table 1 summarizes the effects of the vasodilatory prostaglandins PGE_2 and prostacyclin (PGI_2), as well as the actions of nonsteroidal antiinflammatory drugs (NSAID) on physiologic determinants of blood pressure. Cyclooxygenase inhibition with NSAID has effects opposite to PGE_2 and PGI_2 on the five listed factors of blood pressure control. The contribution of prostaglandins to the control of vascular resistance seems less important in normotensive subjects than in hypertensive subjects, as revealed by the increments in blood pressure in the latter group after administration of NSAID (see below). In both normotensive and hypertensive subjects, infusion of PGE_2 or PGI_2 would be expected to antagonize the vasoconstrictor action of angiotensin and norepinephrine, whereas it is well-established that NSAID potentiate the constrictor and, hence, pressor actions of these compounds. The importance of PGE_2 to reduce sodium chloride reabsorption in the renal tubule and to enhance sodium chloride excretion can be demon-

---

Present address for H.-J. Gröne is Medizinische Klinik, Universität Göttingen, Robert-Koch-Strasse 40, 3400 Göttingen, Federal Republic of Germany.

TABLE 1. *Mechanisms of prostaglandin control of blood pressure*

Mechanism	PGE_2 and PGI_2	NSAID
Vascular resistance	↓	↑
Vasoreactivity to ANG II and NE	↓	↑
NaCl excretion	↑	↓
Renin secretion	↑	↓
Cardiac output	↑	↓

Abbreviations: NSAID, nonsteroidal antiinflammatory drugs; ANG II, angiotensin II; NE, norepinephrine.

strated in subjects who have avid sodium chloride reabsorption. NSAID, by virtue of reducing renal medullary synthesis of PGE_2, causes positive sodium balance, weight gain, and some expansion of plasma volume. Taken together with these changes of vascular resistance, vascular responsiveness to pressor hormones, and sodium chloride excretion, inhibition of prostaglandin synthesis would be expected to raise blood pressure. However, it should be noted that there are two actions of PGE_2 and PGI_2 that increase blood pressure, i.e., stimulation of renin secretion and cardiac output. Reduction of renal and cardiovascular prostaglandin synthesis with cyclooxygenase inhibitors reduces renin secretion and generally decreases cardiac output. Since the antihypertensive actions of prostaglandins predominate over these prohypertensive actions, the usual consequences of prostaglandin inhibition with NSAID are increments in blood pressure, whereas administration of PGE_2 or PGI_2 intravenously reduces blood pressure (5,28).

PROSTAGLANDIN SYNTHESIS IN HUMAN ESSENTIAL HYPERTENSION

The majority of studies of *in vivo* prostaglandin synthesis in essential hypertension have focused on renal synthesis, as measured by urinary excretion. Table 2

TABLE 2. *Renal PGE_2 excretion in human essential hypertension*

Author (ref.)	Observation
Abe et al., 1977 (1)	↓ Basal and stimulated urine PGE_2[a]
Tan et al., 1978 (30)	↓ Basal and stimulated urine PGE_2
Weber et al., 1979 (34)	↓ Basal and stimulated urine PGE_2
Ruilope et al., 1982 (23)	↓ Urine PGE_2 in low-renin patients
Lebel and Grose, 1982 (11)	Normal urine PGE_2
Campbell et al., 1982 (3)	Normal urine PGE_2
Rathaus et al., 1983 (22)	↓ Urine PGE_2 in low-renin patients

[a]Furosemide stimulation.

summarizes most of the pertinent literature on the renal synthesis and excretion of PGE_2 in human essential hypertension. Until 1982, there was unanimity amongst investigators that renal excretion of PGE_2 was diminished under both basal as well as furosemide-stimulated conditions in patients with essential hypertension. These data fit with the hypothesis that renal underproduction of PGE_2 reduced sodium excretion and may have contributed to either the genesis or the maintenance of hypertension. Other studies have since appeared that did not fully confirm the earlier results, reporting normal PGE_2 excretion or reductions of urine PGE_2 only in low-renin patients. Although some of the differences may be attributable to artifact caused by the inclusion of male subjects, a recent study that included only female hypertensives continued to demonstrate reduced urinary PGE_2 in essential hypertension (27). Since prostaglandins are autacoids, one must question whether they have a circulating or systemic role; nonetheless, increased plasma levels of PGE_2 have been reported in patients with borderline and with sustained essential hypertension (12,24).

EFFECTS OF CYCLOOXYGENASE INHIBITORS ON THE CONTROL OF BLOOD PRESSURE

In normotensive subjects, the acute intravenous or oral administration of indomethacin, a potent cyclooxygenase inhibitor, has substantial effects not only on blood pressure but also on total peripheral resistance and the cardiac index (Table 3). Acute inhibition of vascular and renal prostaglandin synthesis with indomethacin raised mean arterial blood pressure 8 to 10 mm Hg. These increments of blood pressure underestimated the extent of the vasoconstriction, since increments of total peripheral resistance ranged from 20 to 35%. This vasoconstriction, which was most prominent in renal and splanchnic vascular beds, was accompanied by decrements of cardiac output that moderated the extent of the blood-pressure increments (Table 3). Chronic administration of indomethacin or other NSAID has little effect on blood pressure in normotensive and untreated hypertensive patients

TABLE 3. *Acute effects of indomethacin on cardiovascular indices*

Author (ref.)	Mean BP	Hemodynamics
Nowak and Wennmalm (N)[a] (18)	↑ 10 mm Hg	TPR[d], 20% ↑ CI[e], slight ↓
Hermiller et al. (PH)[b] (9)	↑ 8 mm Hg	TPR, 25% ↑ CI, 15% ↓
Safar et al. (EH)[c] (24)	↑ 9 mm Hg	TPR, 35% ↑ CI, 20% ↓

[a]Normal.
[b]Pulmonary hypertension.
[c]Essential hypertension.
[d]Total peripheral resistance.
[e]Cardiac index.

(4,8,13,36). Although several studies have noted small increments in blood pressure ranging from 5 to 12 mm Hg (15,23), most investigators have been unable to document significant changes of blood pressure. This may be attributable to chronic depression of cardiac output, reduction of renin secretion, and alterations of baroreceptor function with decreased alpha-adrenergic tone. No chronic studies of the effects of NSAID have been reported in which hemodynamic indices such as cardiac index and total peripheral resistance have been measured. It is noteworthy that normotensive subjects who are pretreated with a NSAID have enhanced blood pressure responses to angiotensin II (17,32) and arginine vasopressin (7).

PROSTAGLANDIN INHIBITION IN ANTIHYPERTENSIVE THERAPY

Although inhibition of cyclooxygenase with NSAID has negligible effects on most normotensive and untreated hypertensive patients, blood pressure generally increases when NSAID are combined with antihypertensive therapy. Table 4 summarizes this literature. In every reported study, indomethacin, in doses ranging from 75 to 200 mg/day, administered orally for periods ranging from 3 days to 6 weeks, reduced the efficacy of diverse types of antihypertensive therapy. The changes in blood pressure were always statistically significant, and the increments of blood pressure were variable. Table 4 lists only the average changes in either mean or systolic and diastolic pressure, and it should be noted that several authors have commented that the increments in blood pressure may exceed 30 mm Hg systolic and 25 mm Hg diastolic when prostaglandin-inhibitory drugs have been added to antihypertensive therapy (15,33). This negative interaction between NSAID and antihypertensive drugs is not specific for any category of drug and has been reported with diverse types of diuretics, beta blockers, alpha-adrenergic mimetic compounds, vasodilators, and converting-enzyme inhibitors. It is quite unlikely that all of these heterogeneous antihypertensive drugs stimulate prostaglandin synthesis

TABLE 4. *Effects of prostaglandin inhibition on antihypertensive therapy*

Author (ref.)	Antihypertensive therapy	ΔBP	NSAID
Patak, 1975 (19)	Furosemide	18[a]	Indomethacin, 200 mg/day
Durao, 1977 (6)	Propranolol; pindolol	14/13[b]	Indomethacin, 100 mg/day
Lopez-Overjero, 1978 (13)	Thiazide; propranolol	7	Indomethacin, 200 mg/day
Watkins, 1980 (33)	Thiazide; propranolol	16/9	Indomethacin, 100 mg/day
Abe, 1981 (2)	Captopril[c]	10	Indomethacin, 75–150 mg/day
Wing, 1981 (35)	Mixed[d]	16/6	Indomethacin, 75 mg/day
Mills, 1982 (15)	Mixed	9/2	Indomethacin, 75 mg/day
Salvetti, 1983 (25)	Atenolol	11/7	Indomethacin, 200 mg/day

[a]Mean BP change, mm Hg.
[b]Systolic/diastolic, mm Hg.
[c]Low-renin hypertension only.
[d]Diuretics, beta blockers, methylDOPA, vasodilators, clonidine.
NSAID, nonsteroidal antiinflammatory drugs.

as their mechanism of action. A preferable explanation is that inhibition of renal and vascular PGE_2 and PGI_2 simply makes it more difficult for the antihypertensive therapy to alter the balance of cardiovascular forces in favor of a reduction in blood pressure. The effects of NSAID on blood-pressure control in treated hypertensives are complex, as can be surmised from Table 1. Although vascular resistance may have increased in most of the reported cases, this hemodynamic parameter has unfortunately not been measured in any of the studies summarized in Table 4. Some reports have noted reductions of sodium chloride secretion and weight gain. Virtually all reports have also documented significant decreases in plasma renin activity and plasma aldosterone when indomethacin was combined with antihypertensive therapy, and these latter changes would serve to offset the prohypertensive effects of increased vascular resistance and positive sodium balance. The deleterious effects of indomethacin on the hypotensive action of captopril seem restricted to low-renin hypertensives, since normal and high-renin patients had similar blood pressures when treated with captopril or captopril plus indomethacin (2). It is perhaps clinically important to note that Mills et al. (15) found no effect of aspirin at 1,950 mg daily on antihypertensive blood-pressure control and, consequently, aspirin may be the preferable antiinflammatory agent when this category of compounds is indicated in the treated hypertensive.

EFFECTS OF POLYUNSATURATED FATTY ACIDS ON BLOOD PRESSURE

Polyunsaturated fatty acids are the precursors of prostaglandin synthesis and act as the substrates for the cyclooxygenase enzyme (Fig. 1). Prostaglandins with one, two, and three double bonds belong to the monoenoic, dienoic, and trienoic series, respectively. Most attention has been paid to the normally prevalent dienoic prostaglandins, which are synthesized from arachidonic acid. Most arachidonic acid is not ingested as such but is synthesized by chain elongation and desaturation of the 18-carbon fatty acid linoleic acid. Linoleic acid can also act as the precursor for dihomo-gamma-linolenic acid, which in turn is cyclooxygenated to the monoenoic prostaglandins. The trienoic prostaglandins are formed from eicosapentaenoic acid, which can either be ingested as such or as the precursor linolenic acid. Safflower and sunflower oils are rich sources of linoleic acid, whereas fish oils such as cod

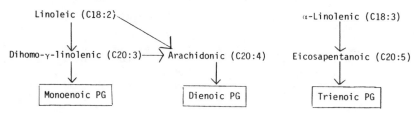

FIG. 1. Fatty acid precursors of prostaglandins (PG) with one, two, and three double bonds (monoenoic, dienoic, and trienoic, respectively). Arachidonic acid conversion to dienoic prostaglandins and thromboxane predominates in humans on a normal diet.

liver oil and menhaden oil are the most abundant sources of eicosapentaenoic acid. Eicosapentaenoic acid competes with arachidonic acid for the cyclooxygenase enzyme and hence can reduce the synthesis of the dienoic prostaglandins and thromboxane A_2. In addition, eicosapentaenoic acid yields PGE_3 and PGI_3, which are vasodilatory, whereas thromboxane A_3 is relatively inactive as a vasoconstrictor and platelet-aggregating material. Since essential fatty acid deficiency has only been studied in experimental animal models of hypertension, this discussion will focus on dietary supplementation with either linoleic acid or eicosapentaenoic acid as means of lowering blood pressure in both normotensive and hypertensive subjects. Table 5 summarizes some of the reported studies of the effects of polyunsaturated fatty acids on blood pressure control in normotensive and hypertensive humans. There is unanimity among these reports that either dietary supplementation with polyunsaturated fatty acids or reduction of saturated fatty acids, so that the polyunsaturated to unsaturated ratio approaches unity, will reduce blood pressure. The extent of the blood-pressure reduction was variable but generally ranged from 5 to 10 mm Hg systolic and diastolic. The specific explanation for the hypotensive action of polyunsaturated fat supplements is unknown, since the investigations with linoleic acid or sunflower oil did not document increased production of dienoic prostaglandins and the investigations with fish oils and eicosapentaenoic acid did not measure trienoic prostaglandins. Lorenz and co-workers, in a careful study of the effects of cod liver oil, 20 ml twice daily, documented that the increased dietary eicosapentaenoic acid altered platelet membrane phospholipids and reduced platelet aggregation and release of thromboxane. Urinary dienoic prostaglandins also decreased (14). These studies point out the potential efficacy of polyunsaturated fatty acid supplements as a means of reducing not only blood pressure but possibly also platelet adhesiveness and *in vivo* aggregability. The possible synergistic action of linoleic or eicosapentaenoic acid with diuretics and other antihypertensive drugs has not been tested.

TABLE 5. *Polyunsaturated fatty acids and control of blood pressure*

Author (ref.)	Subjects	Fatty acid	ΔBP
Vergroesen et al. (31)	EH	Sunflower oil	↓ BP
Stern et al. (29)	EH	Linoleic	↓ BP
Rao et al. (21)	EH		↓ BP
Ianoco et al. (10)	EH; N	P/S = 1; linoleic[a]	↓ BP
Puska et al. (20)	EH; N	P/S = 1; linoleic	↓ BP
Sanders et al. (26)	N	Cod liver oil	↓ BP
Mortensen et al. (16)	N	Eicosapentaenoic	↓ BP
Lorenz et al. (14)	N	Cod liver oil	↓ BP

[a]Polyunsaturated/saturated ratio and increased linoleic acid.
Abbreviations: EH, essential hypertension; N, normotensives.

SUMMARY

In normotensive and hypertensive humans, prostaglandins, particularly PGE_2 and PGI_2, affect blood pressure through control of vascular resistance, salt excretion, cardiac output, and renin secretion. The majority of studies of human essential hypertension have documented diminished renal synthesis and, hence, urinary excretion of PGE_2. The acute administration of indomethacin inhibits prostaglandin synthesis and increases total peripheral resistance as well as mean blood pressure, with a countervailing decrease of cardiac index. The important vasodilatory and natriuretic roles of PGE_2 and PGI_2 are most apparent in hypertensive patients receiving antihypertensive therapy. The concomitant use of NSAID attenuates blood-pressure control in all reported studies using indomethacin. Consequently, potent NSAID should be avoided during treatment of hypertensive patients, and aspirin may be the safest NSAID in these circumstances. Interesting data are accumulating on the beneficial effects of polyunsaturated fatty acids, particularly linoleic acid and eicosapentaenoic acid, as dietary means to reduce blood pressure. All reported studies have documented small 5 to 10 mm Hg decrements of blood pressure with dietary supplementation with these fatty acids and conversion of the ratio of polyunsaturated to saturated fatty acids toward unity.

ACKNOWLEDGMENTS

This work was supported by the National Institutes of Health, HL 02563. H.-J. Gröne was a recipient of a fellowship from Deutsche Forschungsgemeinschaft. Linda Goldberg provided excellent secretarial and editorial assistance.

REFERENCES

1. Abe, K., Yasujima, M., Chiba, S., Irokawa, N., Ito, T., and Yoshinaga, K. (1977): Effect of furosemide on urinary excretion of prostaglandin E in normal volunteers and patients with essential hypertension. *Prostaglandins*, 14:513–521.
2. Abe, K. (1981): The kinins and prostaglandins in hypertension. *Clin. Endocrinol. Metab.*, 10:577–605.
3. Campbell, W. B., Holland, O. B., and Adams, B. V. (1982): Urinary excretion of prostaglandin E_2, prostaglandin $F_{2\alpha}$ and thromboxane B_2 in normotensive and hypertensive subjects on varying sodium intakes. *Hypertension*, 4:735.
4. Donker, A. J. M., Arisz, L., and Brentjens, J. R. H. (1976): The effect of indomethacin on kidney function and plasma renin activity in man. *Nephron*, 17:288.
5. Dunn, M. J. (1983): Renal prostaglandins. In: *Renal Endocrinology*, edited by M. J. Dunn, pp. 1–74. Williams & Wilkins, Baltimore.
6. Durao, B., Martins Prata, M., and Pires Goncalves, L. M. (1977): Modification of antihypertensive effect of β-adrenoreceptor-blocking agents by inhibition of endogenous prostaglandin synthesis. *Lancet*, II:1005–1007.
7. Glänzer, K., Prüssing, B., Düsing, R., and Kramer, H. J. (1982): Hemodynamic and hormonal responses to 8-arginine-vasopressin in healthy man: Effects of indomethacin. *Klin. Wochenschr.*, 60:1234–1239.
8. Güllner, H. G., Gill, J. R., Bartter, F. C., and Düsing, R. (1980): The role of the prostaglandin system in the regulation of renal function in normal women. *Am. J. Med.*, 69:718–723.
9. Hermiller, J. B., Bambach, D., Thompson, M. J., Huss, P., Fontana, M. E., Magorien, R. D.,

Unverferth, D. V., and Leier, C. V. (1982): Vasodilators and prostaglandin inhibitors in primary pulmonary hypertension. *Ann. Intern. Med.*, 97:480–489.

10. Iacono, J. M., Dougherty, R. M., and Puska, P. (1982): Reduction of blood pressure associated with dietary polyunsaturated fat. *Hypertension*, 4(suppl. III):III-34–III-42.

11. Lebel, M., and Grose, J. H. (1982): Renal prostaglandins in borderline and sustained essential hypertension. *Prostaglandins Leukotrienes Med.*, 8:409–418.

12. London, G. M., Hornych, A., Safar, M. E., Levenson, J. A., and Simon, A. C. (1982): Plasma prostaglandins PGE_2 and $PGF_{2\alpha}$, total effective vascular compliance and renal plasma flow in essential hypertension. *Nephron*, 32:118–124.

13. Lopez-Ovejero, J. A., Weber, M. A., Drayer, J. I. M., Sealey, J. E., and Laragh, J. H. (1978): Effects of indomethacin alone and during diuretic or β-adrenoreceptor-blockade therapy on blood pressure and the renin system in essential hypertension. *Clin. Sci. Mol. Med.*, 55:203s–205s.

14. Lorenz, R., Spengler, U., Fischer, S., Duhm, J., and Weber, P. C. (1983): Platelet function, thromboxane formation and blood pressure control during supplementation of the Western diet with cod liver oil. *Circulation*, 67:504–511.

15. Mills, E. H., Whitworth, J. A., Andrews, J., and Kincaid-Smith, P. (1982): Non-steroidal anti-inflammatory drugs and blood pressure. *Aust. N. Z. J. Med.*, 12:478–482.

16. Mortensen, J. Z., Schmidt, E. B., Nielsen, A. H., and Dyerberg, J. (1983): The effect of N-6 and N-3 polyunsaturated fatty acids on hemostasis, blood lipids and blood pressure. *Thromb. Haemostas. (Stuttgart)*, 50:543–546.

17. Negus, P., Tannen, R. L., and Dunn, M. J. (1976): Indomethacin potentiates the vasoconstrictor actions of angiotensin II in normal man. *Prostaglandins*, 12:175–180.

18. Nowak, J., and Wennmalm, A. (1978): Influence of indomethacin and of prostaglandin E_1 on total and regional blood flow in man. *Acta Physiol. Scand.*, 102:484–491.

19. Patak, R. V., Mookerjee, B. K., Bentzel, C. J., Hysert, P. E., Babej, M., and Lee, J. B. (1975): Antagonism of the effects of furosemide by indomethacin in normal and hypertensive man. *Prostaglandins*, 10:649–659.

20. Puska, P., Nissinen, A., Vartiainen, E., Dougherty, R., Mutanen, Iacono, J., Korhonen, H. J., Pietinen, P., Leino, U., Moisio, S., and Huttunen, J. (1983): Controlled, randomised trial of the effect of dietary fat on blood pressure. *Lancet*, I:1–5.

21. Rao, R. H., Rao, U. B., and Srikantia, S. C. (1981): Effect of polyunsaturated-rich vegetable oils on blood pressure in essential hypertension. *Clin. Exp. Hypertension*, 3:27.

22. Rathaus, M., Korzets, Z., and Bernheim, J. (1983): The urinary excretion of prostaglandins E_2 and $F_{2\alpha}$ in essential hypertension. *Eur. J. Clin. Invest.*, 13:13–17.

23. Ruilope, L., Garcia Robles, R., Barrientos, A., Bernis, C., Alcazar, J., Tresguerres, J. A. F., Mancheno, E., Millet, V. G., Sancho, J., and Rodicio, J. L. (1982): The role of urinary PGE_2 and renin–angiotensin–aldosterone system in the pathogenesis of essential hypertension. *Clin. Exper. Hyper.*, A4:989–1000.

24. Safar, M. E., Hornych, A. F., Levenson, J. A., Simon, A. C., London, G. M., Bariety, J. L., and Milliez, P. L. (1981): *Clin. Sci.*, 61:323s–325s.

25. Salvetti, A., Pedrinelli, R., and Magagna, A. (1983): The influence of indomethacin on some pharmacologic actions of atenolol. In: *Prostaglandins and the Kidney*, edited by M. J. Dunn, C. Patrono, and G. Cinotti, pp. 287–295. Plenum Medical Book Company, New York.

26. Sanders, T. A. B., Vickers, M., and Haines, A. P. (1981): Effect on blood lipids and haemostasis of a supplement of cod-liver oil, rich in eicosapentaenoic and docosahexaenoic acids, in healthy young men. *Clin. Sci.*, 61:317–324.

27. Sato, K., Abe, M., Seino, M., Yasujima, M., Chiba, S, Sato, M., Haruyama, T., Hiwatari, M., Goto, T., Tajima, J., Tanno, M., and Yoshinaga, K. (1983): Reduced urinary excretion of prostaglandin E in essential hypertension. *Prostaglandins, Leukotrienes Med.*, 11:188–197.

28. Smith, M. C., and Dunn, M. J. (1981): Renal kallikrein, kinins, and prostaglandins in hypertension. In: *Hypertension*, edited by B. M. Brenner and J. Stein, pp. 168–202. Churchill Livingstone, New York.

29. Stern, B., Heyden, S., Miller, D., Latham, G., Klimas, A., and Pilkington, K. (1980): Intervention study in high school students with elevated blood pressures. *Nutr. Metab.*, 24:137–147.

30. Tan, S. Y., Bravo, E., and Mulrow, P. J. (1978): Impaired renal prostaglandin E_2 biosynthesis in human hypertensive states. *Prostaglandins Med.*, 1:76–85.

31. Vergroesen, A. J., Fleischman, A. I., Comberg, H.-U., Heyden, S., and Hames, C. G. (1978):

The influence of increased dietary linoleate on essential hypertension in man. *Acta Biol. Med. Germ.*, 37:879–883.

32. Vierhapper, H., Waldhäusl, W., and Nowotny, P. (1981): Effect of indomethacin upon angiotensin-induced changes in blood pressure and plasma aldosterone in normal man. *Eur. J. Clin. Invest.*, 11:85–89.

33. Watkins, J., Abbott, E. C., Hensby, C. N., Webster, J., and Dollery, C. T. (1980): Attenuation of hypotensive effect of propranolol and thiazide diuretics by indomethacin. *Br. Med. J.*, 281:702–705.

34. Weber, P. C., Scherer, B., Held, E., Siess, W., and Stoffel, H. (1979): Urinary prostaglandins and kallikrein in essential hypertension. *Clin. Sci.*, 57:259s–261s.

35. Wing, L. M. H., Bune, A. J. C., Chalmers, J. P., Graham, J. R., and West, M. J. (1981): The effects of indomethacin in treated hypertensive patients. *Clin. Exp. Pharmacol. Physiol.*, 8:537–541.

36. Ylitalo, P., Pitkäjärvi, T., Metsä-Ketelä, T., and Vapaatalo, H. (1978): The effect of inhibition of prostaglandin synthesis on plasma renin activity and blood pressure in essential hypertension. *Prostaglandins Med.*, 1:479–488.

Advances in Prostaglandin, Thromboxane, and
Leukotriene Research, Vol. 13, edited by G. G. Neri
Serneri, et al. Raven Press, New York © 1985.

Effects of Acute Hydration on Urinary Kallikrein Production in Hypertensive Patients

G. Masotti, R. Sciagrà, F. Trotta, S. Castellani, and G. G. Neri Serneri

Clinica Medica I, University of Florence, 50134 Florence, Italy

The renal kallikrein-kinin system represents a homeostatic mechanism which, through prostaglandin mediation, is involved in the regulation of renal vascular resistance (3) and volume excretion. An alteration of this system has often been considered as a possible pathogenetic mechanism of essential hypertension (9). However, in some reports urinary kallikrein has been found to be reduced in hypertensive patients (4,7,9) and in other reports no statistical differences were found from controls (5,6).

The present study was designed to verify whether in hypertensive patients the response of the kallikrein-kinin system is defective in front of a condition able to strongly stimulate the renal homeostasis, such as volume expansion (1).

MATERIALS AND METHODS

Ten patients were studied (7 females; 3 males) with II WHO grade essential hypertension (mean age 41.5 ± 8 years) and 10 control normotensive subjects matched for age (mean age 42.7 ± 6.6 years), sex, body weight, and smoking habits.

No subject presented with diabetes, cardiac or renal disease and none had taken any drugs in the previous three weeks. After 5 days of standard 108 mEq sodium, 80 mEq potassium diet, fasting subjects were introduced a vesical catheter and lay in a supine position for 3 hr before and throughout the experiment. Urine was collected 2 hr before (baseline sample) and 1 hr during volume expansion (500 ml 5% glucose i.v. infusion). Urinary kallikrein was measured, as a reliable index of renal kallikrein-kinin system, by a radioenzymatic method (2) and urinary sodium was measured by a flame photometer.

RESULTS

In the two groups, urinary volume was not statistically different in baseline conditions and was potently and equally stimulated by volume expansion (Table 1). In addition, sodium excretion was similarly stimulated in the two groups (Fig. 1). In hypertensive patients baseline values of urinary kallikrein were significantly lower than in controls (0.32 ± 0.09 esterase units (EU)/hr vs. 0.73 ± 0.26 EU/hr, $p < 0.001$). Volume expansion showed a stimulus able to induce a significant and consistent increase of urinary kallikrein both in control and hypertensive patients (Fig. 2). In hypertensive patients the absolute increase was also greater so that

TABLE 1. *Urinary volume (ml/min)*

	Baseline	During 1 hr volume expansion (500 ml 5% glucose i.v. infusion)
Controls	0.97 ± 0.22	5.26 ± 2.5
Patients with essential hypertension	0.79 ± 0.29	6.15 ± 3.04

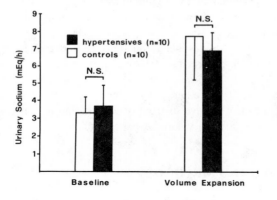

FIG. 1. Effects of volume expansion (500 ml 5% glucose i.v. infusion) on urinary sodium excretion (mEq/hr).

FIG. 2. Effects of volume expansion (500 ml 5% glucose i.v. infusion) on urinary kallikrein excretion (EU/hr).

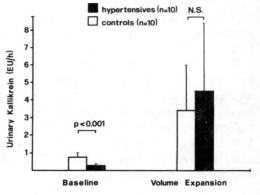

after glucose infusion there were no more statistical differences between the two groups.

CONCLUSIONS

The present results indicate pure volume expansion as a physiologic condition able to stimulate the kallikrein-kinin system independently from variations of sodium intake as employed in previous investigations (1).

In baseline conditions, urinary kallikrein excretion is depressed in essential hypertension, therefore supporting similar previous observations (3,4–9) and opposing those reporting no differences from controls (5,6). However, the increase in kallikrein excretion after volume expansion as great as in controls does not support the hypothesis that an impairment of this system is of pathogenetic importance in essential hypertension. This consideration is limited by the small number of hypertensive patients examined and by their electrolyte balance showing a normal baseline and stimulated sodium excretion. Hypertensive patients with sodium retention should be examined before drawing definitive conclusions, since the pathogenetic relevance of the kallikrein-kinin system for hypertension could be limited to situations characterized by a defective sodium excretion.

REFERENCES

1. Abe, K., Sato, M., Imay, I., Haruyama, T., Sato, K., Hiwatari, M., Kasai, Y., and Yashinaga, K. (1981): Renal kallikrein-kinin: Its relation to urinary prostaglandins and renin-angiotensin-aldosterone in man. *Kidney Int.*, 19:869–880.
2. Beaven, V. H., Pierce, J. V., and Pisano, J. J. (1971): A sensitive isotopic procedure for the assay of esterase activity: Measurement of human urinary kallikrein. *Clin. Chim. Acta*, 32:67–73.
3. Carretero, O. A., and Scicli, A. G. (1980): The renal kallikrein-kinin system. *Am. J. Physiol.*, 238:247–255.
4. Elliot, A. H., and Nuzum, F. R. (1934): Urinary excretion of a depressor substance (kallikrein of Frey and Kraut) in arterial hypertension. *Endocrinology*, 18:462–474.
5. Holland, O. B., Chud, J. M., and Brauenstein, H. (1980): Urinary kallikrein excretion in essential and mineral corticoid hypertension, *J. Clin. Invest.*, 65:347–356.
6. Lawton, W. J., and Fitz, A. E. (1980): Abnormal urinary kallikrein in hypertension is not related to aldosterone or plasma renin activity. *Hypertension*, 2:787–793.
7. Lechi, A., Covi, G., Corgnati, A., Arosio, E., Zatti, M., and Scuro, L. A. (1978): Urinary kallikrein excretion and plasma renin activity in patients with essential hypertension and primary aldosteronism. *Clin. Sci. Mol. Med.*, 55:51–55.
8. Levy, S. B., Lilley, J. J., Frigon, R. P., and Stone, R. A. (1977): Urinary kallikrein and plasma renin activity as determinants of renal blood flow: The influence of race and dietary sodium intake. *J. Clin. Invest.*, 60:129–138.
9. Margolius, H. S., Horwitz, D., Pisano, J. J., and Keiser, H. R. (1974): Urinary kallikrein excretion in hypertensive man. Relationship to sodium intake and sodium retaining steroids. *Circ. Res.*, 35:820–825.

Advances in Prostaglandin, Thromboxane, and Leukotriene Research, Vol. 13, edited by G. G. Neri Serneri, et al. Raven Press, New York © 1985.

Urinary Kallikrein in Mild to Moderate Essential Hypertension

*F. Franchi, *G. Strazzulla, *A. Scardi, *P. Lo Sapio, *G. Fabbri, **M. Mannelli, and †C. Curradi

*Istituto di Clinica Medica IV (Cattedra di Patologia Speciale Medica II), **Servizio di Endocrinologia USL 10/D-Florence, and †Istituto di Patologia Medica e Farmacologia Clinica, University of Florence, 50134 Florence, Italy

Various reports indicate that urinary kallikrein excretion was either decreased or normal in patients with essential hypertension (1,4,5,8). Its significance is not clear in the pathophysiology of high blood pressure. The present study was designed to reexamine the urinary excretion of kallikrein and its relationship to natriuresis and to the renin–angiotensin–aldosterone system. Two groups were evaluated: those with early essential hypertension (hemodynamically defined), and age-matched normotensive subjects. The stimulating effect of furosemide was then assessed in hypertensives.

PATIENTS AND METHODS

Sixteen untreated hospitalized patients [13 males, 3 females, mean age 57 ± 2.5 (SD) years] with mild to moderate (World Health Organization I–II) essential hypertension (mean blood pressure, MBP: 125 ± 16.8 mm Hg) and normotensive hospitalized patients (6 males, 4 females, mean age 52 ± 4 SD) were studied. A strict dietary control was imposed. All hypertensives underwent radionuclide angiocardiography (99mTc) in order to assess their cardiovascular profile. Informed consent was obtained from all participants.

In 24-hr urine samples, kallikrein, creatinine, sodium, and aldosterone were measured. At the end of the collection period, plasma renin activity (PRA) and plasma creatinine values were obtained. PRA was measured both in the supine (PRA_1) and standing (PRA_2) positions. The esterolytic activity of urinary kallikrein was estimated using a fluorogenic peptide substrate following the technique of Kato et al. (3). Values of urinary kallikrein activity are expressed in terms of nanomoles methylcoumarylamide (AMC) liberated per minute, with relation to the collection period. Sodium and creatinine clearance were measured by standard methods. Urinary aldosterone and PRA were evaluated by radioimmunoassay.

In 14 of the 16 hypertensive patients, two 6-hr urinary collections (1 to 7 p.m.) were then carried out. PRA_1 and PRA_2 were measured after both collection periods. Prior to the second collection, 40 mg furosemide was administered intravenously.

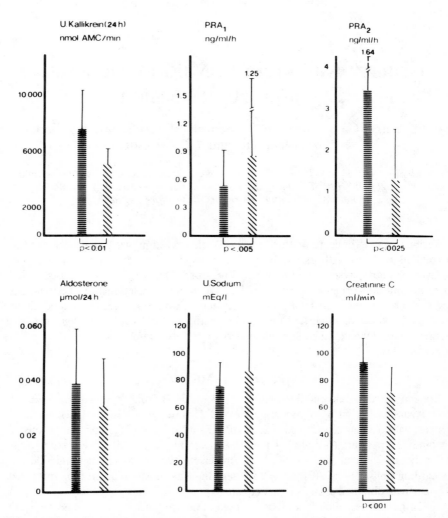

FIG. 1. Mean values ± SD under basal conditions. Horizontal bars indicate the normotensives; oblique bars indicate the hypertensives. U. = urinary, PRA = plasma renin activity, C. = clearance, AMC = methylcoumarylamide.

The urine samples were evaluated for kallikrein, aldosterone, and sodium excretion.

RESULTS

In basal conditions, hypertensive patients showed a slight increase in the systemic vascular resistance index (SVRI = 3371 ± 501 dyne·sec·cm⁵·m²) with a normality of left ventricular function indexes. Urinary kallikrein activity (Fig. 1) was de-

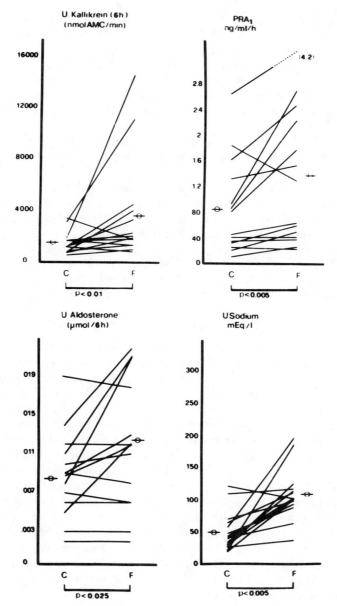

FIG. 2. Single and mean values before (C) and after (F) 40 mg i.v. furosemide in 14 hypertensives. Abbreviations are the same as in Fig. 1.

creased, although with a high dispersion of values, in these patients in respect to normotensive individuals (5166 ± 2092 versus 7712 ± 2789 nmole AMC/min, $p < 0.01$). Furthermore, the PRA_2 was reduced in the hypertensives, as was the creatinine clearance, with respect to the normotensives (1.31 ± 1.24 versus 3.54 ± 1.64 ng/ml·hr; 72.3 ± 18.5 versus 94.8 ± 18.7 ml/min; $p < 0.0025$ and $p < 0.01$, respectively). The creatinine clearance, however, was within the lower limits of the normal range. PRA_1 was higher in the hypertensives (0.86 ± 1.25 versus 0.54 ± 0.38; $p < 0.005$).

No correlation has been found between urinary kallikrein excretion and the following: urinary volume, creatinine clearance, natriuresis, aldosterone excretion, PRA_1, PRA_2, MBP, and SVRI.

After intravenous furosemide (Fig. 2), the hypertensive participants showed a significant increase, with respect to normal controls, in urinary kallikrein (3742 ± 3058 versus 1531 ± 871 nmole AMC/min, $p < 0.025$), PRA_1 and PRA_2 (1.37 ± 1.14 and 1.87 ± 1.47 versus 0.85 ± 0.72 and 1.16 ± 0.76 ng/ml·hr, $p < 0.005$ and $p < 0.01$, respectively), urinary aldosterone (0.011 ± 0.006 versus 0.008 ± 0.004 μmole/6 hr, $p < 0.025$), and natriuresis (107 ± 36 versus 51.2 ± 30 mEq/liter, $p < 0.0005$). The only linear relation found was that between the change in percent urinary kallikrein and the change in percent natriuresis ($r = 0.58$, $p < 0.05$).

DISCUSSION

The reduced mean urinary kallikrein excretion (although with a high dispersion of values), found in basal condition in our early hypertensive patients, is not in complete agreement with the normal urinary kallikrein excretion of mild or labile essential hypertension as reported by other authors (4,6). Our findings suggest that a subnormal kallikrein excretion is not secondary to the hypertensive process. In fact, none of our hypertensives showed any definite impairment of renal and cardiac functions. Furthermore, no correlation was found between urinary kallikrein and hemodynamic indexes. The role of the renal kallikrein–kinin system in the pathophysiology of essential hypertension is still unknown and needs further definition.

Furosemide stimulates kallikrein excretion (7,9). Therefore, the synthesis of glandular kallikrein in the first stages of essential hypertension is probably preserved. This finding, along with the positive correlation between kallikrein and sodium excretion, may indicate that part of the prompt natriuretic and antihypertensive effects of furosemide is mediated by means of an increased activity in the renal kallikrein–kinin system. The lack of any correlation between urinary kallikrein and aldosterone confirms that aldosterone is not the mediator of the acute increase of urinary kallikrein (2).

REFERENCES

1. Carretero, O. A., and Scicli, A. G. (1978): The renal kallikrein–kinin system in human and experimental hypertension. *Klin. Wochenschr.*, 56(suppl.I):113–125.
2. Carretero, O. A., and Scicli, A. G. (1983): The renal kallikrein–kinin system. In: *Renal Endocrinology*, edited by M. J. Dunn, pp.96–113. Williams & Wilkins, Baltimore.

3. Kato, H., Adachi, N., Iwanaga, S., Abe, K., Takada, K., Kimura, T., and Sakakibara, S. (1980): A new fluorogenic substrate method for the estimation of kallikrein in urine. *J. Biochem.*, 87:1127–1132.

4. Lawton, W. S., and Fritz, A. E. (1977): Urinary kallikrein in normal renin essential hypertension. *Circulation*, 56:856–859.

5. Mersey, J., Williams, G., Emanuel, R., Dluhy, R. G., Wong, P. Y., and Moore, T. S. (1979): Plasma bradykinin levels and urinary kallikrein excretion in normal renin essential hypertension. *J. Clin. Endocrinol. Metab.*, 48:642–647.

6. Overlack, A., Stumpe, K. O., Zywzok, W., Ressel, C., and Krück, F. (1978): Renale kallikreinausscheidung bei normotonikern und hypertonikern unter unterschiedlicher kochsalzzufuhr. *Verh. Dtsch. Ges. Inn. Med.*, 84:810–813.

7. Seino, M., Abe, K., Irokawa, N., Ito, T., Yasujima, M., Sakurai, Y., Chiba, S., Saito, K., Ritz, K., Kusaka, T., Miyazaki, S., and Yoshinaga, K. (1978): Effect of furosemide on urinary kallikrein excretion in patients with essential hypertension. *Tohoku J. Exp. Med.*, 124:197–203.

8. Weber, P. C., Scherer, E., Held, E., Siess, W., and Stoffel, H. (1979): Urinary prostaglandins and kallikrein in essential hypertension. *Clin. Sci.*, 57:259s–261s.

9. Zschiedrich, H., Fleckenstein, P., Geiger, R., Fink, E., Sinterhauf, K., Philipp, T., Distler, A., and Wolff, H. P. (1980): Urinary kallikrein in normotensive subjects and in patients with essential hypertension. *Clin. Exp. Hypertension*, 2:693–708.

Advances in Prostaglandin, Thromboxane, and Leukotriene Research, Vol. 13, edited by G. G. Neri Serneri, et al. Raven Press, New York © 1985.

Urinary 6-Keto-PGF$_{1\alpha}$ After Captopril and Indomethacin: Possible Contribution of PGI$_2$ to the Antihypertensive Mechanism of ACE Inhibitors

*P. Minuz, **M. Degan, **G. Covi, †C. Lechi, *G. P. Velo, and **A. Lechi

*Istituto di Farmacologia, **Clinica Medica, and †Cattedra di Chimica e Microscopia Clinica, University of Verona, Verona, Italy

The mechanism of action of angiotensin-converting enzyme (ACE) inhibitors essentially consists of a decreased production of angiotensin II and, consequently, of a reduction of peripheral and renal vasoconstriction, of aldosterone production, and maybe of the effects of angiotensin II on the central nervous system. However, this mechanism does not completely explain the antihypertensive activity of these drugs, which is not always related to plasma renin activity. Since ACE is also a kininase II, many authors have suggested that ACE inhibitors could act through an inhibition of kinin metabolism and therefore an amplification of their vasodilator and antihypertensive effects (5). Moreover, it is well known that the antihypertensive effect of kinins is partially mediated by prostaglandins (PGs), particularly prostacyclin (PGI$_2$) (3), and therefore, prostaglandin synthetase inhibitors could reduce the efficacy of ACE inhibitors in lowering blood pressure. The aim of this study was to evaluate the effect of the inhibition of prostaglandin synthesis on the urinary excretion of prostacyclin metabolite 6-keto-PGF$_{1\alpha}$ in patients treated with captopril.

Eight patients with mild or moderate essential hypertension (1–2 World Health Organization) aged 22 to 55 years, mean age 37, were treated for 1 week with captopril at 50 mg t.i.d. After day 4 of treatment, the patients received in addition 50 mg t.i.d. indomethacin. The patients had not been treated before the study with other antihypertensive drugs and did not take any drugs in the previous 2 weeks. They received a standard hospital diet (about 140 mEq NaCl/day).

Before treatment and at days 4 and 7 of treatment, blood pressure, heart rate, plasma renin activity (PRA), and plasma aldosterone in supine and upright position were determined. The 24-hr urine collections were also taken at the same time. Urinary excretion of kallikrein and 6-keto-PGF$_{1\alpha}$ was determined. Urinary 6-keto-

TABLE 1. *Modification of plasma renin activity, plasma aldosterone, mean arterial pressure, urinary kallikrein and urinary 6-keto-PGF$_{1\alpha}$ after treatment with captopril and captopril plus indomethacin*

Parameter	Condition	Basal	Difference	Captopril	Difference	Captopril + indomethacin
PRA (ng/ml · hr)	Supine	0.41 ± 0.34		0.49 ± 0.40		0.30 ± 0.23
	Upright	1.00 ± 0.54		3.75 ± 4.75	*	0.85 ± 0.73
Aldosterone (pg/ml)	Supine	91.8 ± 31.8		72.5 ± 40.9		68.7 ± 30.8
	Upright	130.0 ± 36.5		110.0 ± 53.7		121.4 ± 54.3
Mean arterial pressure (mm Hg)	Supine	145 ± 22.6	**	116 ± 18.3	**	130 ± 17.5
	Upright	146 ± 22.6	***	122 ± 15.8	***	130 ± 16.9
Urinary kallikrein (μmole/24 hr)		10.5 ± 2.17		10.0 ± 4.32		7.22 ± 4.41
Urinary 6-keto-PGF$_{1\alpha}$ (ng/24 hr)		442.5 ± 155.3		439.8 ± 170.1	*	251.2 ± 57.3

Values are expressed as mean ± standard deviation.
Significance of difference between data in adjacent columns: * $p < 0.05$; ** $p < 0.01$; *** $p < 0.005$.

$PGF_{1\alpha}$, plasma renin activity, and plasma aldosterone were measured by radioimmunoassay, and urinary kallikrein by colorimetric assay.

RESULTS

Mean arterial pressure decreased significantly after captopril, but this effect was almost totally abolished by indomethacin administration (Table 1).

PRA, in upright position, increased after captopril and returned to basal levels after indomethacin. Plasma aldosterone levels and urinary kallikrein excretion were not significantly modified by either treatment. Urinary 6-keto-$PGF_{1\alpha}$ was significantly reduced after treatment with both captopril and indomethacin.

DISCUSSION

The inhibition of prostaglandin synthesis could favor a hypertensive effect by enhancing the vascular sensitivity to pressor hormones like catecholamines or angiotensin and by inducing salt retention. This effect is particularly evident for ACE inhibitors, and our data indicate that the antihypertensive activity of captopril was almost completely abolished by prostaglandin inhibitors such as indomethacin. Other authors have shown a similar effect after indomethacin or other cyclooxygenase inhibitors, and this phenomenon was heightened when associated with a high salt intake (1). Captopril might act through a mechanism that is not only dependent on the renin–angiotensin system but also mediated, at least in part, by prostaglandins. Our data do not show any variation in 6-keto-$PGF_{1\alpha}$ urinary excretion during treatment with captopril, and this seems inconsistent with an increase in the synthesis of this compound. Other authors, however, have observed an increase in the plasma levels of prostaglandins or their metabolites after acute captopril administration. Moreover, a direct captopril-induced prostaglandin release was observed *in vitro* in rabbit renomedullary interstitial cells (2,4,6).

It is possible that the determination of urinary 6-keto-$PGF_{1\alpha}$ may not represent the most direct expression of a vascular and/or renal phenomenon. Moreover, the data are controversial and a correlation between prostaglandin and kinin level variations and the antihypertensive effect of the drug has not always been demonstrated.

Finally, it is important in the clinical practice to be aware that nonsteroidal antiinflammatory drugs can substantially reduce the antihypertensive action of captopril.

REFERENCES

1. Goldstone, R., Martin, K., Zipser, R., and Horton, R. (1981): Evidence for a dual action of converting enzyme inhibitor on blood pressure in normal man. *Prostaglandins*, 22:587–598.
2. Moore, T. J., Crantz, F. R., Hollenberg, N. K., Koletsky, R. J., Leboff, M. S., Swartz, S. L., Levine, L., Podolsky, S., Dluhy, R. G., and Williams, G. H. (1981): Contribution of prostaglandins to the antihypertensive action of captopril in essential hypertension. *Hypertension*, 3:168–173.
3. Mullane, K. M., and Moncada, S. (1980): Prostacyclin release and the modulation of some vasoactive hormones. *Prostaglandins*, 20:25–49.

4. Mullane, K. M., and Moncada, S. (1980): Prostacyclin mediates the potentiated hypotensive effect of bradykinin following captopril treatment. *Eur. J. Pharmacol.*, 66:355–365.
5. Swartz, S. L., Williams, G. H., Hollenberg, N. K., Moore, T. J., and Dluhy, R. G. (1979): Converting enzyme inhibition in essential hypertension: the hypotensive response does not reflect only reduced angiotensin II formation. *Hypertension*, 1:106–111.
6. Zusman, R. M. (1981): Captopril stimulates prostaglandin E_2 synthesis *in vitro*: Possible mechanism of antihypertensive action. *Clin. Res.*, 29:362A.

Advances in Prostaglandin, Thromboxane, and
Leukotriene Research, Vol. 13, edited by G.G. Neri
Serneri, et al. Raven Press, New York © 1985.

Altered Renal Prostaglandin Production after Sodium Loading in Hypertensive Patients

G. G. Neri Serneri, S. Castellani, L. Scarti, F. Trotta, R. Sciagrà, and G. Masotti

Clinica Medica I, University of Florence, 50134 Florence, Italy

Renal prostaglandins (PG) are of primary importance in the regulation of renal vascular resistance since they modulate the vasconstrictor response to pressor stimuli such as AII (8) and adrenergic activation (7). Moreover, renal prostaglandins participate in the regulation of volume excretion by the kidney (4). Therefore, an impaired prostaglandin synthesis could be a possible mechanism of hypertension.

In the present study, production of renal prostaglandins was studied in hypertensive patients both in baseline conditions and after a stimulus, such as acute sodium loading, which strongly challenges water and sodium homeostasis by the kidney.

MATERIALS AND METHODS

Seven healthy females aged 25 to 46 years and 7 females affected by essential hypertension aged 26 to 48 years were studied. Male subjects had been excluded in order to avoid urinary contamination by prostaglandin of extrarenal origin (9). All subjects were nonsmokers, did not present with diabetes or renal diseases, and had not taken antihypertensive or cyclooxygenase inhibitory drugs in the previous three weeks. After 5 days of standard 108 mEq Na, 80 mEq potassium diet, fasting subjects were infused i.v. with 150 mEq of Na in 150 ml solution in 10 min and maintained a supine position throughout the experiment. Urines were collected during 3 hr before and 2, 4, 8, and 12 hr after the infusion and stored at $-20°C$ until the assay. Urinary PGE_2 and $PGF_{2\alpha}$ were measured by radioimmunoassay (RIA) according to Ciabattoni et al. (1) after extraction and purification. Statistical analysis of the data was performed by analysis of variance and Student's t-test. Results are given as mean $\pm$ SD.

RESULTS

Baseline urinary PGE_2 excretion in hypertensive women was lower than in controls without reaching statistical significance and $PGF_{2\alpha}$ was significantly greater ($p < 0.001$).

Hypertonic sodium loading induced, during the 12 hr of observation, completely different effects in the two groups (Fig. 1). In normotensive patients, the increase of both PGE_2 and $PGF_{2\alpha}$ was sustained and lasted for 8 hr. In hypertensive patients, sodium loading did not induce any significant variations of PGE_2 excretion compared to baseline values but greatly increased $PGF_{2\alpha}$ (Fig. 1). These differences

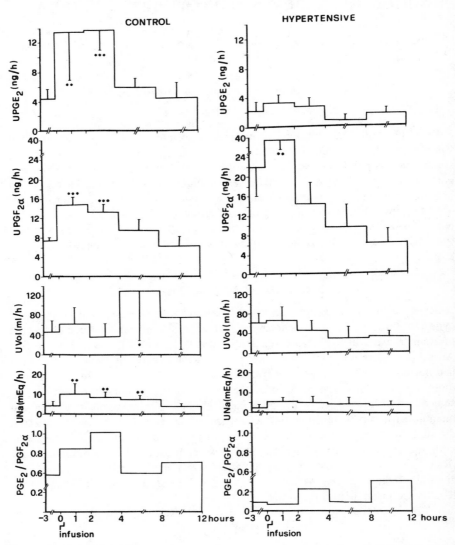

FIG. 1. Effects of a 100 mEq Na i.v. infusion in 150 ml in 10 min on urine (U) PGs, U Na, and U volume during a 12 hr period in 7 healthy females and 7 female patients affected by essential hypertension (mean values ± SD). Each value after infusion was tested against the value before infusion (* = $p<0.05$; ** = $p<0.01$; *** = $p<0.001$).

are particularly evident in the first 2 hr after sodium loading (Fig. 2). However, the stimulating effect of sodium loading on prostaglandin excretion in hypertensive patients is short lasting, as shown from the average hourly excretion calculated in the 12 hr period, when the majority of infused sodium was excreted (Fig. 3). Whereas in normotensive controls the excretion was significantly greater for both

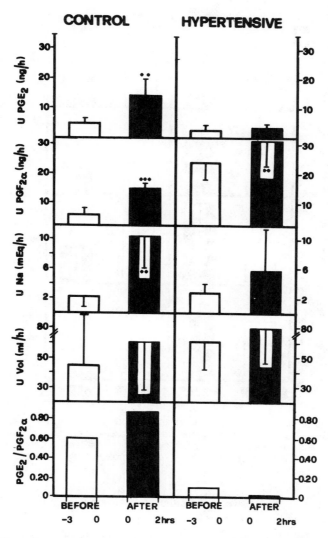

FIG. 2. Effects of a 100 mEq Na i.v. infusion in 150 ml in 10 min on urine (U) PGs, U Na, and U volume (mean values ± SD for 7 healthy females and 7 female patients affected by essential hypertension) during the first 2 hr after infusion. Each value after infusion was tested by the paired Student's *t*-test against the value before infusion (** = $p < 0.01$; *** = $p < 0.001$).

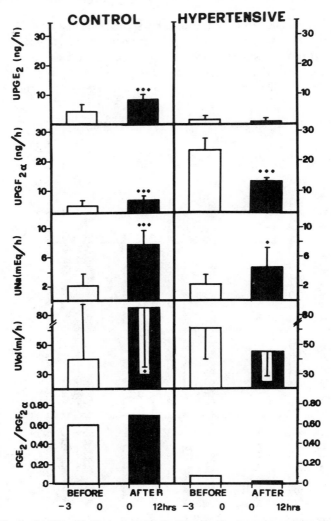

FIG. 3. Effects of a 100 mEq Na i.v. infusion in 150 ml in 10 min on the average hourly excretion of urine (U) PGs, U Na, and U volume calculated on the entire 12 hr period of observation in 7 healthy females and 7 female patients affected by essential hypertension (mean values ± SD). Each value after infusion was tested against the value before infusion (* = $p<0.05$; ** = $p<0.01$; *** = $p<0.001$).

prostaglandins, in hypertensive patients the hourly average excretion of $PGF_{2\alpha}$ was even lower than baseline values ($p<0.001$). Concerning sodium excretion, controls were found to eliminate in 12 hr 80% of the infused sodium, and hypertensive patients only 50% ($p<0.01$). No relationship was found by means of variance analysis in the 12 hr time course between sodium water diuresis and excretion of the two prostaglandins for both control and hypertensive patients.

DISCUSSION

Present results not only confirm previous observations (10) of a defective renal PGE_2 formation in hypertensive patients but also show for the first time a significantly higher excretion of $PGF_{2\alpha}$ emphasized by sodium loading.

The mechanism of diversion of renal prostaglandin synthesis towards $PGF_{2\alpha}$ in essential hypertension cannot be inferred from the present study, but could be tentatively interpreted as a consequence of a higher activity of 9-keto-reductase, an enzyme particularly active in the kidney that is stimulated by a high sodium tissue content (11). Formation of renal PGE_2 in hypertensive patients seems to be particularly depressed since it does not increase even after acute sodium loading, a condition known to be a potent stimulator of renal prostaglandins (5). The sodium-induced increase of $PGF_{2\alpha}$ itself is limited in time as if prostaglandin-forming potential by the hypertensive kidney would be in some way "exhausted".

Present results do not offer any data on the role of the defective renal prostaglandin synthesis in essential hypertension. They only suggest that PGE_2 seems not to be directly involved in the defective sodium excretion observed in hypertensive patients under study. However, the defect of a prostaglandin such as PGE_2 that mediates the renal autoregulation and favors volume excretion (3,6) together with diversion towards $PGF_{2\alpha}$ that constricts blood vessels, especially veins (2) and augments adrenergic nervous activity (3), seem to be factors able to worsen the increased vascular resistance typical of essential hypertension.

REFERENCES

1. Ciabattoni, G., Pugliese, F., Spaldi, M., Cinotti, G. A., and Patrono, C. (1979): Radioimmunoassay of prostaglandin E_2 and F_{2alpha} in human urine. *J. Endocrinol. Invest.*, 2:173–182.
2. Ducharme, D. W., Weeks, J. R., and Montgomery, R. G. (1968): Studies on the mechanism of the hypertensive effect of prostaglandin F_{2alpha}. *J. Pharmacol. Exp. Ther.*, 160:1–10.
3. Frame, M. H. (1976): A comparison of the effects of prostaglandins A_2, E_2 and F_{2alpha} on the sympathetic neuroeffector system of the isolated rabbit kidney. In: *Advances in Prostaglandin and Thromboxane Research, Vol. 1*, edited by B. Samuelsson, and R. Paoletti, pp. 368–373. Raven Press, New York.
4. Grantham, J. J., and Orloff, J. (1968): Effect of prostaglandin E_1 on the permeability response of the isolated collecting tubule to vasopressin, adenosine 3'5'-monophosphate, and theophylline. *J. Clin. Invest.*, 47:1154–1161.
5. Kaye, Z., Zipser, R. D., Majeda, S., Zia, P. K., and Horton, R. (1979): Renal prostaglandins and sodium balance in normal man. *Prostaglandins Med.*, 2:123–131.
6. Kramer, H. J., Backer, A., Hinzen, S., and Dusing, R. (1978): Effects of inhibition of prostaglandin synthesis on renal electrolyte excretion and concentrating ability in healthy man. *Prostaglandins Med.*, 1:341–349.
7. Malik, K. U., and McGiff, J. C. (1975): Modulation by prostaglandins of adrenergic transmission in isolated perfused rabbit and rat kidney. *Circ. Res.*, 36:599–609.
8. McGiff, J. C., Crowshaw, K., Terragno, H. A., and Lonigro, A. J. (1970): Release of a prostaglandin-like substance into renal venous blood in response to angiotensin II. *Circ. Res.*, 26(I):121–130.
9. Patrono, C., Wennmalm, A., Ciabattoni, G., Nowak, J., Pugliese, F., and Cinotti, G. (1979):

Evidence for an extrarenal origin of urinary prostaglandin E_2 in healthy men. *Prostaglandins*, 18:623–629.

10. Tan, S. J., Sweet, P., and Mulrow, P. J. (1978): Impaired renal production of prostaglandin E_2: A newly identified lesion in human essential hypertension. *Prostaglandins*, 15:139–149.

11. Weber, P. C., Larsson, C., and Scherer, D. (1977): Prostaglandin E_2-9-keto-reductase as a mediator of salt-intake-related prostaglandin-renin interaction. *Nature*, 266:65–66.

Advances in Prostaglandin, Thromboxane, and
Leukotriene Research, Vol. 13, edited by G. G. Neri
Serneri, et al. Raven Press, New York © 1985.

Thromboxane and Leukotrienes in Clinical and Experimental Transplant Rejection

*M. L. Foegh, **M. R. Alijani, **G. B. Helfrich,
†B. S. Khirabadi, ‡M. H. Goldman, ‡R. R. Lower,
and †P. W. Ramwell

*Department of Medicine, Division of Nephrology, **Department of Surgery, Division of
Transplantation, †Department of Physiology and Biophysics, Georgetown University
Medical Center, Washington, D.C. 20007; and ‡Division of Cardiac Surgery,
Medical College of Virginia, Richmond, Virginia 23298

Organ transplantation is a challenging field where most technical, surgical problems have been resolved; however, there is now better appreciation of the limitations of historical immunology to long-term graft survival. Knowledge of arachidonic acid metabolism provides a valuable opportunity to relate and strengthen these two key areas. There are several reasons for believing arachidonate products have a highly significant role in transplantation. First, the activation of arachidonate metabolism appears to be an early and perhaps immediate step following cell activation. Second, the products have powerful immunologically active properties in their own right (7,8). Consequently these products can be used as indicators with a causal role. Third, the qualitatively opposite effects of some of the products (5) opens the possibility of using some metabolites in a cytoprotective role while interdicting the pathogenic products. Fourth, the availability of many existing and new drugs that affect the arachidonate system permits ready experimental evaluation of the contributions of arachidonate products to transplant rejection. This, in turn, permits better insight into the existing treatment modalities and enables their use to be more effective.

CELLS INVOLVED IN REJECTION

During organ rejection, the allograft is invaded by a variety of inflammatory cells. The cellular composition of both cardiac and renal allografts has been determined during rejection by several investigators with largely concordant results (11,18,19). The first cells to invade the untreated experimental allograft are lymphocytes and monocytes. This is then followed by a blastogenic response *in situ*. In recent publications, Hayry and his collaborators reported on the presence of T-cell subsets in a rejecting renal allograft in the rat (10,11). When the cells of the allograft were dispersed and were analyzed with monoclonal antibodies directed to the lymphoid subsets, the majority of the infiltrating cells were T cells. Within the T-cell subsets, the T suppressor/cytotoxic cells (T_8) predominated. Also present in the lymphoid infiltrate was a sizable population of B cells. At later stages, mononuclear phagocytes dominated the inflammatory picture. Invasion of polymorphonucleocytes (PMN) is mainly seen in hyperacute rejection. The involvement of platelets in hyperacute rejection is well documented (15), but the association of platelets with acute rejection has not been studied in detail.

Studies with indium-labeled platelets and neutrophils in patients clearly demonstrated that platelets accumulate in the allograft at a very early stage of rejection; furthermore, the platelets reoccur in the circulation following successful reversal of the rejection. It is reasonable to anticipate that during kidney allograft rejection, platelet-derived products such as thromboxane B_2 (TXB_2) may be excreted in the urine (3,6). It was, however, surprising to find the same pattern of urinary immunoreactive thromboxane B_2 ($iTXB_2$) where the graft is located elsewhere (4,13), as on the abdominal vessels in the experimental cardiac allograft rejection model of Ono and Lindsey (15a). Two questions arise from these findings: (a) will urine $iTXB_2$ be an indicator of human cardiac allograft rejection, and (b) does the parent compound TXA_2 have a causal role in allograft rejection?

However, activation of all these different cell types entails release of arachidonic acid and subsequent formation of lipoxygenase as well as cyclooxygenase products. Moreover, the cell type determines the pattern of the elicited arachidonate products rather than the tissue or organ. A major arachidonate metabolite of platelets and human monocytes and macrophages is thromboxane, whereas PMN mainly synthesize leukotrienes. Table 1 shows the capacity for thromboxane synthesis of different human blood elements and peritoneal macrophages. Lymphocytes appear not to possess cyclooxygenase activity and probably not 5-lipoxygenase activity (9). Nevertheless, the lymphocytes release arachidonic acid on stimulation, and the arachidonate may be used by monocytes/macrophages for thromboxane synthesis (9).

POTENTIAL IMMUNOLOGICAL PROPERTIES OF THROMBOXANE AND LEUKOTRIENES

The immunological properties of thromboxane and leukotrienes are still largely unexplained, but what is known is in accordance with the proposition that these arachidonate products promote rejection as seen in Fig. 1, whereas prostacyclin (PGI_2) and prostaglandin E_2 (PGE_2) possess "antirejection" properties. These protective effects of PGI_2 and PGE_2 have been demonstrated in both experimental models and in patients, as recently reviewed by Shaw (17). The immunosuppressive activity of thromboxane synthase inhibitors, the benzimidazoles, were first mentioned by Paget et al. in 1969 (16), long before the discovery of the thromboxanes. Also, imidazoles, which are weak TXA_2 synthase inhibitors, have been shown to be immunosuppressive. It will be recalled that azathioprine consists of 6-mercaptopurine linked to imidazole. The immunosuppressive properties are normally

TABLE 1. *TXB₂ release stimulated by calcium ionophor (A23187)*

Cell	Thromboxane release (ng/10⁶ cells · 30 min)
Platelets[a]	10
Macrophages	4
Eosinophils	1
Polymorphonuclear leukocytes	0.1
Lymphocytes	0

[a]Determined following thrombin-induced aggregation.

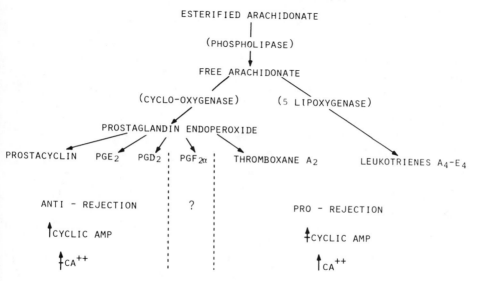

FIG. 1. Diagram of arachidonic acid metabolites and their putative pro- and antirejection properties.

ascribed to the 6-mercaptopurine, which is released from imidazole in the liver; however, in some early experiments in dog kidney allografts, azathioprine prolonged graft survival more than 6-mercaptopurine (2). Furthermore, *in vitro* experiments suggest that imidazole inhibits cell-mediated immunity through inhibition of TXA_2 synthesis. Cell-mediated immunity is also inhibited by PGI_2 and to a lesser degree PGE_2 (14).

The immunological importance of the leukotrienes (LT) has barely been studied, since until recently their availability has been strictly limited. Recent work now implicates at least indirectly the involvement of the 5-lipoxygenase products. These products (LTB_4) appear to stimulate Ca^{2+} uptake in PMN, for example. The importance of calcium has been shown in lymphocyte response to mitogens (1). Leukotriene B_4 also increases cyclic guanylate monophosphate in lymphocytes. In addition, LTB_4, LTC_4, and LTD_4 are reported capable of replacing the requirement for interleukin 2 for interferon production (12). This is of interest because interferon appears to be of central importance in mediation and modulation of immunologic activities such as induction of natural killer cell activity and cytotoxic T-cell activity, as well as expression of both class I and class II antigens with the major histocompatibility complex. In conclusion, thromboxane and leukotrienes may promote allograft rejection through stimulation of lymphocytes and macrophages, as well as by vasoconstriction, platelet and leukocyte aggregation, and increased vascular permeability.

THROMBOXANE: AN EARLY INDICATOR OF REJECTION

Urine iTXB₂ Monitoring of Human Renal Allograft Rejection

In kidney transplant patients, we have shown that urine $iTXB_2$ is an early indicator of allograft rejection (3,5). A typical pattern of changes in urine $iTXB_2$ as compared to serum creatinine and serum B_2 microglobulins is shown in Fig. 2. Our recent data analysis of 90 patients reveals that urinary $iTXB_2$ is a reliable indicator and is somewhat better than serum B_2 microglobulins.

It is reasonable to anticipate that a compound synthesized in the kidney may occur in the urine in measurable amounts. However, it is questionable whether

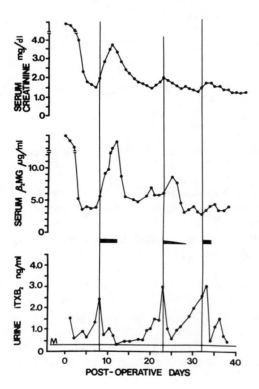

FIG. 2. Daily values of serum creatinine, serum beta₂-microglobulin (β_2-MG), and urine $iTXB_2$ in a kidney transplant patient. Day 0 is the day of transplantation. Horizontal line (M) is the mean of the lowest value of the transplant patients; solid bar, treatment with i.v. methylprednisolone; vertical line, diagnosis of rejection.

TXA_2 synthesized in other organs would occur in the urine as $iTXB_2$. Thus, the finding that deep venous thrombosis was associated with large increases in urine $iTXB_2$ (6) was encouraging in this respect and increased the confidence that cardiac allograft rejection might be associated with increased excretion of $iTXB_2$ in the urine.

Urine $iTXB_2$ in a Rat Cardiac Transplant Model

In order to establish this postulate more firmly, a heterotopic cardiac allograft rat model (4,13) was monitored by determining the daily values of urine $iTXB_2$. Different histoincompatible strains were studied (Table 2). Some were modified with immunosuppressive drugs. Isograft and sham-operated animals acted as controls. Depending on the histoincompatibility of the animals and the immunosuppressants used, the cardiac graft survival ranged from 6 days to more than 20 days. In all the histoincompatible combinations, an increase in urine $iTXB_2$ excretion was found to occur prior to rejection, as judged by cessation of heart beats. Figure 3 shows an example of the changes seen in urine $iTXB_2$ excretions during cardiac rejection in an ACI to Lewis combination as compared to changes in urine $iTXB_2$ in rats receiving an isograft in a Lewis to Lewis combination.

Urine $iTXB_2$ in Human Heart Transplantation

Following this successful experiment, we were then more confident in attempting to deal with the far more complex clinical situation by documenting changes in urine $iTXB_2$ in cardiac transplant patients during rejection. In 12 consecutive heart transplant patients, 17 rejection episodes were diagnosed. In 16 of these episodes, an elevation was measured in urine $iTXB_2$ values. However, increases in $iTXB_2$ were also seen during other periods, representing either undiagnosed rejection or a false–positive $iTXB_2$. Figure 4 illustrates urine $iTXB_2$ values from 2 patients,

TABLE 2. *Histocompatible strains of rats used in the cardiac transplant model*

Donor[a]	Recipient	Immunosuppressant	Daily dose (mg/kg)	Day of rejection
ACI	Lewis	None		6
B-N	Fisher	None		11
B-N	Fisher	Azathioprine	2	14
		Prednisone	2	
B-N	Fisher	Cyclosporin A	15	9–>20
ACI	L × B-N F_1	Cyclosporin A	15	>20
L × B-N F_1	Lewis	Azathioprine	5	11
		OKY-1581	10	
L × B-N F_1	Lewis	Azathioprine	5	9
L × B-N F_1	Lewis	Azathioprine	5	14
		L 640035	50	

[a]Brown-Norway, B-N; Lewis × Brown-Norway F_1 hybrid, L × B-N F_1.

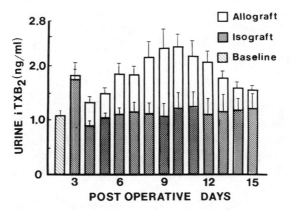

FIG. 3. Daily levels of urine iTXB$_2$ in rat cardiac heterotopic transplantation (ACI to Lewis and Lewis to Lewis). A gradual increase in iTXB$_2$ is seen from day 4 to a maximum at days 8–11, followed by a diminution. The iTXB$_2$ from rats receiving an isograft remains unchanged from day 4.

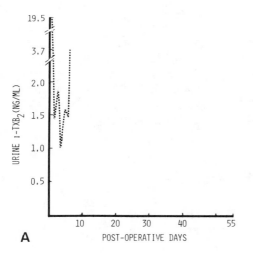

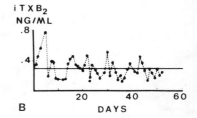

FIG. 4. Daily values of urine iTXB$_2$ cardiac transplant patients. **A:** One patient did not experience any rejection. **B:** The other patient died of acute rejection on day 7.

one who did not exhibit any rejection and where urine iTXB$_2$ remained low, and one who died on day 7 of accelerated rejection associated with continuously high iTXB$_2$ values. Figure 5 demonstrates interesting cyclical fluctuations in urine iTXB$_2$. High urinary iTXB$_2$ values were observed prior to initiation of rejection, after which there is a drop in urine iTXB$_2$ for the remaining period. This change is coincident with the abrupt fall in electrocardiogram (EKG) voltage. The cause of the prominent rhythmic fluctuations of iTXB$_2$ has not yet been identified.

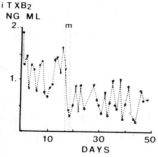

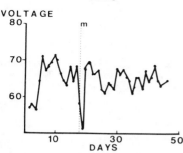

FIG. 5. Daily values of urine iTXB$_2$ and EKG voltage in a cardiac transplant patient where rejection was diagnosed (indicated by a vertical dotted line) and treated with i.v. methylprednisolone at 1 g daily for 3 days (m).

We conclude from these studies of human cardiac and renal allograft rejection and rat cardiac allograft rejection that the rejection phenomenon is associated with increased excretion of iTXB$_2$ and its metabolites, such as 2,3-dinor-TXB$_2$. This supports the proposition that iTXB$_2$ may be employed as an immunological monitor in allograft rejection. The relative contributions of intragraft and extragraft TXA$_2$ sources remain to be determined.

EVIDENCE FOR CAUSAL ROLE OF THROMBOXANE AND LEUKOTRIENES IN ALLOGRAFT REJECTION

We have performed recently two types of experiments in the rat heterotopic cardiac allograft model (Lewis Brown-Norway F$_1$ to Lewis). An increased (but not significant) allograft survival was observed with administration of the thromboxane synthase inhibitor OXY 1581 (Ono Pharmaceutical, Japan) in a dosage of 5 mg/kg s.c. twice daily (Table 2) in the presence of azathioprine. However, in a second study using the same histoincompatible strain, a new receptor antagonist of the smooth-muscle contractile arachidonate cyclooxygenase products (3-hydroxy-methyl-dibenzo[b,f]thiopin-5,5-dioxide; L-640,035; Merck Frost, Canada) was administered orally (50 mg/kg daily) in combination with azathioprine. A significant increase in allograft survival was observed (Table 2).

CONCLUSIONS

Our findings in cardiac and renal allograft transplant recipients and the animal cardiac heterograft model show that thromboxane is an early indicator of allograft rejection. Our preliminary work indicates that it is possible to interdict selective arachidonate products to promote allograft survival. Thus, leukotrienes, thromboxane, and the other smooth muscle contracting eicosanoids may have a causal role in allograft rejection.

ACKNOWLEDGMENTS

This work was supported by grants from the National Institutes of Health (AM30499), the National Kidney Foundation, and the American Heart Association (84-1147).

REFERENCES

1. Blitstein-Willinger, E., and Diamantstein, T. (1978): Inhibition by isoptin (a calcium antagonist) of the mitogenic stimulation of lymphocytes prior to the S-phase. *Immunology*, 34:303–307.
2. Calne, R. Y. (1961): Inhibition of the rejection of renal homografts in dogs by purine analogues. *Transplant Bull.*, 28:65–81.
3. Foegh, M L., Alijani, M., Helfrich, G. B., Schreiner, G. E., and Ramwell, P. W. (1984): Urine thromboxane as an immunological monitor in kidney transplant patients. *Transplant Proc.*, 16:1603–1605.
4. Foegh, M. L., Alijani, M., Khirabadi, B. S., Shapiro, R., Goldman, M. H., Lower, R. R., and Ramwell, P. W. (1984): Monitoring of rat heart allograft rejection by urinary thromboxane. *Transplant Proc.*, 16:1606–1608.
5. Foegh, M., and Ramwell, P. (1983): Implications of products in the arachidonic acid cascade. *In: Prostaglandins and Related Substances*, edited by C. Pace-Asciak and E. Granstrom, pp. XIII–XIX. Elsevier, Amsterdam.
6. Foegh, M. L., Zmudka, M., Cooley, C., Winchester, J. E., Helfrich, G. B., Ramwell, P. W., and Schreiner, G. E. (1981): Urine i-TXB$_2$ in renal allograft rejection. *Lancet*, II:431–434.
7. Ford-Hutchinson, A., Bray, M., Doig, M., Shipley, M., and Smith, M. (1980): Leukotriene B; A potent chemokinetic and aggregating substance released from polymorphonuclear leukocytes. *Nature (Lond.)*, 286:264–265.
8. Goldyne, M. E., and Stobo, J. D. (1981): Immunoregulatory role of prostaglandins and related lipids. *CRC Crit. Rev. Immunol.*, 2:189–223.
9. Goldyne, M. E., and Stobo, J. D. (1983): T-Lymphocytes as a source of arachidonic acid for the synthesis of eicosanoids by human monocytes/macrophages. *Adv. Prostaglandin, Thromboxane Leukotriene Res.*, 12:39–43.
10. Hayry, P. (1983): Lymphoid cell subclasses in rejecting renal allograft in the rat. *Cell. Immunol.*, 77:187–195.
11. Hayry, P., Von Willebrand, E., and Soots, A. (1979): *In situ* effector mechanisms in rat kidney allograft rejection. *Scand. J. Immunol.*, 10:95–108.
12. Johnson, H. M., and Tomes, B. A. (1984): Leukotrienes: Positive signals for regulation of gamma-interferon production. *J. Immunol.*, 132:413–416.
13. Khirabadi, B. S., Foegh, M. L., and Ramwell, P. W. (1985): Thromboxane in rat cardiac allograft rejection. *Transplantation*, 39:6–8.
14. Leung, K. H. and Mihich, E. (1980): Prostaglandin modulation of development of cell-mediated immunity in culture. *Nature (Lond.)*, 288:597–600.
15. Matthew, T. H., Lewers, D. T., Hogan, G. P., Rubio-Paez, D., Alter, H. J., Antonovych, T., Bauer, H., Maher, J. F., and Schreiner, G. E. (1971): The induction of vascular renal allograft rejection by leukocyte sensitization. *J. Lab. Clin. Med.*, 77:396–409.
15a. Ono, K., and Lindsey, E. S. (1969): Improved technique of heart transplantation in rats. *J. Thorac. Cardiovasc. Surg.*, 57:225.
16. Paget, J., Kisner, K., Stone, R. L., and DeLong, D. C. (1967): Heterocyclin substituted ureas. I: Immunosuppression and virus inhibition by benzimidazoleureas. *J. Med. Chem.*, 12:1010–1012.

17. Shaw, J. F. L. (1983): Prostaglandins and transplantation. *I.R.C.S. Med. Sci.*, 11:95–96.
18. Strom, T. B., Tilney, N. L., Carpenter, C. B., and Busch, G. J. (1975): Identity of cytotoxic capacity of cells infiltrating renal allografts. *N. Engl. J. Med.*, 191:1257.
19. Tilney, N., Strom, T., Macpherson, S., and Carpenter, C. (1976): Studies on infiltrating host cells harvested from acutely rejecting rat cardiac allografts. *Surgery*, 79:209–217.

Advances in Prostaglandin, Thromboxane, and
Leukotriene Research, Vol. 13, edited by G. G. Neri
Serneri, et al. Raven Press, New York © 1985.

Drugs Affecting the Prostaglandin Synthetic Pathway and Rat Heart Allograft Survival

J. F. L. Shaw and R. A. Greatorex

Department of Surgery, Whittington Hospital, London N19 5NF, England

Prostaglandins may be involved in the control of the immune system (1) and may be involved in several of the processes concerned with allograft rejection. Drugs affecting different parts of the prostaglandin and leukotriene biosynthetic pathway were tested for their ability to modify the rejection of heterotopic DA(RT1^a) rat hearts in PVG(RT1^c) rat recipients. Cessation of palpable graft beat was taken as the endpoint of graft survival. The method of Heron (2) was used for heart transplantation. Drugs were generally administered by subcutaneous injection every 8 hr until the time of rejection. Wilcoxon rank sum analysis for unpaired data was used for analysis of differences between control and experimental graft survival times.

Previous experiments (3) have demonstrated that aspirin and sodium salicylate both lead to prolongation of graft survival in this model. The results of the present experiments are presented in Table 1.

Graft survival was not influenced by an increase of prostaglandin precursor supply (Intralipid, Naudicelle), by leukotriene synthesis inhibition (BW755C, hydrocortisone), or by low doses of prostaglandin E$_1$. Graft survival was shortened by the use of a cyclooxygenase inhibitor (Timegadine) ($p < 0.05$). A thromboxane synthetase inhibitor (UK-38,485), a thromboxane receptor antagonist (EIP), and a 5-hydroxytryptamine (5-HT$_2$) receptor antagonist (Ketanserin) were without effect on graft survival. It is concluded that the immunosuppressive activity of nonsteroidal antiinflammatory agents may be independent of changes in prostaglandin metabolism.

REFERENCES

1. Goodwin, J. S., and Webb, D. R. (1980): Regulation of the immune response by prostaglandins. *Clin. Immunol. Immunopathol.*, 15:106–122.
2. Heron, I. (1971): A technique for accessory cervical heart transplantation in rabbits and rats. *Acta Pathol. Microbiol. Scand.*, 79:366–372.
3. Shaw, J. F. L. (1983): Comparison of the effects of acetylsalicylic acid and sodium salicylate on prolongation of rat cardiac allograft survival and on inhibition of rat platelet aggregation. *Transplantation*, 36:33–36.

TABLE 1. *DA to PVG heart survival time with various treatment schedules*

Drug used	Graft survival (days)	Median	Difference versus control
None: saline (0.2 ml/day)	6,7,7,7,7,7,8,8,8,8,9	7.4	—
Intralipid 20% (5 ml/day)	†,†,7,7,7	7.0	NS
Naudicelle (500 mg/kg · day)	6,6,6,7,8	6.4	NS
Hydrocortisone (1.2 mg/kg · day)	7,7,8,8,†,†	7.5	NS
BW755C (100 mg/kg · day)	6,7,8,8,8	7.6	NS
Aspirin (200 mg/kg · day)	8,8,9,9,10,10,11,11,11,14, 63,6/12	10.5	$p < 0.01$
Salicylate (200 mg/kg · day)	11,11,13,28,48,60,>4/12, >6/12,>6/12,>6/12, >6/12,>6/12	90	$p < 0.01$
Timegadine (50 mg/kg · day)	6,6,6,7,7	6.3	$p < 0.05$
Timegadine (200 mg/kg · day)	6,6,6,6,7	6.3	$p < 0.05$
Surgam (tiaprofenic acid) (200 mg/kg · day)	†,†,†,†,†	—	—
UK-38,485 (20 mg/kg · day)	7,7,7,8,8,8,8,8,9,10	8.0	NS
UK-38,485 (200 mg/kg · day)	7,7,8,8,8	7.7	NS
EIP (1 mg/kg · day)	6,7,7,7,8	7.0	NS
PGE$_1$ (10 µg/kg · day)	7,8,8,8,9	8.0	NS
Ketanserin (40 mg/kg · day)	7,7,7,8,8,8	7.3	NS

† = Rats died before grafts rejected; NS = not significant.

Advances in Prostaglandin, Thromboxane, and Leukotriene Research, Vol. 13, edited by G. G. Neri Serneri, et al. Raven Press, New York © 1985.

Eicosanoids as Regulators of Pancreatic Islet Hormone Secretion

Sumer Belbez Pek and Mary F. Walsh

Department of Internal Medicine, The University of Michigan, Ann Arbor, Michigan 48109

The endocrine pancreas is a complex organ, secreting several hormones synthesized in different types of cells. Some of these hormones interact. At times, this interaction is in the form of counterregulation at the level of target tissues, resulting in opposing biological effects. Insulin lowers the level of glucose in the circulation by inhibiting gluconeogenesis and glycogenolysis and by promoting the transport of glucose into cells and its anaerobic glycolysis. On the other hand, glucagon raises circulating glucose by promoting gluconeogenesis and glycogenolysis. At other times, the interaction of the pancreatic islet hormones occurs within the islets as paracrine events. Somatostatin inhibits the secretion of both insulin and glucagon, glucagon stimulates insulin release, and insulin may inhibit glucagon release. This two-tier interaction of islet hormones demands that their secretion is regulated in an integrated manner; indeed, some such mechanisms (circulating level of nutrients, neurotransmitters) have been identified. Products formed in the specific oxidative metabolism of arachidonic acid locally regulate biological events in a variety of organ systems. Research conducted during the last decade suggests that these eicosanoids play a significant modulatory role in the regulation of secretion of pancreatic islet hormones in an integrating manner.

The major mechanism for the release of arachidonic acid from any membrane-bound phospholipid to the cytosol is deacylation activated by phospholipase A_2, a calcium-dependent enzyme. Glucose activates this enzyme, probably because it induces influx of calcium into cells. Evidence has been presented that in isolated pancreatic islets exogenous phospholipase A_2 activates insulin secretion (48). Islet cells possess phospholipase A_2 activity (20). Phospholipase C-induced hydrolysis, with participation of two other enzymes, also liberates arachidonic acid from phosphatidylinositol, thus providing the substrate for specific pathways of oxidative metabolism (3). Exogenous phospholipase C stimulates insulin release (48). Metabolic activity consistent with the presence of phospholipase C in islets has been documented as well (10). Yamamoto et al. (50) demonstrated in isolated rat islets that bromophenacylbromide (BPB), which is an inhibitor of phospholipase, inhibited insulin release induced by a phorbol ester. We observed in the isolated, perfused rat pancreas that BPB inhibited arginine-induced secretion of insulin and glucagon (46).

The first recognized, biologically important specific oxidative pathway of arachidonate metabolism was the one activated by cyclooxygenase, the products of which are dienoic prostaglandins (PGs) and thromboxane (TX) (4). Johnson et al. (17) and Burr and Sharp (6) first showed that administered PGE_1 stimulates insulin release. Using the isolated perfused rat pancreas, we demonstrated that insulin release occurs in a biphasic manner in response to PGE_1, PGE_2, and $PGF_{2\alpha}$ and that these PGs augment biphasic release of insulin induced by arginine (30–32). We documented that in vitro, PGE_2 can evoke insulin release at a concentration as low as 10^{-9} M in the presence of 5 mM glucose, fumarate, glutamate, and pyruvate (31); this concentration is of physiological significance. Nishi et al. (28) also observed in the isolated rat pancreas that PGE_1 stimulated insulin release. We were the first to show that administered PGE_1, PGE_2, and $PGF_{2\alpha}$ also stimulate biphasic release of glucagon and augment arginine-induced glucagon release, and that the release of glucagon in response to PGs precedes that of insulin (30–32). PGs are selective in their effects on islet hormone secretion: prostacyclin (PGI_2) and TX have little or no effect on insulin or glucagon release, while PGD_2 stimulates mainly glucagon secretion (1,29). Matsuyama et al. (23) confirmed the stimulatory effect of PGD_2 on glucagon release from the rat pancreas and demonstrated that at certain concentrations of glucose it can also stimulate insulin release. We also have shown that the immediate precursor of dienoic PGs, cyclic endoperoxide PGH_2, stimulates the release of both hormones (29), which is likely to result from pancreatic conversion of PGH_2 to PGs that are secretagogues (2). These in vitro studies indicate that certain exogenous PGs directly stimulate the release of insulin and glucagon. PGE_1 also stimulated somatostatin release from the isolated rat pancreas (28). The results of in vivo studies frequently contradict the in vitro findings on insulin secretion. Basal plasma levels of insulin and particularly the glucose-induced increases in plasma insulin were blunted by the administration of PGE_1, dimethyl-PGE_1, PGE_2, and PGA_1 to human subjects, dogs, or rats (11,14,19,35,38,39,41). Indirect mechanisms may have been operative in vivo. There is no discrepancy with respect to glucagon secretion; PGs induce glucagon release also in vivo (15,40).

Prostaglandins principally function as local regulators. Thus, documentation of the capability of the pancreas and particularly of the pancreatic islets to produce PGs was essential in order to assign to endogenous PGs a regulatory role in the secretion of pancreatic hormones. Release of prostaglandin-like activity from the isolated rat pancreas upon administration of arachidonic acid was observed by Hamamdzic and Malik (16). In isolated rat islets, Clements and Rhoten (10), Kelly and Laychock (18), and Evans et al. (12) provided evidence for the biosynthesis of several PGs, using labeled precursor methods. In a system of cultured neonatal rat pancreatic cells, which comprises more than 50% fibroblasts, Metz et al. (25) observed the release of immunoreactive PGE. We demonstrated that the isolated perfused rat pancreas releases immunoreactive PGE_2 and to a lesser extent $PGF_{2\alpha}$ and TXB_2 (stable metabolite of TXA_2) (44), and that isolated rat islets produce large amounts of immunoreactive PGE_2, to a lesser extent $PGF_{2\alpha}$, and 6-keto-$PGF_{1\alpha}$ (a stable metabolite of PGI_2), and very little or no TXB_2 (43). Thus, the evidence is conclusive, although not comprehensive, that the endocrine as well as the exocrine pancreas produces PGs, and that PGE_2 appears to be the dominant product.

The interrelationships of endogenous PGs and pancreatic islet hormone secretion have been explored, mainly by employing drugs that inhibit the cyclooxygenase enzyme. The results of studies on the effects of cyclooxygenase inhibitors on insulin release *in vivo* or *in vitro* are confusing; inhibition, stimulation, or no effects have been reported (36). In the *in vivo* studies, extrapancreatic events may have perturbed the picture. Robertson (36) proposed that PGE interacts with glucose in a unique way so that glucose-induced insulin release needs to be differentiated from other forms of insulin release to resolve the controversy of the influence of endogenous PGs on insulin secretion. The results of several studies, including our own (22,47), are not consistent with this paradigm. In pancreatic islets we observed that mild to moderate inhibition of PG biosynthesis by several chemically distinct cyclooxygenase inhibitors is consistently accompanied by inhibition of insulin release; at near maximal inhibition of PG synthesis, insulin secretion is frequently no longer inhibited. We proposed that when cyclooxygenase is inhibited profoundly in islets, arachidonate may be metabolized in other pathways to products that stimulate insulin release and mask the effect of reduction in PG synthesis. The information on the role of endogenous PGs in glucagon secretion is difficult to interpret as well; under various *in vivo* and *in vitro* conditions, cyclooxygenase inhibitors were found to inhibit, promote, or have no effect on glucagon secretion (21). In the isolated perfused pancreas or isolated islets, we observe most frequently an inhibition of glucagon secretion and occasionally no change in secretion in response to cyclooxygenase inhibitors (22,43,46).

The recognition of the lipoxygenase pathways of arachidonate metabolism followed that of the cyclooxygenase pathway by many years (5,34). Several types of lipoxygenase enzymes induce hydroxylation and peroxide formation of the arachidonate chain at carbon atom 5, 12, or 15, leading to formation of 5-, 12-, or 15-hydroperoxyeicosatetraenoic (HPETE) and hydroxyeicosatetraenoic (HETE) acids. These compounds exert biological effects, but their physiological significance is an unsettled issue. The 5-lipoxygenase pathway is of particular importance, since biologically significant leukotrienes (LTs) are produced in this pathway. LTA_4, the unstable intermediate compound, is further metabolized to LTB_4 or enzymatically conjugated with cysteine or glutathione to form LTC_4, LTD_4, and LTE_4. LTs are powerful local regulators of diverse biological events of physiological and pathophysiological significance. The identity of the long-recognized slow-reacting substance of anaphylaxis (SRS-A) has now been established as mainly LTC_4. A role for LTs in the regulation of the secretion process has been recognized. Particularly, lipoxygenase-pathway products appear to play a key role in the activation of the release of lysosomal enzymes from the polymorphonuclear leukocytes (27). Recent evidence indicates that lipoxygenase products exert a stimulatory effect on the secretion of insulin. The stimulated release of insulin from isolated islets, cultured pancreatic cells, or perfused intact pancreas is inhibited by nordihydroguaiaretic acid, 5,8,11,14-eicosatetraenoic acid or BW755c, which are inhibitors of lipoxygenases (26,47,50). The inhibitory effect of lipoxygenase inhibitors on insulin release was particularly evident when insulin secretion had been stimulated by agents that activate phospholipase A_2, or when exogenous arachidonate had been added, thus providing substrate for lipoxygenase (26,49,50). Our studies with the lipoxygenase inhibitors did not indicate a role for endogenous lipoxygenase products in the regulation of secretion of glucagon. In labeled precursor studies, pancreatic islets were shown to produce fatty acid derivatives which had high-pressure liquid chromatographic (HPLC) patterns of HETE and HPETE acids (18). Subsequently, Metz et al. (24) and Turk et al. (45) demonstrated the production of 12-HETE from radiolabeled arachidonic acid. Using the labeled precursor and HPLC methodology, we now have preliminary evidence that freshly isolated rat pancreatic islets produce LTB_4, LTC_4, possibly other LTs, and 12-HETE (Fig. 1), and that a continuously cultured, insulin-producing homogenous rat islet-cell line produces LTB_4, LTC_4, possibly other LTs, and 5-HETE (Fig. 2). Thus, the lipoxygenase metabolic pathways exist in islet cells. Using the isolated perfused rat pancreas, we have shown (33) that LTB_4, LTC_4, and, to a lesser extent, LTD_4 and LTE_4, all products of the 5-lipoxygenase pathway, stimulate insulin release but have little or no effect on glucagon release (Fig. 3).

Capdevila et al. (7) reported a novel oxidative metabolic pathway of arachidonate in rat liver microsomes that is dependent on the presence of NADPH, oxygen, and cytochrome P-450. Chacos et al. (9) identified the products of this oxidative metabolism as 5,6-, 8,9-, 11,12-, and 14,15-epoxyeicosatrienoic acids (EETs). Capdevila and his collaborators refer to this metabolic pathway of arachidonate as the "epoxygenase" pathway. The same group (8) demonstrated the presence of EETs in the microsomal fraction of rat hypothalamic median eminence; exogenous 5,6-EET stimulated the release of somatostatin from nerve terminals of the median eminence. Snyder et al. (42) observed the release of luteinizing hormone from isolated rat anterior pituitary cells in response to EETs, particularly to 5,6-EET. Most recently, Capdevila's group (13) demonstrated in isolated rat pancreatic islets that, among the exogenous EETs tested, only 5,6-EET stimulated insulin release; this analog had no effect on glucagon release. The 8,9-, 11,12-, and 14,15-EETs stimulated glucagon release selectively. Products of the epoxygenase pathway are yet to be identified in islets; the nature of the enzymatic regulation of the pathway suggests that they will be found.

Now, as compared to our view 10 years ago, a much more elaborate and meaningful picture emerges with respect to the role of arachidonate metabolism in the regulation of secretion of pancreatic islet hormones. The substrate is stored in the cell membrane and rapidly released into the cytosol upon activation of membrane-associated phospholipases in response to membrane-reactive stimuli, most importantly calcium, glucose, and certain hormones. Free arachidonate can then enter the three specific oxidative metabolic pathways. The products in each of these pathways differ with respect to their efficacy in influencing the secretion of islet

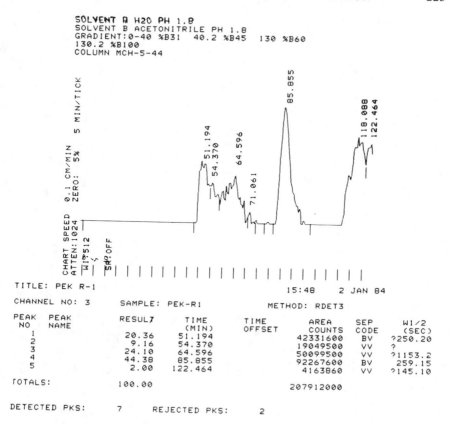

SOLVENT A H2O PH 1.8
SOLVENT B ACETONITRILE PH 1.8
GRADIENT:0-40 %B31   40.2 %B45   130 %B60
130.2 %B100
COLUMN MCH-5-44

TITLE: PEK R-1   15:48   2 JAN 84

CHANNEL NO: 3   SAMPLE: PEK-R1   METHOD: RDET3

PEAK NO	PEAK NAME	RESULT	TIME (MIN)	TIME OFFSET	AREA COUNTS	SEP CODE	W1/2 (SEC)
1		20.36	51.194		42331600	BV	?250.20
2		9.16	54.370		19049500	VV	?
3		24.10	64.596		50099500	VV	?1153.2
4		44.38	85.855		92267600	BV	259.15
5		2.00	122.464		4163860	VV	?145.10
TOTALS:		100.00			207912000		

DETECTED PKS: 7   REJECTED PKS: 2

FIG. 1. HPLC profile of radioactive eicosanoids produced in freshly isolated rat pancreatic islets incubated with ^{3}H-arachidonate. Elution times (min) of major peaks are printed on the graph and quantified as areas of radioactivity (counts, and % of total) in the table. The 51- and 54-min peaks are estimated to correspond to LTB_4 and LTC_4, the broader region (until 72 min) to other LTs, and the 85-min peak to 12-HETE. Peaks with elution times greater than 100 min are due likely to residual ^{3}H-arachidonate.

hormones; however, as a whole, the net result is amplification of hormone secretion. There is considerable selectivity in terms of which hormone is to be affected, and there is considerable difference with respect to potency to exert an effect on the secretion of a given hormone. Thus, shifts in arachidonate metabolism result in selective amplification of the secretion of insulin or glucagon. Diversion of the substrate from one pathway, the products of which exert a minor amplifying effect on insulin secretion, to another pathway, which produces powerful stimulators of insulin (e.g., inhibition of cyclooxygenase with drugs leading to increased activity in the lipoxygenase pathway) would strengthen the arachidonate-associated amplification of insulin secretion. The metabolism of arachidonate in the specific oxidative pathways represents an amplifying unit to "fine-tune" islet hormone secretion;

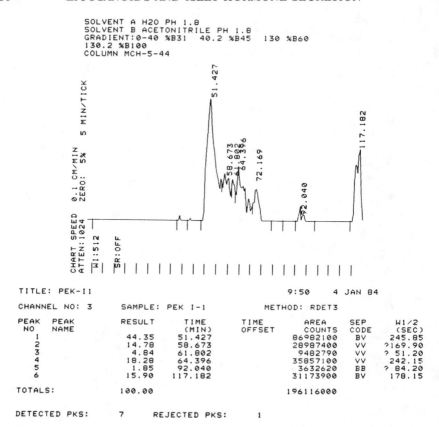

SOLVENT A H2O PH 1.8
SOLVENT B ACETONITRILE PH 1.8
GRADIENT:0-40 %B31   40.2 %B45   130 %B60
130.2 %B100
COLUMN MCH-5-44

TITLE: PEK-II   9:50   4 JAN 84

CHANNEL NO: 3   SAMPLE: PEK I-1   METHOD: RDET3

PEAK NO	PEAK NAME	RESULT	TIME (MIN)	TIME OFFSET	AREA COUNTS	SEP CODE	W1/2 (SEC)
1		44.35	51.427		86982100	BV	245.85
2		14.78	58.673		28987400	VV	?169.90
3		4.84	61.802		9482790	VV	? 51.20
4		18.28	64.396		35857100	VV	242.15
5		1.85	92.040		3632620	BB	? 84.20
6		15.90	117.182		31173900	BV	178.15

TOTALS: 100.00   196116000

DETECTED PKS: 7   REJECTED PKS: 1

FIG. 2. HPLC profile of radioactive eicosanoids produced by insulin-secreting rat islet tumor cells maintained in continuous culture, incubated with ³H-arachidonate. Refer to legend of Fig. 1 for elution times; the 92-min peak corresponds to 5-HETE.

exclusive attention to any one of these pathways while ignoring the others results in erroneous conclusions. A key question is, what happens when the amplifying unit malfunctions? Can it lead to a disease such as diabetes mellitus? We and others are just starting a comprehensive evaluation of specific arachidonate metabolism in islets; the answers should be forthcoming. The existing reports exclusively on the role of prostaglandins in glucose homeostasis or in defective secretion of insulin in response to glucose (37) are not conclusive.

We believe that arachidonate metabolism is a significant, quick-response modulator of islet function, amplifying the signals for secretion in favor of insulin, glucagon, or both. A delayed, "tonic-modulatory" component may also exist. A comprehensive evaluation of all pathways of metabolism is likely to generate new knowledge with respect to physiology and pathophysiology of islet hormone secretion.

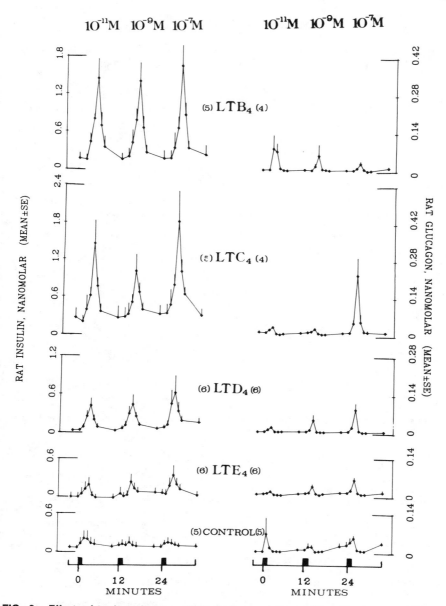

FIG. 3. Effects of 1-min perfusions with 10^{-11}, 10^{-9}, and 10^{-7} M LTB$_4$, LTC$_4$, LTD$_4$, and LTE$_4$ and the basic perfusion solution alone (control) on the release of insulin *(left panel)* and glucagon *(right panel)* from the isolated rat pancreas, as measured in 1-min fractions of pancreatic venous effluent. Perfusion solutions contained 5.6 mM glucose at all times but no protein. (Reprinted with the permission of the National Academy of Sciences, ref. 33.)

ACKNOWLEDGMENTS

The authors are indebted to Dr. John Pike and Dr. Frank Fitzpatrick of the Upjohn Company, Kalamazoo, Michigan, for their long-lasting support by providing prostanoids and reagents for prostanoid assays, and to Dr. Joshua Rokach of Merck Frosst Canada Inc., Pointe Claire, Quebec, Canada, for the generous gift of leukotrienes. The work was supported in part by the U.S. Public Health Service grants AM 21192, AM 07245, and AM 20572 through the National Institute of Arthritis, Diabetes, Digestive and Kidney Diseases.

REFERENCES

1. Akpan, J. O., Hurley, M. C., Pek, S., and Lands, W. E. M. (1979): The effects of prostaglandins on secretion of glucagon and insulin by the perfused rat pancreas. *Can. J. Biochem.*, 57:540–547.
2. Akpan, J. O., Hurley, M. C., Pek, S., and Lands, W. E. M. (1981): Dissociation of vascular resistance with endocrine pancreas secretion: The effects of epoxymethano analogs of PGH_2. *Prostaglandins Med.*, 7:473–481.
3. Bell, R. L., Kennerly, D. A., Stanford, N., and Majerus, P. W. (1979): Diglyceride lipase: A pathway for arachidonate release from human platelets. *Proc. Natl. Acad. Sci. U.S.A.*, 76:3238–3241.
4. Bergström, S., and Samuelsson, B. (1965): Prostaglandins. *Annu. Rev. Biochem.*, 34:101–108.
5. Borgeat, P., and Samuelsson, B. (1979): Transformation of arachidonic acid by rabbit polymorphonuclear leukocytes. *J. Biol. Chem.*, 254:2643–2646.
6. Burr, I. M., and Sharp, R. (1974): Effects of prostaglandin E_1, and epinephrine on the dynamics of insulin release *in vitro*. *Endocrinology*, 94:835–839.
7. Capdevila, J., Chacos, N., Werringloer, J., Prough, R. A., and Estabrook, R. W. (1981): Liver microsomal cytochrome P-450 and the oxidative metabolism of arachidonic acid. *Proc. Natl. Acad. Sci. U.S.A.*, 78:5362–5366.
8. Capdevila, J., Chacos, N., Falck, J. R., Manna, S., Negro-Vilar, A., and Ojeda, S. R. (1983): Novel hypothalamic arachidonate products stimulate somatostatin release from the median eminence. *Endocrinology*, 113:421–423.
9. Chacos, N., Falck, J. R., Wixtrom, C., and Capdevila, J. (1982): Novel epoxides formed during the liver cytochrome P-450 oxidation of arachidonic acid. *Biochem. Biophys. Res. Commun.*, 104:916–922.
10. Clements, R. S., Jr., and Rhoten, W. B. (1976): Phosphoinositide metabolism and insulin secretion from isolated rat pancreatic islets. *J. Clin. Invest.*, 57:684–691.
11. Dodi, G., Santoro, M. G., and Jaffe, B. M. (1978): Effect of a synthetic analog of PGE_2 on exocrine and endocrine pancreatic function in the rat. *Surgery*, 83:206–213.
12. Evans, M. H., Pace, C. S., and Clements, R. S. Jr. (1983): Endogenous prostaglandin synthesis and glucose-induced insulin secretion from the adult rat pancreatic islet. *Diabetes*, 32:509–515.
13. Falck, J. R., Manna, S., Moltz, J., Chacos, N., and Capdevila, J. (1983): Epoxyeicosatrienoic acids stimulate glucagon and insulin release from isolated rat pancreatic islets. *Biochem. Biophys. Res. Commun.*, 114:743–749.
14. Giugliano, D., and Torella, R. (1978): Prostaglandin E_1 inhibits glucose-induced insulin secretion in man. *Prostaglandins Med.*, 1:165–174.
15. Giugliano, D., Torella, R., Sgambato, S., and D'Onofrio, F. (1978): Prostaglandin E_1 increases basal glucagon in man. *Pharmacol. Res. Commun.*, 10:813–821.
16. Hamamdzic, M., and Malik, K. U. (1977): Prostaglandins in adrenergic transmission of isolated perfused rat pancreas. *Am. J. Physiol.*, 232:E201–E209.
17. Johnson, D. G., Fujimoto, W. T., and Williams, R. H. (1973): Enhanced release of insulin by prostaglandins in isolated pancreatic islets. *Diabetes*, 22:658–663.
18. Kelly, K. L., and Laychock, S. G. (1981): Prostaglandin synthesis and metabolism in isolated pancreatic islets of the rat. *Prostaglandins*, 21:759–769.
19. Konturek, S. J., Mikos, E. M., Krol, R., Wierzbicki, Z., and Dobrzanska, M. (1978): Effect of methylated prostaglandin E_2 analogue on insulin secretion in man. *Prostaglandins*, 15:591–602.

20. Laychock, S. G. (1982): Phospholipase A_2 activity in pancreatic islet cells is calcium-dependent and stimulated by glucose. *Cell Calcium*, 3:43–54.
21. Luyckx, A. S., and Lefebvre, P. J. (1983): Prostaglandins and glucagon secretion. *Handbook Exp. Pharmacol.*, 66/II:83–98.
22. MacAdams, M. R., Pek, S. B., and Lands, W. E. M. (1984): The effect of flurbiprofen, a potent inhibitor of prostaglandin synthesis, on insulin and glucagon release from isolated pancreas. *Endocrinology*, 114:1365–1370.
23. Matsuyama, T., Horie, H., Namba, M., Nonaka, K., and Tarui, S. (1983): Glucose-dependent stimulation by prostaglandin-D_2 of glucagon and insulin in perfused rat pancreas. *Life Sci.*, 32:979–982.
24. Metz, S. A., Fujimoto, W. Y., and Robertson, R. P. (1983): A role for the lipoxygenase pathway of arachidonic acid metabolism in glucose- and glucagon-induced insulin secretion. *Life Sci.*, 32:903–910.
25. Metz, S. A., Robertson, R. P., and Fujimoto, W. Y. (1981): Inhibition of prostaglandin E synthesis augments glucose-induced insulin secretion in cultured pancreas. *Diabetes*, 30:551–557.
26. Metz, S., VanRollins, M., Strife, R., Fujimoto, W., and Robertson, R. P. (1983): Lipoxygenase pathway in islet endocrine cells. Oxidative metabolism of arachidonic acid promotes insulin release. *J. Clin. Invest.*, 71:1191–1205.
27. Naccache, P. H., Molski, T. F. P., Becker, E. L., Borgeat, P., Picard, S., Vallerand, P., and Sha'afi, R. I. (1982): Specificity of the effect of lipoxygenase metabolites of arachidonic acid on calcium homeostasis in neutrophils. *J. Biol. Chem.*, 257:8608–8611.
28. Nishi, S., Seino, Y., Seino, S., Tsuda, K., Takemura, J., Ishida, H., and Imura, H. (1982): Prostaglandin E_1: Stimulation of somatostatin and insulin responses to glucose from the isolated perfused rat pancreas. *Prostaglandins Leukotrienes Med.*, 8:593–597.
29. Pek, S., Lands, W. E. M., Akpan, J. O., and Hurley, M. C. (1980): Effect of prostaglandins H_2, D_2, I_2 and thromboxane on *in vitro* secretion of glucagon and insulin. *Adv. Prostaglandin Thromboxane Res.*, 8:1295–1298.
30. Pek, S., Tai, T.-Y., Crowther, R., and Fajans, S. S. (1976): Glucagon release precedes insulin release in response to common secretagogues. *Diabetes*, 25:764–770.
31. Pek, S., Tai, T.-Y., and Elster, A. (1978): Stimulatory effects of prostaglandins E-1, E-2, and F-2-alpha on glucagon and insulin release *in vitro*. *Diabetes*, 27:801–809.
32. Pek, S., Tai, T.-Y., Elster, A., and Fajans, S. S. (1975): Stimulation by prostaglandin E-2 of glucagon and insulin release from isolated rat pancreas. *Prostaglandins*, 10:493–502.
33. Pek, S. B., and Walsh, M. F. (1984): Leukotrienes stimulate insulin release from the rat pancreas. *Proc. Natl. Acad. Sci. U.S.A.*, 81:2199–2202.
34. Radmark, O., Malmsten, C., Samuelsson, B., Goto, G., Marfat, A., and Corey, E. J. (1980): Leukotriene A: Isolation from human polymorphonuclear leukocytes. *J. Biol. Chem.*, 255:11828–11831.
35. Robertson, R. P. (1974): *In vivo* insulin secretion: Prostaglandin and adrenergic interrelationships. *Prostaglandins*, 6:501–508.
36. Robertson, R. P. (1983): Hypothesis: PGE, carbohydrate homeostasis, and insulin secretion: A suggested resolution of the controversy. *Diabetes*, 32:231–235.
37. Robertson, R. P. (1983): Prostaglandins, glucose homeostasis, and diabetes mellitus. *Annu. Rev. Med.*, 34:1–12.
38. Robertson, R. P., Gavareski, D., Porte, D. Jr., and Bierman, E. L. (1974): Inhibition of *in vivo* insulin secretion by prostaglandin E_1. *J. Clin. Invest.*, 54:310–315.
39. Robertson, R. P., and Guest, R. J. (1978): Reversal by methysergide of inhibition of insulin secretion by prostaglandin in the dog. *J. Clin. Invest.*, 62:1014–1019.
40. Sacca, L., and Perez, G. (1976): Influence of prostaglandins on plasma glucagon levels in the rat. *Metabolism*, 25:127–130.
41. Sacca, L., Perez, G., Rengo, F., Pascucci, I., and Condorelli, M. (1975): Reduction of circulating insulin levels during the infusion of different prostaglandins in the rat. *Acta Endocrinol.*, 79:266–274.
42. Snyder, G. D., Capdevila, J., Chacos, N., Manna, S., and Falck, J. R. (1983): Action of luteinizing hormone-releasing hormone: Involvement of novel arachidonic acid metabolites. *Proc. Natl. Acad. Sci. U.S.A.*, 80:3504–3507.
43. Spangler, R. S., and Pek, S. B. (1983): Effects of cyclooxygenase inhibition on prostaglandin

production and insulin and glucagon secretion by isolated rat islets. *Adv. Prostaglandin Thromboxane Leukotriene Res.*, 12:291–297.

44. Spangler, R. S., Walsh, M. F., and Pek, S. B. (1984): Apparent lack of a role of pancreatic prostaglandins in the action of somatostatin on secretion of insulin and glucagon. *Hormone Metab. Res. (in press)*

45. Turk, J., Kotagal, N., and Greider, M. (1983): Arachidonic acid metabolism in isolated pancreatic islets from the rat. *Diabetes*, 32(suppl. 1):139A.

46. Walsh, M. F., and Pek, S. B. (1984): Possible role of endogenous arachidonic acid metabolites in stimulated release of insulin and glucagon from the isolated perfused rat pancreas. *Diabetes*, 33:929–936.

47. Walsh, M. F., and Pek, S. B. (1984): Effects of lipoxygenase and cyclooxygenase inhibitors on glucose-stimulated insulin secretion from the isolated perfused rat pancreas. *Life Sci.*, 34:1699–1706.

48. Yamamoto, S., Nakaki, T., Nakadate, T., and Kato, R. (1983): Insulinotropic effects of exogenous phospholipase A_2 and C in isolated pancreatic islets. *Eur. J. Pharmacol.*, 86:121–124.

49. Yamamoto, S., Nakadate, T., Nakaki, T., Ishii, K., and Kato, R. (1982): Prevention of glucose-induced insulin secretion by lipoxygenase inhibitor. *Eur. J. Pharmacol.*, 78:225–227.

50. Yamamoto, S., Nakadate, T., Nakaki, T., Ishii, K., and Kato, R. (1982): Tumor promoter 12-*o*-tetradecanoylphorbol-13-acetate-induced insulin secretion: Inhibition by phospholipase A_2- and lipoxygenase-inhibitors. *Biochem. Biophys. Res. Commun.*, 105:759–765.

Advances in Prostaglandin, Thromboxane, and Leukotriene Research, Vol. 13, edited by G. G. Neri Serneri, et al. Raven Press, New York © 1985.

Thromboxane- and ADP-Independent Aggregation and Exposure of Fibrinogen Receptors on Platelets from Patients with Familial Hypercholesterolemia

A. M. Cerbone, G. Di Minno, A. Postiglione, F. Cirillo, M. Pannain, P. L. Mattioli, and M. Mancini

Istituto di Medicina Interna e Malattie Dismetaboliche, II Facoltà di Medicina e Chirurgia, University of Naples, 80131 Naples, Italy

Patients with hypercholesterolemia exhibit an increased risk of thromboembolic episodes *in vivo* associated with a variety of platelet abnormalities *in vitro* (4). These include increased sensitivity to several aggregating agents, increased synthesis of thromboxane, and increased secretion of nucleotides. Evidence is accumulating that platelet aggregation involves exposure of receptors for fibrinogen on the platelet surface (1–3,5,6,8,9,11,12) and that secreted ADP (3,10,12) and thromboxane (2,3,10) expose such receptors on normal platelets. In this report we show that, following stimulation with thrombin or collagen, hyperaggregable platelets from patients with homozygous familial hypercholesterolemia (hmz FH) aggregate and bind significantly more fibrinogen than control platelets when prostaglandin/thromboxane formation is suppressed (aspirin) and secreted ADP is scavenged (apyrase).

SUBJECTS AND METHODS

Nine FH patients (5 females, 4 males, 7–36 years old) and 10 control subjects matched for sex and age were studied. None of the controls had a history of disease known to alter platelet aggregation. Neither FH patients nor controls had taken any medication for at least 10 days before donating blood. There was no difference between FH [109.9 ± 10.6 mg/dl (SEM)] and control (112 ± 12.5 mg/dl) subjects in total triglyceride levels and in very low density lipoprotein (VLDL) triglycerides (79.5 ± 6.1 mg/dl for FH patients and 79.2 ± 11.6 mg/dl for controls). None of the subjects tested had fasting plasma glucose concentrations higher than 92 mg/dl. Diagnosis of FH in hypercholesterolemic patients was based on (a) a plasma cholesterol level consistently higher than 500 mg/dl with low density lipoprotein (LDL) cholesterol always higher than 450 mg/dl, (b) appearance of xanthomata in the first decade of life, and (c) presence of marked hypercholesterolemia in both parents.

Platelet aggregation, secretion, thromboxane formation, and ^{125}I-fibrinogen binding in the presence or in the absence of aspirin were determined as previously described (3) in washed platelet suspensions from all the volunteers and the patients.

RESULTS AND DISCUSSION

In the presence of fibrinogen, the minimal concentrations of ADP, collagen, arachidonic acid (AA), or thrombin that caused 50% light transmittance (AC_{50}) were significantly ($p<0.01$) lower in suspensions from FH patients than in those from controls. In parallel, thromboxane synthesis in response to given concentrations of collagen, thrombin, or AA was significantly higher ($p<0.05$) in platelets from FH than in those from controls. As expected, aspirin (1 mM) suppressed thromboxane synthesis in response to all the stimuli and aggregation in response to AA. However, even in the presence of aspirin, the AC_{50} levels for ADP, collagen, or thrombin with FH platelets were significantly lower ($p<0.05$) than with control platelets. The combination of apyrase (500 µg/ml) plus aspirin suppressed ADP- or AA-induced aggregation of control and FH platelets and inhibited by about 70% and 80%, respectively, the aggregation of control platelets exposed to thrombin (10 mU/ml) or collagen (1 µg/ml), whereas inhibition of aggregation of FH platelets was about 17% and 37%, respectively. It also appeared that FH platelets bound significantly ($p<0.01$) more fibrinogen than those from normals. Preincubation of platelets with aspirin (1–4 mM) plus apyrase (500–2000 µg/ml) sufficed to suppress the binding to normal platelets, but it reduced that to FH platelets by only 75 to 80%. The aggregation and the binding of fibrinogen in response to U-46619 (a stable analog of prostaglandin endoperoxides/thromboxane A_2) was quantitatively similar in platelets from normal and FH patients. This suggests that FH platelets exhibit normal sensitivity to cyclic endoperoxides/thromboxane A_2. Analysis of the binding data of a monoclonal antibody (B79.7) to the platelet receptor for fibrinogen showed that this receptor is the same in platelets from normal and FH patients both in the presence and in the absence of aspirin plus apyrase and before and after exposure to thrombin, collagen, or arachidonic acid.

REFERENCES

1. Bennet, J. S., and Vilaire, G. (1979): Exposure of platelet fibrinogen receptors by ADP and epinephrine. *J. Clin. Invest.*, 64:1393–1401.
2. Bennet, J. S., Vilaire, G., and Burch, J. W. (1981): A role for prostaglandins and thromboxanes in the exposure of platelet fibrinogen receptors. *J. Clin. Invest.*, 68:981–987.
3. Di Minno, G., Thiagarajan, P., Perussia, B., Martinez, J., Shapiro, S., Trinchieri, G., and Murphy, S. (1983): Exposure of platelet fibrinogen binding sites by collagen, arachidonic acid and ADP. Inhibition by a monoclonal antibody to the glycoprotein IIb–IIIa complex. *Blood*, 61:140–148.
4. Harlan, J. M., and Harker, L. A. (1981): Hemostasis, thrombosis and thromboembolic disorders. The role of arachidonic acid metabolites in platelet–vessel wall interaction. *Med. Clin. North Am.*, 65:855–879.
5. Hawiger, J., Parkinson, S., and Timmons, S. (1980): Prostacyclin inhibits mobilization of fibrinogen-binding sites on human ADP and thrombin treated platelets. *Nature (Lond.)*, 283:195–197.
6. Kornecki, E., Niewiarowski, S., Morinelli, T. A., and Kloczewiak, M. (1981): Effect of chy-

motrypsin and adenosine diphosphate on the exposure of fibrinogen receptors on normal human and Glanzmann's thrombasthenic platelets. *J. Biol. Chem.*, 256:5696–5701.

7. Marguerie, G. A., Plow, E. F., and Edgington, T. S. (1979): Human platelets possess an inducible and saturable receptor specific for fibrinogen. *J. Biol. Chem.*, 254:5357–5363.

8. Mustard, J. F., Kinlough-Rathbone, R. L., Packham, M. A., Perry, D. W., Harfenist, E. J., and Pai, K. R. M. (1979): Comparison of fibrinogen association with normal and thrombasthenic platelets on exposure to ADP or chymotrypsin. *Blood*, 54:987–993.

9. Niewiarowski, S., Budzynski, A. Z., Morinelli, T. A., Budzynski, T. M., and Steward, G. J. (1981): Exposure of fibrinogen receptors on human platelets by proteolytic enzymes. *J. Biol. Chem.*, 256:917–925.

10. Peerschkle, E. (1983): Induction of human platelet fibrinogen receptors by epinephrine in the absence of released ADP. *Blood*, 60:71–76.

11. Peerschke, E. I., Zucker, M. B., Grant, R. A., Egan, J. J., and Johnson, M. M. (1980): Correlation between fibrinogen binding to human platelets and platelet aggregability. *Blood*, 55:841–847.

12. Plow, E. F., and Marguerie, G. A. (1980): Induction of the fibrinogen receptor on human platelets by epinephrine and the combination of epinephrine and ADP. *J. Biol. Chem.*, 256:917–925.

Advances in Prostaglandin, Thromboxane, and Leukotriene Research, Vol. 13, edited by G. G. Neri Serneri, et al. Raven Press, New York © 1985.

Platelets, Endothelium, and Vessel Injury

*J. F. Mustard, *R. L. Kinlough-Rathbone, and **M. A. Packham

*Department of Pathology, McMaster University, Hamilton, Ontario L8N 3Z5;
and **Department of Biochemistry, University of Toronto,
Toronto, Ontario M5S 1A8, Canada*

This chapter is directed primarily to factors influencing platelet interaction with injured vessels and the part played by prostaglandins and related products in this process. In the first section, the role of platelets in the development of atherosclerosis, and the clinical complications of atherosclerosis, such as strokes and myocardial infarction, are considered. In the second section, the role of prostaglandins and of other products of arachidonic acid that influence platelet interaction with the normal and damaged arterial wall is discussed.

PLATELETS AND VASCULAR DISEASE

The early stages of the development of atherosclerosis are characterized by focal intimal thickening of arteries, particularly around vessel orifices and branches (51). The explanation for the focal characteristics of these early lesions has not been established, but involves altered blood flow, accumulation of lipid, interaction of formed elements (particularly white cells and possibly platelets), and probably some form of injury or alteration of endothelial cells (55). Although the full spectrum of atherosclerosis can be produced in animals by repeated vessel injury, it seems likely that the formation of the early lesions is caused in a number of ways and that no single mechanism is responsible. For example, certain viruses such as Marek's virus can alter the vessel wall (46), producing intimal thickening and lipid accumulation without obvious injury to the endothelium, and without white-cell or platelet interaction with the vessel wall. This is probably a direct effect of the virus on the smooth muscle cells in the vessel wall. In addition, hypercholesterolemia causes the focal accumulation of lipids and macrophages and the formation of foam cells in the intima which, in the early stages, is probably not dependent on endothelial injury and platelet accumulation (26,34). All of these concepts have been reviewed in a number of articles (45,55,63).

When platelets interact with exposed subendothelium following injury of the endothelium in normal vessels, the platelets release chemotactic and mitogenic factors that cause smooth muscle cell migration and proliferation in the intima. The importance of this process in the development of the early lesions of atherosclerosis is unclear, but repeated injury of the endothelium of large arteries in experimental animals produces intimal thickening and the development of lesions that mimic the spectrum of lesions found in human atherosclerosis (49). It is known that platelets interact with connective-tissue constituents in the subendothelium (59). Platelets adhere to several forms of fibrillar collagen, and collagen induces the release of the contents of platelet granules. The interaction of platelets with collagen also leads to the activation of phospholipases (probably phospholipase A_2), with the freeing of arachidonic acid and the formation from it of thromboxane A_2 (TXA_2) and products of the lipoxygenase pathway. Platelets also can adhere to basement membrane, but this platelet interaction appears to be less strong than their interaction with fibrillar collagen and there is little release of the contents of platelet granules or activation of the arachidonate pathway. Platelets interact with microfibrils, and it has been reported that in the presence of von Willebrand factor, microfibrils induce platelet aggregation (21). Von Willebrand's factor may be involved in platelet adherence to the connective tissue in vessel walls in circumstances in which the shear rates are high, such as occur in the microcirculation (44). Considerably more work is necessary to define the extent to which the various components of connective tissue are exposed, how platelets interact with these components, and the roles of proteins such as fibronectin, thrombospondin, and the von Willebrand factor. Small endothelial lesions can occur without platelets adhering to the subendothelium (61), and even when large sections of endothelium are removed there are some areas that are not covered with platelets; large platelet aggregates or thrombi do not form on the subendothelium of normal large arteries unless blood flow is disturbed (53).

The development of more advanced lesions of atherosclerosis involves the organization of mural thrombi (9,18,33,71). Thrombi may form repeatedly at the same site, and the resulting lesion will have a layered appearance. The development of focal stenotic lesions may, in some circumstances, involve recurrent episodes of vessel injury and mural thrombosis. Such thrombi are initially composed largely of platelets, and it may be that the initiation and growth of these thrombi are influenced by products of the arachidonate pathway such as TXA_2 and prostacyclin (PGI_2). Under some experimental conditions, thrombus growth has been shown to be enhanced by inhibition of PGI_2 formation (35). However, these studies were done under circumstances in which there was extensive generation of thrombin and stasis, so that the experimentally-induced thrombi were not analogous to the thrombi that form in areas of disturbed flow in the high-flow, pulsatile systems of arteries. The evidence that atherosclerotic vessel walls may produce less PGI_2 than normal vessels (47,70) raises the possibility that if the endothelium is injured at sites of stenotic lesions, a lack of PGI_2 may lead to enhanced thrombosis. In other studies, however, normal or increased PGI_2 production has been observed with atherosclerotic vessels (41,69).

It is clear that platelets and thrombosis contribute to the development of advanced focal atherosclerotic lesions, but the relative importance of thrombosis in the progression of atherosclerotic lesions is not known. However, there is no evidence from studies with inhibitors of thrombus formation that drugs with this effect have caused the regression of atherosclerotic lesions in man.

Platelets and the Clinical Complications of Atherosclerosis

The mechanisms involved in the clinical complications of atherosclerosis are becoming better understood, but the relative importance of the different mechanisms is not known. It is now fairly well established that focal arterial spasm can occur in diseased coronary arteries (2,42,43). Individuals who die suddenly from ischemic heart disease seldom have occlusive thrombi in their coronary arteries, although they have extensive atherosclerosis (7,14). It is thought that some of the ischemic episodes that cause sudden death may be due to coronary artery spasm. In contrast to subjects dying suddenly, individuals who die with myocardial infarction have a high probability of having occlusive thrombi in their coronary arteries (7,14,62). Recent studies have indicated that lysis of thrombi in individuals who are developing myocardial infarction can significantly improve the clinical course of these individuals (65).

There are other mechanisms that may be involved in causing the clinical complications of atherosclerosis, such as tears in diseased vessel walls so that flaps of tissue can temporarily block blood flow (54), and possibly abnormalities in the myocardial metabolism (57) associated with diminished blood flow that contributes to impaired cardiac function and ventricular fibrillation.

The majority of cardiac problems associated with atherosclerosis of the coronary artery appear to be due to spasm of the coronary artery and thrombosis. Experimentally it has been shown that the smooth muscle cells in a region of focal, intimal thickening are hypersensitive to vasoconstrictive stimuli (66). Furthermore, although it was believed for a number of years that atherosclerotic vessels are rigid, there is now direct evidence from angiographic studies that atherosclerotic vessels can go into spasm (42). Since vessel injury that involves severing or puncturing of blood vessels is associated with contraction and the formation of a hemostatic plug, it is not surprising that injury to a diseased artery could be associated with constriction and thrombosis. PGI_2 appears to be involved in controlling vessel tone following injury to normal blood vessels (3,4); the importance of PGI_2 in diseased blood vessels, however, is not clear. TXA_2 and leukotrienes can certainly cause vasoconstriction (20,64), but a role for them in arterial spasm is not established. The role of the endothelium in controlling vessel tone deserves consideration, since when the endothelium is stimulated it can form PGI_2, and a number of studies have shown that the endothelium can also be stimulated by a number of agents to release a nonprostaglandin factor that causes smooth muscle cell relaxation (25).

The relationship between spasm and thrombosis is important. There is now good reason to believe that many episodes of angina (particularly variant, or unstable, angina) are secondary to spasm. Although some spasm may be neurogenic in origin, it is thought that most coronary artery spasm is focal, raising the possibility that local events such as vessel injury may be a key factor in its development (12).

In an area of severe stenosis, flow may cause injury to the endothelium at the sites where there is a high shear rate (the proximal side of the stenosis) (27). Distally, the disturbed flow could promote the accumulation of chemical mediators that could stimulate both thrombosis and spasm (53). In theory, spasm that is sufficient to impair the blood supply to the distal myocardium could cause ventricular fibrillation and death. In other circumstances, if sudden death does not occur, the spasm could persist long enough to enhance the development of thrombosis. Even if the vessel relaxes, an occlusive thrombus could persist and cause myocardial infarction. Furthermore, if the vessel relaxes and the thrombus is dislodged and fragmented, the fragments could embolize the distal circulation, causing ventricular fibrillation and sudden death (30,32). Thus the range of responses of diseased coronary arteries to stimulation or endothelial cell injury could produce most of the pathological events and the clinical manifestations of coronary artery disease.

Platelets could contribute to spasm through products released from their granules (such as ADP and serotonin) and through the formation of TXA_2.

The effects of flow control the development of occlusive thrombi (53). In areas of severe stenosis, the shear rates are high enough to induce platelet aggregation, probably without significant injury of endothelial cells (23). This type of platelet aggregation appears to be dependent on products formed when the arachidonate pathway is activated, since it can be inhibited by aspirin (22). In areas of disturbed flow, such as distal to a stenosis, the altered flow permits platelet adherence to the wall and the accumulation of chemical factors that promote platelet aggregation and thrombosis, such as ADP and thrombin (53).

Thrombosis is initiated not only by the adherence of platelets to subendothelial connective tissue but also by thrombin, which converts fibrinogen to fibrin. The latter mechanism is responsible for the initiation of some thrombi in vessels in which the intima is thickened, as in atherosclerosis. In addition to causing the release of the contents of platelet granules and activating the arachidonate pathway, thrombin can cause platelet aggregation independently of released ADP or TXA_2 formation (53). Collagen also causes the release of ADP from platelets independently of the activation of the arachidonate pathway. Thrombin or ADP, with released serotonin acting synergistically to augment their effects, can cause platelet aggregation independently of the arachidonate pathway. The role of platelet activating factor (PAF) in thrombus formation is not clear, but the amounts formed by human platelets are probably too small to have much effect on the function of platelets.

PROSTAGLANDINS, PLATELETS, ATHEROSCLEROSIS, AND CLINICAL COMPLICATIONS

There has been speculation that prostaglandins are important in the development of atherosclerosis and its clinical complications (47).

The results from early studies indicated that the capacity of the atherosclerotic vessel to form prostaglandins appears to be diminished in comparison with normal vascular tissue (47,58,70). However, more recent studies have failed to confirm these earlier observations (41,69). Products of lipid peroxidation have been reported to inhibit the prostaglandin pathway, and the accumulation of lipids in atherosclerotic plaques could contribute to the formation of lipid peroxides (48). It has been observed that there is a positive correlation between the apparent increased levels of lipid peroxides and the severity of atherosclerotic lesions (28). In atherosclerotic rabbits (16), it was found that arterial rings from these animals had a decreased capacity to form PGI_2. The investigators suggested that this was caused by the effects of chronic exposure to lipid peroxides. At present, the results from the different studies make it difficult to come to a firm conclusion about the capacity of atherosclerotic vessels to form PGI_2.

Prostaglandins could influence the migration and proliferation of smooth muscle cells, the cellular metabolism of lipids, and possibly the synthesis of connective tissue. Furthermore, low-density lipoprotein (LDL) has been found to inhibit PGI_2 synthesis by cells in tissue culture (56). There are several studies showing that aspirin treatment inhibits the development of diet-induced atherosclerosis in monkeys (60) and pigs (10,38). This effect is not caused by inhibition of platelet adhesion to the subendothelium, since aspirin does not influence the extent of adherence under physiological conditions (15). This effect of aspirin on experimental atherosclerosis could indicate that products of arachidonate metabolism influence the development of atherosclerotic lesions, possibly by increasing the amount of the products of the lipoxygenase pathway or by inhibiting PGI_2 formation. However, other nonsteroidal antiinflammatory drugs are less effective (1). It has also been shown that salicylate activates fibrinolysis through an effect on leukocytes (50).

There have been many studies of the role of prostaglandins, TXA_2, and leukotrienes in the interaction of platelets and white blood cells with the vessel wall and the contribution that platelets make to the migration and proliferation of smooth muscle cells. Although it was proposed that PGI_2 prevents platelets from adhering to the endothelium (29), direct experimental testing of this hypothesis has shown that PGI_2 is not responsible for preventing platelet adhesion to normal endothelium (13,15). Although platelets appear to be able to adhere to altered endothelium (13), this is not a common occurrence. It has been shown that high concentrations of PGI_2 significantly inhibit platelet adhesion to the subendothelium, but it is unlikely that plasma concentrations of PGI_2 required for this effect are ever achieved in either normal or diseased states (6,17,31). There has been speculation that high concentrations may be achieved locally on the vessel surface, but in vessels denuded of endothelium it is doubtful that local concentrations could be sustained for a period of time sufficiently long to keep platelets from adhering to injured vessel walls, which remain attractive to platelets for 6 to 8 hr after the removal of the endothelium (37). Administration of aspirin to inhibit PGI_2 production by the deendothelialized rabbit aorta does not cause increased platelet adherence to the subendothelium (15). It appears that tissues usually produce prostaglandins only in short bursts following stimulation (17), so that local, sustained formation in concentrations sufficient to inhibit thrombus formation at an injury site may not occur.

The interaction of platelets with subendothelial tissues occurs independently of activation of the platelet arachidonate pathway (15,36). It is not generally appreciated that platelets that adhere to collagen release their granule contents through a pathway that is not dependent on the formation of TXA_2. Platelets that have been treated with aspirin to inhibit the cyclooxygenase still adhere to connective tissues such as collagen, and the adherent platelets release their granule contents. The results of studies showing that aspirin treatment inhibits platelet accumulation on the subendothelium are primarily studies in which the extent of platelet aggregation that occurs on top of the initial platelet layer that forms when the subendothelium is exposed is inhibited, rather than the initial accumulation of platelets on the exposed subendothelium.

In the later stages of the development of atherosclerosis, platelet–fibrin thrombi can play a major part (9,18). Since TXA_2 is important in platelet aggregation and the release of the contents of platelet granules, it could be argued that in circumstances in which the production of TXA_2 is enhanced, platelet aggregation and thrombosis will be more extensive. Platelets in individuals with hypercholesterolemia or some forms of diabetes are hypersensitive to aggregating agents, and this appears to be mediated through increased activation of the arachidonate pathway (5,11). One explanation for this is that the lipid composition of the platelet membranes is changed and this modifies the pathways that are involved in the release of arachidonic acid and its metabolism. Changing the fatty acid composition of diets of humans or experimental animals can change the fatty acid composition of the platelets and their function (19,67). Diets enriched in eicosapentaenoic acid are associated with platelets that respond less strongly to stimulation, and this is thought to be an explanation of the observation that Eskimos, who eat diets rich in eicosapentaenoic acid, appear to have a lower incidence of atherosclerosis and its complications such as heart attacks (19). In addition to having effects on platelets, these diets are likely to affect prostaglandin production by the vessel wall.

Clinical Complications of Atherosclerosis

As discussed earlier, it has been shown experimentally that vessels with intimal thickening caused by the proliferation of smooth muscle cells are more sensitive than normal vessels to agents that contract vessel walls (66). Furthermore, studies in man are compatible with the sites of focal atherosclerosis being most sensitive to spasm (42). Both TXA_2 and PGI_2 may have significant effects on spasm of coronary arteries, but other agents such as serotonin and histamine can also change coronary artery tone. Failure of vessel walls to produce PGI_2 could reduce the ability of the coronary artery to relax when it is stimulated to contract. At present we have very little information about the relationship of PGI_2 production to the ability of the coronary arteries to contract or relax. Experimentally it has been shown that inhibitors of cyclooxygenase cause vessels to be more sensitive to agents that cause contraction (66). On the other hand, however, attempts to relieve coronary artery spasm in subjects with unstable angina by infusions of PGI_2 have been unsuccessful (8). This may indicate that PGI_2 produced by the vessel wall is more important than PGI_2 in plasma in controlling vessel spasm. In addition, studies with inhibitors of the cyclooxygenase (24) support the hypothesis that PGI_2 formation by smooth muscle cells in the vessel wall is likely to be important in the control of spasm and clinical manifestations such as angina.

At present, it is not known whether spasm in stenotic, diseased coronary arteries facilitates thrombus formation, although there are case reports that support this concept (12,68). As discussed in the first part of this review, it is likely that spasm in a stenotic coronary artery would facilitate the development of thrombosis. Theoretically, therefore, one could have spasm, myocardial ischemia, and complications such as ventricular fibrillation and death without observable thrombosis in the coronary arteries. Alternatively, if the spasm lasts long enough for a thrombus to form, and the individual does not die immediately, the artery could be blocked by an occlusive thrombus that persists after relaxation of the contracted artery. If death occurs subsequently, it would be attributable to myocardial infarction caused by the occlusive thrombus. These points concerning spasm, thrombosis, and prostaglandins are of some importance in trying to interpret the results of clinical trials using drugs such as aspirin for the secondary prevention of myocardial infarction.

In trials of the effect of aspirin in post myocardial infarction patients, there was no reduction or significant increase in the incidence of sudden death (52); an increase might have been expected if the doses of aspirin had been sufficient to inhibit PGI_2 formation by the vessel wall and, assuming PGI_2 is important in preventing spasm of coronary arteries, make them more susceptible to spasm. The recent study (39) showing that a low dose of aspirin reduced the incidence of myocardial infarction in individuals who had unstable angina, but did not influence the frequency of angina attacks (40), may indicate that the dose of aspirin that was used had little effect on the production of PGI_2 by the vessel wall, but inhibited the contribution of the platelets to thrombus formation by inhibiting TXA_2 formation. Experimentally, platelet-rich thrombi form in the areas of high shear in severely stenosed vessels. This platelet aggregation is dependent on TXA_2 formation, and the formation of the platelet aggregates can be inhibited by aspirin and other nonsteroidal antiinflammatory drugs (22,23). Theoretically, therefore, one might expect that spasm, superimposed on a severe stenosis, would cause platelet aggregation at the stenotic sites; in low doses, aspirin would be expected to inhibit the extent of platelet aggregation at the site, but not have much effect on the extent of spasm.

It is apparent that further study is needed to determine the relationships among spasm, vessel injury, thrombosis, and the role of prostaglandins, particularly those formed by the vessel wall, in controlling arterial tone.

SUMMARY

Injury to the endothelial lining of arteries is an important mechanism in both the early and late stages of the development of atherosclerosis. Platelets can contribute to the early lesions by releasing factors that cause smooth muscle cell migration and proliferation. In the later stages, the formation of large platelet–fibrin thrombi that become organized into the vessel wall contributes to the development of focal atherosclerotic narrowing of arteries.

Injury to the vessel wall can also be a factor in causing spasm of coronary arteries, particularly at sites of stenosis. The spasm may cause ischemia, anginal pain, and, in some individuals, ventricular fibrillation and death. In other individuals, the spasm may not cause death but may persist long enough for an occlusive thrombus to form and cause myocardial infarction.

The events leading to thrombosis involve not only the release of arachidonic acid and the formation of TXA_2, but other pathways that are independent of the arachidonate pathway. In some circumstances thrombin (which causes platelet aggregation and release that are largely independent of the arachidonate pathway and TXA_2 formation) is the primary stimulus causing the initiation and growth of the thrombus.

The role of products of the arachidonate pathway in causing spasm is not understood. PGI_2 produced by the vessel wall could be important in preventing or minimizing coronary artery spasm. The best way to prevent the development of atherosclerosis and its clinical complications is to prevent or minimize injury of the endothelium.

REFERENCES

1. Bailey, J. M., and Butler, J. (1973): Anti-inflammatory drugs in experimental atherosclerosis, Part 1. Relative potencies for inhibiting plaque formation. *Atherosclerosis*, 17:515–522.
2. Bertrand, M. E., LaBlanche, J. M., Tilmant, P. Y., Thieuleux, F. A., Delforge, M. R., Carre, A. G., Asseman, P., Berzin, B., Libersa, C., and Laurent, J. M. (1982): Frequency of provoked coronary arterial spasm in 1089 consecutive patients undergoing coronary arteriography. *Circulation*, 65:1299–1306.
3. Blajchman, M. A., Senyi, A. F., Hirsh, J., Surya, Y., Buchanan, M., and Mustard, J. F. (1979): Shortening of the bleeding time in rabbits by hydrocortisone caused by inhibition of prostacyclin generation by the vessel wall. *J. Clin. Invest.*, 63:1026–1035.
4. Buchanan, M. R., Blajchman, M. A., Dejana, E., Mustard, J. F., Senyi, A. F., and Hirsh, J. (1979): Shortening of the bleeding time in thrombocytopenic rabbits after exposure of jugular vein to high aspirin concentration. *Prostaglandins Med.*, 3:333–342.
5. Carvalho, A. C. A., Colman, R. W., and Lees, R. S. (1974): Platelet function in hyperlipoproteinemia. *N. Engl. J. Med.*, 290:434–438.
6. Cazenave, J.-P., Dejana, E., Kinlough-Rathbone, R. L., Richardson, M., Packham, M. A., and Mustard, J. F. (1979): Prostaglandins I_2 and E_1 reduce rabbit and human platelet adherence without inhibiting serotonin release from adherent platelets. *Thromb. Res.*, 15:273–279.
7. Chandler, A. B., Chapman, I., Erhardt, L. R., Roberts, W. C., Schwartz, C. J., Sinapius, D., Spain, D. M., Sherry, S., Ness, P. M., and Simon, T. L. (1974): Coronary thrombosis in myocardial infarction. Report of a workshop on the role of coronary thrombosis in the pathogenesis of acute myocardial infarction. *Am. J. Cardiol.*, 34:823–833.
8. Chierchia, S., Patrono, C., Crea, F., Ciabattoni, G., De Caterina, R., Cinotti, G. A., Distante, A., and Maseri, A. (1982): Effects of intravenous prostacyclin in variant angina. *Circulation*, 65:470–477.

9. Clark, E., Graef, T., and Chasis, H. (1936): Thrombosis of the aorta and coronary arteries with special reference to the "fibrinoid" lesions. *A.M.A. Arch. Pathol.*, 22:183–212.
10. Clopath, P. (1980): The effect of acetylsalicylic acid (ASA) on the development of atherosclerotic lesions in miniature swine. *Br. J. Exp. Pathol.*, 61:440–443.
11. Colwell, J. A., Winocour, P. D., Lopes-Virella, M., and Halushka, P. V. (1983): New concepts about the pathogenesis of atherosclerosis in diabetes mellitus. *Am. J. Med.*, 75:67–80.
12. Conti, C. R. (1983): Coronary-artery spasm and myocardial infarction. *N. Engl. J. Med.*, 309:238–239.
13. Curwen, K. D., Gimbrone, M. A., Jr., and Handin, R. I. (1980): *In vitro* studies of thromboresistance: The role of prostacyclin (PGI_2) in platelet adhesion to cultured normal and virally transformed human vascular endothelial cells. *Lab. Invest.*, 42:366–374.
14. Davies, M. J., Woolf, N., and Robertson, W. B. (1976): Pathology of acute myocardial infarction with particular reference to occlusive coronary thrombi. *Br. Heart J.*, 38:659–664.
15. Dejana, E., Cazenave, J.-P., Groves, H. M., Kinlough-Rathbone, R. L., Richardson, M., Packham, M. A., and Mustard, J. F. (1980): The effect of aspirin inhibition of PGI_2 production on platelet adherence to normal and damaged rabbit aortae. *Thromb. Res.*, 17:453–464.
16. Dembinska-Kiec, A., Gryglewska, T., Zmuda, A., and Gryglewski, R. (1977): The generation of prostacyclin by arteries and by the coronary vascular bed is reduced in experimental atherosclerosis in rabbits. *Prostaglandins*, 14:1025–1034.
17. Dollery, C. T., Barrow, S. E., Blair, I. A., Lewis, P. J., MacDermot, J., Orchard, M. A., Ritter, J. M., Robinson, C., Shepherd, G. L., Waddell, K. A., and Allison, D. J. (1983): Role of prostacyclin. In: *Atherosclerosis. Mechanisms and Approaches to Therapy*, edited by N. E. Miller, pp. 105–123. Raven Press, New York.
18. Duguid, J. B. (1946): Thrombosis as a factor in the pathogenesis of coronary atherosclerosis. *J. Pathol. Bacteriol.*, 58:207–212.
19. Dyerberg, J., Bang, H. O., Stoffersen, E., Moncada, S., and Vane, J. R. (1978): Eicosapentaenoic acid and prevention of thrombosis and atherosclerosis? *Lancet*, 2:117–119.
20. Ellis, E. F., Oelz, O., Roberts, L. J., II, Payne, N. A., Sweetman, B. J., Nies, A. S., and Oates, J. A. (1976): Coronary artery smooth muscle contraction by a substance released from platelets: evidence that it is thromboxane A_2. *Science*, 193:1135–1137.
21. Fauvel, F., Grant, M. E., Legrand, Y. J., Souchon, H., Tobelem, G., Jackson, D. S., and Caen, J. P. (1983): Interaction of blood platelets with a microfibrillar extract from adult bovine aorta: Requirement for von Willebrand factor. *Proc. Natl. Acad. Sci. U.S.A.*, 80:551–554.
22. Folts, J. D., Crowell, E. B. Jr., and Rowe, G. G. (1976): Platelet aggregation in partially obstructed vessels and its elimination with aspirin. *Circulation*, 54:365–370.
23. Folts, J. D., Gallagher, K., and Rowe, G. G. (1982): Blood flow reductions in stenosed canine coronary arteries: vasospasm or platelet aggregation? *Circulation*, 65:248–255.
24. Friedman, P. L., Brown, E. J., Jr., Gunther, S., Alexander, R. W., Barry, W. H., Mudge, G. H., Jr., and Grossman, W. (1981): Coronary vasoconstrictor effect of indomethacin in patients with coronary-artery disease. *N. Engl. J. Med.*, 305:1171–1175.
25. Furchgott, R. F. (1983): Role of endothelium in responses of vascular smooth muscle. *Circ. Res.*, 53:557–573.
26. Gerrity, R. G. (1981): The role of the monocyte in atherogenesis. I. Transition of blood-born monocytes into foam cells in fatty lesions. *Am. J. Pathol.*, 103:181–190.
27. Gertz, S. D., Uretsky, G., Wajnberg, R., Navot, N., and Gotsman, M. S. (1981): Endothelial cell damage and thrombus formation after partial arterial constriction: relevance to the role of coronary artery spasm in the pathogenesis of myocardial infarction. *Circulation*, 63:476–486.
28. Glavind, J., Hartmann, S., Clemmesen, J., Jessen, K. E., and Dam, H. (1952): Studies on the role of lipoperoxides in human pathology. II. The presence of peroxidized lipids in the atherosclerotic aorta. *Acta Pathol. Microbiol. Scand.*, 30:1–6.
29. Gryglewski, R. J., Bunting, S., Moncada, S., Flower, R. J., and Vane, J. R. (1976): Arterial walls are protected against deposition of platelet thrombi by a substance (prostaglandin X) which they make from prostaglandin endoperoxides. *Prostaglandins*, 12:685–713.
30. Haerem, J. W. (1974): Mural platelet microthrombi and major acute lesions of main epicardial arteries in sudden coronary death. *Atherosclerosis*, 19:529–541.
31. Higgs, E. A., Moncada, S., Vane, J. R., Caen, J. P., Michel, H., and Tobelem, G. (1978): Effect of prostacyclin (PGI_2) on platelet adhesion to rabbit arterial subendothelium. *Prostaglandins*, 16:17–22.

32. Jørgensen, L., Rowsell, H. C., Hovig, T., Glynn, M. F., and Mustard, J. F. (1967): Adenosine diphosphate-induced platelet aggregation and myocardial infarction in swine. *Lab. Invest.*, 17:616–644.
33. Jørgensen, L., Rowsell, H. C., Hovig, T., and Mustard, J. F. (1967): Resolution and organization of platelet-rich mural thrombi in carotid arteries of swine. *Am. J. Pathol.*, 51:681–719.
34. Joris, I., Zand, T., Nunnari, J. J., Krolikowski, F. J., and Majno, G. (1983): Studies on the pathogenesis of atherosclerosis I. Adhesion and emigration of mononuclear cells in the aorta of hypercholesterolemic rats. *Am. J. Pathol.*, 113:341–358.
35. Kelton, J. G., Hirsh, J., Carter, C. J., and Buchanan, M. R. (1978): Thrombogenic effect of high-dose aspirin in rabbits. Relationship to inhibition of vessel wall synthesis of prostaglandin I_2-like activity. *J. Clin. Invest.*, 62:892–895.
36. Kinlough-Rathbone, R. L., Cazenave, J.-P., Packham, M. A., and Mustard, J. F. (1980): Effect of inhibitors of the arachidonate pathway on the release of granule contents from platelets adherent to collagen. *Lab. Invest.*, 42:28–34.
37. Kinlough-Rathbone, R. L., Groves, H. M., and Mustard, J. F. (1983): Factors influencing vessel wall reactivity following injury. *Thromb. Haemostas.*, 50:380.
38. Kim, D. N., Lee, K. T., Schmee, J., and Thomas, W. A. (1983): Anti-proliferative effect of pryidinolcarbamate and of aspirin in the early stages of atherogenesis in swine. *Atherosclerosis*, 48:1–13.
39. Lewis, H. D., Davis, J. W., Archibald, D. G., Steinke, W. E., Smitherman, T. C., Doherty, J. E., Schnaper, H. W., Le Winter, M. M., Linares, E., Pouget, J. M., Sabharwal, S. C., Chesler, E., and De Mots, H. (1983): Protective effects of aspirin against acute myocardial infarction and death in men with unstable angina. Results of a Veterans' Administration Cooperative Study. *N. Engl. J. Med.*, 309:396–403.
40. Lewis, H. D., Jr., Davis, J. W., and Archibald, D. G. (1984): Aspirin and the risk of myocardial infarction. *N. Engl. J. Med.*, 310:122–123.
41. Majerus, P. W. (1983): Arachidonate metabolism in vascular disorders. *J. Clin. Invest.*, 72:1521–1525.
42. Maseri, A., and Chierchia, S. (1982): Coronary artery spasm: Demonstration, definition, diagnosis, and consequences. *Prog. Cardiovasc. Dis.*, 25:169–192.
43. Maseri, A., L'Abbate, A., Baroldi, G., Chierchia, S., Marzilli, M., Ballestra, A. M., Severi, S., Parodi, O., Biagini, A., Distante, A., and Pesola, A. (1978): Coronary vasospasm as a possible cause of myocardial infarction. A conclusion derived from the study of "preinfarction" angina. *N. Engl. J. Med.*, 299:1271–1277.
44. Meyer, D., and Baumgartner, H. R. (1983): Role of von Willebrand factor in platelet adhesion to the subendothelium. *Br. J. Haematol.*, 54:1–9.
45. Miller, N. E. (1983): High density lipoprotein, atherosclerosis, and ischaemic heart disease. In: *Atherosclerosis: Mechanisms and Approaches to Therapy*, edited by N. E. Miller, pp. 153–168. Raven Press, New York.
46. Minick, C. R., Fabricant, C. G., Fabricant, J., and Litrenta, M. M. (1979): Atheroarteriosclerosis induced by infection with a herpesvirus. *Am. J. Pathol.*, 96:673–706.
47. Moncada, S. (1983): Prostacyclin. In: *Atherosclerosis: Mechanisms and Approaches to Therapy*, edited by N. E. Miller, pp. 55–75. Raven Press, New York.
48. Moncada, S., Gryglewski, R. J., Bunting, S., and Vane, J. R. (1976): A lipid peroxide inhibits the enzyme in blood vessel microsomes that generates from prostaglandin endoperoxides the substance (prostaglandin X) which prevents platelet aggregation. *Prostaglandins*, 12:715–733.
49. Moore, S. (1973): Thromboatherosclerosis in normolipemic rabbits. A result of continued endothelial damage. *Lab. Invest.*, 29:478–487.
50. Moroz, L. A. (1977): Increased blood fibrinolytic activity after aspirin ingestion. *N. Engl. J. Med.*, 296:525–529.
51. Murphy, E. A., Rowsell, H. C., Downie, H. G., Robinson, G. A., and Mustard, J. F. (1962): Encrustation and atherosclerosis: The analogy between early *in vivo* lesions and deposits which occur in extracorporeal circulations. *Can. Med. Assoc. J.*, 87:259–274.
52. Mustard, J. F., Kinlough-Rathbone, R. L., and Packham, M. A. (1983): Aspirin in the treatment of cardiovascular disease: A review. *Am. J. Med.*, 74:43–49.
53. Mustard, J. F., Packham, M. A., and Kinlough-Rathbone, R. L. (1981): Mechanisms in thrombosis. In: *Haemostasis and Thrombosis*, edited by A. L. Bloom and D. P. Thomas, pp. 503–526. Churchill Livingstone, New York.

54. Mustard, J. F., Packham, M. A., and Kinlough-Rathbone, R. L. (1981): Platelets, atherosclerosis, and clinical complications. In: *Vascular Injury and Atherosclerosis*, edited by S. Moore, pp. 79–110. Marcel Dekker, New York.

55. Mustard, J. F., Packham, M. A., and Kinlough-Rathbone, R. L. (1983): Platelets and atherosclerosis. In: *Atherosclerosis: Mechanisms and Approaches to Therapy*, edited by N. E. Miller, pp. 29–43. Raven Press, New York.

56. Nordøy, A., Svensson, B., Wiebe, D., and Hoak, J. C. (1978): Lipoproteins and the inhibitory effect of human endothelial cells on platelet function. *Circ. Res.*, 43:527–534.

57. Oliver, M. F., Kurien, V. A., and Greenwood, T. (1968): Relation between serum-free-fatty acids and arrhythmias and death after acute myocardial infarction. *Lancet*, 1:710–714.

58. Packham, M. A., and Mustard, J. F. (1983): Pharmacology of antiplatelet agents and their role in coronary disease. In: *Myocardial Infarction and Cardiac Death*, edited by E. Margulies, pp. 93–142. Academic Press, New York.

59. Packham, M. A., and Mustard, J. F. (1984): Platelet adhesion. In: *Progress in Hemostasis and Thrombosis, vol. 7*, edited by T. H. Spaet. Grune and Stratton, New York.

60. Pick, R., Chediak, J., and Glick, G. (1979): Aspirin inhibits development of coronary atherosclerosis in cynomolgus monkeys *(Macaca fascicularis)* fed an atherogenic diet. *J. Clin. Invest.*, 63:158–162.

61. Reidy, M. A., and Schwartz, S. M. (1981): Endothelial regeneration III. Time course of intimal changes after small defined injury to rat aortic endothelium. *Lab. Invest.*, 44:301–308.

62. Ridolfi, R. L., and Hutchins, G. M. (1977): The relationship between coronary artery lesions and myocardial infarcts: ulceration of atherosclerotic plaques precipitating coronary thrombosis. *Am. Heart J.*, 93:468–486.

63. Ross, R. (1981): Atherosclerosis: A problem of the biology of arterial wall cells and their interactions with blood components. *Arteriosclerosis*, 1:293–311.

64. Samuelsson, B. (1983): Leukotrienes: Mediators of immediate hypersensitivity reactions and inflammation. *Science*, 220:568–575.

65. Schwarz, F., Faure, A., Katus, H., von Olshausen, K., Hofmann, M., Schuler, G., Manthey, J., and Kubler, W. (1983): Intracoronary thrombolysis in acute myocardial infarction: An attempt to quantitate its effect by comparison of enzymatic estimate of myocardial necrosis with left ventricular ejection fraction. *Am. J. Cardiol.*, 51:1573–1578.

66. Shimokawa, H., Tomoike, H., Nabeyama, S., Yamamoto, H., Araki, H., Nakamura, M., Ishii, Y., and Tanaka, K. (1983): Coronary artery spasm induced in atherosclerotic miniature swine. *Science*, 221:560–562.

67. Thorngren, M., and Gustafson, A. (1981): Effects of 11-week increase in dietary eicosapentaenoic acid on bleeding time, lipids, and platelet aggregation. *Lancet*, II:1190–1193.

68. Vincent, G. M., Anderson, J. L., and Marshall, H. W. (1983): Coronary spasm producing coronary thrombosis and myocardial infarction. *N. Engl. J. Med.*, 309:220–223.

69. Voss, R., ten Hoor, F., and Matthias, F. R. (1983): Prostacyclin production and atherosclerosis of the rabbit aorta. In: *Advances in Prostaglandin, Thromboxane, and Leukotriene Research, vol. 11*, edited by B. Samuelsson, R. Paoletti, and P. Ramwell, pp. 469–474. Raven Press, New York.

70. Warso, M. A., and Lands, W. E. M. (1983): Lipid peroxidation in relation to prostacyclin and thromboxane physiology and pathophysiology. *Br. Med. Bull.*, 39:277–280.

71. Woolf, N., Bradley, J. W. P., Crawford, T., and Carstairs, K. C. (1968): Experimental mural thrombi in the pig aorta. The early natural history. *Br. J. Exp. Pathol.*, 49:257–264.

Advances in Prostaglandin, Thromboxane, and Leukotriene Research, Vol. 13, edited by G. G. Neri Serneri, et al. Raven Press, New York © 1985.

Medical Prevention of Ischemic Stroke

H. J. M. Barnett

Department of Clinical Neurological Sciences, University of Western Ontario, London, Ontario N6A 5A5, Canada

The problem of stroke prevention will be briefly discussed in this chapter in three areas: (a) natural history studies and their bearing on decisions about therapeutic advances; (b) results to date of platelet antiaggregant therapy; and (c) the requirements for future trials.

NATURAL HISTORY STUDIES

The pursuit of natural history studies in cerebrovascular or in cardiovascular disease has been given great stimulus by the advent of randomized clinical trials. Many beneficial spin-offs emerge from large series of similar patients scrutinized with the care needed to conduct a therapeutic study on patients with chronic illness. The data banks of the trials have provided prospective information utilizing the patients in the control groups and in the groups who received totally ineffective medication. They have allowed the statisticians to make sample-size calculations for populations to be entered into studies designed to evaluate subsequent therapeutic strategies. The pathogenesis of the diseases under study has been most carefully surveyed and in a few instances new concepts have emerged. Finally, a scrutiny of this data has focused attention on the accuracy and validity with which the characteristics of patient populations must be defined.

Effect on Risk of Specific Clinical Varieties of Transient Ischemic Attack

The early clinical trials to prevent stroke involved heterogenous groups of patients. Clinical ability to distinguish atherothrombotic varieties of transient ischemic attack (TIA) from those of cardiogenic thromboembolic origin, from lacunar varieties, and even from those due to small intracerebral hematomas was very imperfect. Considering the protean pathogenic mechanisms represented, it is little wonder that the early treatment trials of TIA, largely involving anticoagulants, were inconclusive. These studies frequently, if not invariably, concerned all varieties of TIA lumped together. One early study did attempt to narrow the field of observation down to patients presenting with amaurosis fugax and accompanied by bright retinal embolic plaques (15). The follow-up identified those patients as belonging to a high-risk group for fatal outcome—mostly as a result of myocardial infarction. Of the 208 patients, 15% were dead within 1 year, and 54% in the 7 years of total follow-up.

Another natural history study prospectively looking at a particular variety of TIA was the Canadian Cooperative Study (18). There were 585 patients drawn from a population afflicted with TIA or minor stroke investigated in hospital, of whom 78% were studied by angiography. Entry to the study was denied when the ischemic symptoms occurred in association with potential embolic conditions. Lacunar infarction and stroke due to hemorrhage were judged to be exclusions. The clinical and radiological criteria combined to indicate that they represented a specific group of patients afflicted with atherothrombotic lesions and ischemia due to accompanying thromboemboli. Of the 289 patients who did not receive active therapy, followed for an average of 26 months, the risk of stroke or death was higher in the first year than the later 2 years (Table 1). The average age of these patients was 62.5 years.

Effect on Risk of Gender

In the Canadian study the males were a higher-risk group of patients than were the females in all of the 3 years of follow-up. This increased risk for stroke or death in males after the onset of warning stroke symptoms is noted in all of the available published data on the subject (5). In a hospital-based population study conducted by Dyken (6), the death rate per year of follow-up in 399 patients not given antithrombotic drugs was 12% for males, compared with 4% for the females. In the 310 patients in whom some therapeutic intervention had occurred, the differential risk of death annually for male and female was 10% and 3%, respectively. With endpoints of both stroke and death, calculated on an annual basis, Marshall's study of 64 patients indicated a male versus female risk ratio of 13 versus 7%, respectively (11). In the short American Aspirin Study of 90 control patients, males had a 14% and females a 5% chance of a major endpoint (7); in the Canadian study, this ratio in 289 patients was 12% for males and 6% for

TABLE 1. *Prognosis from Canadian Cooperative Study*[a]

Interval (years)	Percentage of stroke or death		
	Both sexes	Male	Female
1	13	14	11
2	22	24	16
3	30	35	16

[a]The percentage of 289 patients judged at study entry to have had TIA or minor stroke of arterial thromboembolic origin, afflicted with stroke or death after average follow-up of 26 months.
(From the Canadian Cooperative Study Group, ref. 18.)

females. Clearly the phenomenon of a differential prognosis by sex must be included in decisions relating to treatment trials in these patients.

Effect on Risk of Age

Increasing age adds to the risk of stroke, as many national surveys demonstrate. It comes as no great surprise that the prognosis for older patients afflicted with TIA puts them into a higher-risk group. Warlow, conducting the British trial of aspirin in TIA, has identified this relationship in 1,141 patients followed for a total of 5 years: 3% had suffered stroke or death when the initial symptoms occurred under age 50; 6% if between 50 and 59 years; 8% between 60 and 69 years; and 11% if over 70 at entry (C. Warlow, *personal communication*).

Effect on Risk of Uncertain Variables Related to Selection Bias

The multicenter Italian TIA group have identified a lower-risk group of patients than some of the hospital-based studies already outlined (8). Whether they allowed a broader definition or observed a group of patients in a different setting and therefore at a different stage of illness is uncertain. In a follow-up of 48 months, this group reported on the incidence of endpoints of stroke or death in 462 patients. There were 7.7% fatal and nonfatal strokes and 7.1% deaths (including 3.2% of fatal stroke). The population was relatively young, with 19.7% under 45 years of age. A study from Finland represents another population of TIA patients at low risk compared with the majority of the published reports (14). The 314 TIA patients were followed for a mean duration of 7.8 years. Their average age was 49.2 years at the onset of the first TIA. Only 4.7% suffered cerebral infarction during this extended follow-up period, and another 12.7% suffered myocardial infarction. Deaths due to stroke and heart attack combined to involve 10.2% of the group. In both the Italian and the Finnish observations, it appears that the selection bias towards a younger population was one of the reasons for the low-risk situation encountered.

Effect on Risk of Severity of Ischemia

An assumption has been made that a group of individuals afflicted with reversible ischemic neurological deficit (RIND) or minor stroke would be expected to be at higher risk of a subsequent major ischemic event than patients afflicted with TIA alone. If this were correct there would be reason to question the mixture of patients with these deficits in a single trial. From a number of recently published studies, including the data from the Canadian Cooperative Study, and a Mayo Clinic review by Wiebers et al., there is no prognostic difference between these groups (19). The similarity of TIA to RIND and partial nonprogressing stroke (PNS) has been substantiated by computerized tomography (CT) studies, which have identified that 15 to 20% of so-called TIA patients will have appropriate residual CT lesions suggestive of infarction. In our own series, this was corroborated by both a prospective and a retrospective analysis. The retrospective review determined that of 223 consecutive patients admitted and designated as "TIA" patients, 48 (21%) had CT evidence of infarction. A prospective study in which 105 consecutive TIA patients were seen by our neurological resident and then by a consultant required to decide, deliberately prior to CT examination, on the likelihood or not of an infarction demonstrated that 20.9% of TIA patients had "infarction" by the usual radiological criteria. The pathogenesis of the ischemic conditions represented by TIA, RIND, or PNS is the same. The finding of a clinical residual or not relates to the size of the lesion and to its location in an elegant or nonelegant area of the brain. These observations permit the inclusion of patients with ischemic events of varying severity in therapeutic trials.

Effect on Risk of Specific Radiological Entities

Natural history studies are emerging that identify high-risk and lower-risk groups in terms of the site of obstructing or stenosing lesions of some of the cerebral arteries. The prognosis for patients presenting with ischemic events related to stenosis of the intracranial portion of the internal carotid artery (ICA) has proven to be remarkably poor. In two separate studies, involving a total of 110 patients followed for an average of approximately 3 years, stroke occurred in 35 and death from stroke or myocardial infarction in 51 (4,12). The occurrence of neither stroke nor death was evident in only 37 of the 110 patients. Approximately two-thirds were dead or afflicted with a stroke. The outlook for ICA occlusion, once judged to be benign in relation to the territory of the occlusion, is now known from the analysis of the Canadian data to be much less innocent than was thought to be the case (1,3). Five percent per year will suffer a stroke ipsilateral to the occlusion. So little data is available on the natural history of middle cerebral artery (MCA) occlusion and stenosis that it is best to conclude that the prognosis in these conditions remains to be identified by future studies.

In summary, the study of natural history is to be regarded as of consequence for the following reasons:

1. Sample-size calculations for clinical trials can be established based on either general or more specific knowledge.

2. High- and low-risk groups are recognized.

3. Unexpected information emerges that alters preconceived ideas about prognosis. The best immediate example is that noted in patients with occlusion of the internal carotid artery.

4. Data from natural history studies cannot be substituted in clinical trials for proper controls. In the first place the population on which the natural history study was made would never be reliably reproduced in another center. Even in the same center, carried out by the same observers, the changing baseline of stroke mortality and morbidity would deny the value of the previous study as a reliable control (10). With stroke diminishing for several years at the rate of 5% per year, it is evident

that radical changes are affecting the baseline of the risk for stroke in the populations of developed countries.

RESULTS TO DATE OF PLATELET ANTIAGGREGANT THERAPY

The question of anticoagulant therapy will not be addressed in this chapter. Its use in preventing cerebral ischemia is completely unknown because no adequate trials, by modern standards, have ever been conducted. For platelet antiaggregant therapy, six trials that achieve something approaching the gold standard for clinical trials, by at least being doubly blind with randomly assigned treatment or control groups, have been published, and the results are widely known.

Two trials were judged at the time of their design and execution to have been sufficiently large as to achieve a likelihood of showing a benefit. In the Canadian study, 585 patients were assigned to one of four treatment groups and given either 1300 g aspirin/day with placebo, 800 g of sulfinpyrazone per day with placebo, both these active drugs, or finally the placebo of both. A 30% reduction in stroke or death was achieved after an average of 26 months of follow-up. The benefit was significant only in males with a 50% reduction in stroke or death and 51% reduction in stroke or fatal stroke detected by sub-group analysis. Sulfinpyrazone was not any more effective than placebo.

The Collaborative Study reported in 1983 by Bousser et al. (2) entered 600 patients, administered 1200 g daily of aspirin to one-third of the patients, aspirin with persantine to one-third, and placebo to the other third. After 3 years of follow-up of each patient, stroke and stroke death risk were reduced by 50% in the groups given aspirin or aspirin with persantine, with equal benefit in both sexes. No difference was noted between the two groups on the active programs. As in the Canadian study, there were two males for each female in this Paris-based multi-center study.

Two small studies, one of 179 patients (7) and one of 58 patients, followed for 6 months and 24 months, respectively, reported positive benefit for combined endpoints that included TIA reduction; 1300 mg aspirin were compared with placebo. No benefit was detected in two studies of 203 patients and 302 patients, respectively, from Copenhagen (16a) and Toulouse (9), divided into two groups and receiving aspirin or placebo. In the Toulouse study the placebo group received hydergine. The possibility is strong that a negative response in these two studies reflected an insufficient sample size (6).

A number of issues emerge from these trials.

1. The question must be raised whether any of them are large enough to give a credible answer.

2. The question of dose has been raised because of the "yin and yang" issue raised by the thromboxane A_2 and the prostacyclin discovery (13). Many have leaped ahead and recommended a low dose. Until this hypothesis is tested by a clinical trial, one should be skeptical of such quick conclusions.

3. The question of male versus female benefit is unsettled. Either the Canadian study on the basis of too few low-risk patients assigned no benefit when one existed, or it came upon a biological phenomenon for which there is other supporting evidence that has been discussed elsewhere. The Bousser study in finding benefit for females may have done so on the basis of too few low-risk patients and been in error in deciding on a positive benefit. Again the solution must surely lie in a large enough study to overcome this doubt. The British trial will contain nearly 2,000 patients when it is concluded, and with a presumptive ratio of 2:1 male to female they should answer this question. They will also have data on the dose question, as they are comparing 325 mg aspirin with 1,300 mg aspirin and with a third placebo group.

4. There is a need for better drugs. A 50% reduction is satisfying, but there are still too many nonresponders.

5. Many disorders exist for which platelet antiaggregants have never been submitted to a good clinical evaluation. This includes the list given in Table 2. Many of these are logical candidates for platelet antiaggregants. Some of these conditions are too uncommon to be ever assessed by trials, even involving a great many centers. There are other conditions where the problem is that the coagulation cascade has been triggered off or that large thrombi already exist, as in myocardial infarction, pulmonary vein thrombosis, and cerebral sinus and vein thrombosis. Platelet-inhibiting therapy appears to be of dubious rationale in these situations. Data is urgently needed, from good studies, to help the clinician determine the true efficacy or otherwise of anticoagulants in these conditions.

REQUIREMENT FOR FUTURE TRIALS

Making use of our experience with the natural history and the benefit of aspirin in atherothrombotic TIA and minor stroke, deciding to exclude to the best of

TABLE 2. *Platelet antiaggregants—no trials*[a]

Nonarteriosclerotic major arterial lesions
Fibromuscular dysplasia
Postdissection carotid stenosis and aneurysm
Posttraumatic arteriopathy
Postradiation arteriopathy
Preangiogram prophylaxis
Postendarterectomy and extracranial/intracranial anastomosis
Asymptomatic bruit and stenosis
Cardiac valvular lesions
Prolapsing mitral valve
Mitral annulus calcification
Nonbacterial thrombotic endocarditis
Lacunar infarction
Prosthetic heart valves

[a]The likelihood is strong that platelet-induced thrombogenesis causes symptoms in these conditions, but platelet antiaggregants have not been evaluated in any proper trials in patients with these disorders.

clinical ability lacunes, cardiac embolic cases, and hemorrhage, my biostatistical colleague, Wayne Taylor, has prepared a sample-size calculation for any future randomized trial that will attempt to validate a potential new treatment strategy for patients presenting with atherothrombotic TIA and PNS. He has accepted that there is an overall (male and female) risk reduction of 30% and that the mix of males to females will be 2 to 1, as it was in the Canadian and the Bousser studies. Assuming a 30% risk reduction by the new treatment strategy to be evaluated and assigning confidence limits at $\alpha = 0.05$ (one-tailed) and $\beta = 0.10$, he has designed tables for as short as 3 and as long as 8 years of follow-up with 1 to 5 years of case entry. To allow for the mix of males to females, the use or not of aspirin, the variable imposed by the location and amount of disease in the arteries, and the presence of other risk factors, the numbers were estimated for 5-year survivals of 80, 70, and 60% of the controls. The full details are being published (17), but it can be seen from Table 3 that in the usual risk patients, 939 patients would be required in each treatment group, if entry was achieved in a smooth fashion over 3 years and follow-up was excellent for an average of 5 years. Should the new treatment by fortunate circumstance be much more potent at 50% risk reduction, tables have been constructed that indicate how much simpler it could be to conduct a smaller trial to prove efficacy (Table 4).

There is some skepticism about the feasibility of such large trials. However, experience indicates that the techniques of multicenter trials have been refined. A protocol prepared carefully by a team expert in the specific clinical problem, working with biostatisticians, laboratory monitors, and methodologists, can conduct successfully far-flung multicenter trials. The Cooperative Study of Extracranial/Intracranial Arterial Anastomosis, as a possible means of stroke prevention, has been run from London, Canada, and conducted in 58 centers on three continents. The assignment to surgical versus medical therapy has been determined for each patient by a call to a central telephone switchboard at the Data Center in Hamilton,

TABLE 3. *Sample-size calculations[a] for TIA and PNS study—atherothrombotic stroke*

Time spent entering patients (years)	Total trial duration (years)					
	3	4	5	6	7	8
1	748	551	441	372	324	289
2	925	635	490	403	346	305
3	1,227	754	554	443	373	325
4	—	939	641	493	406	348
5	—	—	766	560	446	375

[a]The number of patients that would be required for entry into each of two groups for estimated risk reduction of a new treatment strategy likely to achieve a 30% risk reduction.
Overall 5-year survival = 70% controls, 79% new treatment.
(From Taylor et al., ref. 17.)

TABLE 4. *Smaller sample-size calculations[a] for TIA and PNS study—atherothrombotic stroke*

Time spent entering patients (years)	Total trial duration (years)					
	3	4	5	6	7	8
1	254	187	149	126	109	97
2	314	215	166	136	117	103
3	416	256	187	150	126	110
4	—	318	217	167	137	117
5	—	—	260	189	151	127

[a]The number of patients that would be required for entry into each of two groups for estimated risk reduction of new treatment strategy likely to achieve a 50% risk reduction. Overall 5-year survival = 70% control, 85% experimental. (From Taylor et al., ref. 17.)

Canada; 1419 patients have been randomized. Of these, 730 have been assigned to a medical program and 689 to the surgical cadre. Cross-overs have been uncommon, with 23 receiving surgery despite randomization to the medical treatment and 31 not receiving surgery when this was the assigned category. The patency rate of the anastomosis has been triply checked, by the radiologist in each participating center using the original preoperative and postoperative angiograms, by the neuroradiologist-in-chief in London, Canada, and by a random sampling of this essential part of the data reviewed by nonparticipating members of the radiological and neurosurgical staff at the Mayo Clinic. The surgical work is of highest quality and there is an overall patency rate of 94% (97% in Japan). As of January 31, 1984, 1 year before the end of an average follow-up of 5 years, we know the present status of 100% of the patients entered. None have been lost. Disciplined multicenter studies can and should be done to solve burning issues in clinical treatment.

It is important to remind those who would introduce a new and exciting treatment, whether it be surgical as in the bypass procedure, or medical as in low-dose aspirin: the proof of any therapy is up to the proponent. Furthermore, the only acceptable route with chronic disease is the randomized trial, and many pitfalls and disappointments will emerge before final answers are obtained.

REFERENCES

1. Barnett, H. J. M. (1978): Delayed cerebral ischemic episodes distal to occlusion of major cerebral arteries. *Neurology*, 28:769–774.
2. Bousser, M. G., Eschwege, E., Haguenau, M., Lefauconnier, J. M., Thibult, N., Touboul, D., and Touboul, P. J. (1983): "AICLA" controlled trial of aspirin and dipyridamole in the secondary prevention of atherothrombotic cerebral ischemia. *Stroke*, 14:5–14.
3. Cote, R., Barnett, H. J. M., and Taylor, D. W. (1983): Internal carotid occlusion—A prospective study. *Stroke*, 14:898–902.
4. Craig, D. R., Meguro, K., Watridge, C., Robertson, J. T., Barnett, H. J. M., and Fox, A. J. (1982): Intracranial internal carotid artery stenosis. *Stroke*, 13:825–828.
5. Dyken, M. L. (1981): Antiplatelet aggregating agents in transient ischemic attacks and the relationship of risk factors. In: *Prophylaxis of Venous, Peripheral, Cardiac and Cerebral Vascular*

Diseases with Acetylsalicylic Acid, edited by K. Breddin, D. Loew, K. Uberla, W. Dorndorf, and R. Marx, pp. 141–148. F. K. Schattauer Verlag, Stuttgart.

6. Dyken, M. (1983): Transient ischemic attacks and aspirin, stroke and death; negative studies and type II error (Editorial). *Stroke*, 14:2–4.

7. Fields, W. S., Lemak, N. A., Frankowski, R. F., and Hardy, R. J. (1977): Controlled trial of aspirin in cerebral ischemia. *Stroke*, 8:301–316.

8. Fieschi, C., Mariani, F., Brambilla, G. L., Prencipe, M., Tomasello, F., Argentino, C., Bono, G., Candelise, L., De Zanche, L., Inzitari, D., and Nardini, M. (1983): Italian multicenter study on reversible cerebral ischemic attacks. Population characteristics and methodology. *Stroke*, 14:424–430.

9. Guiraud-Chaumeil, B., Rascol, A., David, J., Boneu, B., Clanet, M., and Bierme, R. (1982): Prevention des recidives des accidents vasculaires cerebraux ischemiques par les anti-agregants plaquettaires. *Rev. Neurol. (Paris)*, 138:367–385.

10. Levy, R. I., and Moskowitz, J. (1982): Cardiovascular research: Decades of progress, a decade of promise. *Science*, 217:121–129.

11. Marshall, J. (1964): The natural history of transient ischemic cerebrovascular attacks. *Q. J. Med.*, 33:309–324.

12. Marzewski, D. J., Furlan, A. J., St. Louis, P., Little, J. R., and Modic, M. T. (1982): Intracranial carotid artery stenosis: Long-term prognosis. *Stroke*, 13:113.

13. Mitchell, J. R. A. (1983): Prostacyclin—Powerful, yes: But is it useful? (Letter to the Editor). *Br. Med. J.*, 287:1824–1826.

14. Muuronen, A., and Kaste, M. (1982): Outcome of 314 patients with transient ischemic attacks. *Stroke*, 13:24–31.

15. Pfaffenback, D. D., and Hollenhorst, R. W. (1973): Morbidity and survivorship of patients with embolic cholesterol crystals in the ocular fundus. *Am. J. Ophthalmol.*, 75:66–72.

16. Reuther, R., and Dorndorf, W. (1978): Aspirin in patients with cerebral ischemia and normal angiograms or non-surgical lesions. The results of a double blind trial. In: *Acetylsalicylic Acid in Cerebral Ischemia and Coronary Heart Disease*, edited by K. Breddin, W. Dorndorf, D. Loew, and R. Marx, pp. 97–106. F. K. Schattauer Verlag, Stuttgart.

16a. Sorensen, P. S., Pedersen, H., Marquardsen, J., Petersson, H., Helteberg, A., Simonsen, N., Munck, O., and Andersen, L. A. (1983): Acetylsalicylic acid in the prevention of stroke in patients with reversible cerebral ischemic attacks. A Danish Cooperative Study. *Stroke*, 14:15–21.

17. Taylor, D. W., Sackett, D. L., and Haynes, R. B. (1984): Sample size calculations for randomized trials in stroke prevention. How many patients do we need. *Stroke*, 15:968–971.

18. The Canadian Cooperative Study Group (1978): A randomized trial of aspirin and sulfinpyrazone in threatened stroke. *N. Engl. J. Med.*, 299:53–59.

19. Wiebers, D. O., Whisnant, J. P., and O'Fallon, W. M. (1982): Reversible ischemic neurologic deficit (RIND) in a community: Rochester, Minnesota, 1955–1974. *Neurology*, 32:459–465.

Advances in Prostaglandin, Thromboxane, and Leukotriene Research, Vol. 13, edited by G. G. Neri Serneri, et al. Raven Press, New York © 1985.

Effects of Dipyridamole Infusion on Local Platelet Aggregation and Local Formation of Thromboxane A_2 in Patients with Pulmonary Hypertension

*G. F. Gensini, *C. Rostagno, **A. Pezza, **F. Fanara, *S. Castellani, *D. Prisco, *P. G. Rogasi, *M. Boddi, and *G. G. Neri Serneri

*Clinica Medica I, University of Florence, 50134 Florence; and **Clinica Tisiologica e delle Malattie dell'Apparato Respiratorio, II Facoltà, University of Naples, Naples, Italy*

Thrombotic lesions were often found at necroscopy in pulmonary arteries of patients suffering from hypoxic pulmonary hypertension (5,10), and platelet aggregating substances infused into pulmonary artery induced pulmonary hypertension in laboratory animals (3a). Moreover, platelet survival time was decreased in hypoxemic patients (9) and increased levels of intraplatelet substances were found in peripheral blood in patients with chronic obstructive pulmonary disease (COPD) (7).

These data, although indicating a relationship between platelet activation and pulmonary hypertension, do not allow us to establish the mechanism(s) leading to platelet activation and the way in which activated platelets cause pulmonary pressure to rise in patients with COPD. In fact, platelet activation might be due to arterial hypoxemia, acidosis, or blood hyperviscosity, all characteristic findings in patients with pulmonary insufficiency.

The aim of this study was to investigate platelet functional parameters and plasma levels of thromboxane (TX) in peripheral blood and at different levels of pulmonary arterial bed in patients with COPD.

PATIENTS AND METHODS

We examined 29 patients (25 men and 4 women; mean age 59.8 years) suffering from COPD and undergoing right cardiac catheterization for diagnostic purposes. The diagnosis of COPD was based on clinical history, physical examination, and pulmonary function tests. Mean arterial P_{O_2} and P_{CO_2} were 68.4 and 43.32, respectively; mean arterial pH was 7.39. Fourteen patients had normal pulmonary pressure [mean pulmonary arterial pressure (MPAP) average values 13.6 mm Hg, range 8–18] and normal pulmonary vascular resistance [(PVR) mean 84.79 ± 28.69 dynes/sec cm^{-5})] whereas 15 had pulmonary hypertension (MPAP average values 35.5 mm Hg range 22–55) with increased PVR (mean 347.76 ± 150.01 dynes/sec cm^{-5}).

Hemodynamic Studies

Right ventricle, pulmonary artery, and pulmonary wedge pressure (PWP) were obtained through a Swan-Ganz catheter and Hewlett-Packard polygraphic recorder. Cardiac output was measured using Fick principle. Arterial blood gases were analyzed using an ABL-1 (Radiometer, DK) gas analyzer. Total pulmonary vascular resistance (TPR) and PVR were calculated according to the following formulae: TPR = MPAP × 80/cardiac output (CO); PVR = (MPAP − PWP) × 80/CO.

Blood Sampling

Blood samples were obtained from right ventricle, pulmonary artery, and arteriolo-capillary vessels through a Swan-Ganz catheter and from an antecubital vein using a siliconized 19-G needle (Abbot, U.S.A.).

Platelet Aggregation

Circulating platelet aggregates were detected according to Wu and Hoak (11). Platelet counts were performed by automatic equipment (PL 100: TOA, Kobe, Japan).

β-Thromboglobulin

β-Thromboglobulin (TG) was assayed in platelet-poor plasma by radioimmunoassay (RIA) according to Ludlam et al. (4) using a commercial kit (β-TG RIA, Radiochemical Centre, Amersham, U.K.).

TXA$_2$

TXA$_2$ was assayed as its stable derivative TXB$_2$ by RIA according to Granström et al. (3) using a commercial kit (TXB$_2$ RIA, Abbot, U.S.A.)

Dipyridamole Infusion

Dipyridamole was administered to 12 patients (7 with increased MPAP and 5 with normal MPAP) by i.v. continuous infusion at a rate of 15 μg/kg/min for 30 min in a fixed volume of 1.5 ml/min of saline. As a control, the same volume of saline was administered to 4 patients with normal MPAP.

Statistical Analysis

Statistical analysis was performed using Student's *t*-test for unpaired data and standard analysis for linear regression.

RESULTS

In patients without pulmonary hypertension, no significant differences were found in platelet aggregates, β-TG and TXB_2 concentrations between peripheral venous blood and the blood withdrawn at the different levels of pulmonary arterial bed. On the contrary, in high mean pulmonary pressure patients (H-MPAP) a significant increase of these values was shown in pulmonary vessels with the highest values reached in arteriolo-capillary blood [39% in arteriolo-capillary vessels vs.

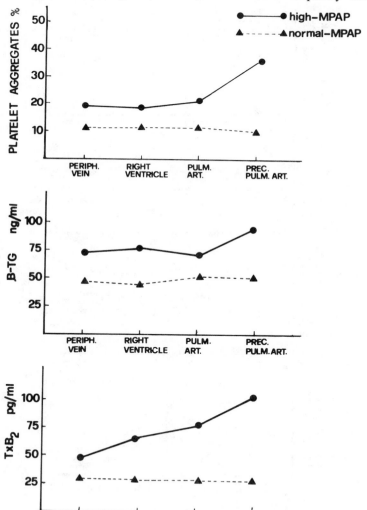

FIG. 1. Platelet aggregates, β-TG, and TXB_2 levels from 4 different sampling sites in patients with normal mean pulmonary pressure and elevated mean pulmonary pressure.

19% in right ventricle for platelet aggregates ($p < 0.005$) and 89 ng/ml vs. 82 ng/ml for β-TG, respectively].

TXB$_2$ levels were significantly higher in pulmonary vessels of H-MPAP patients and a characteristic gradient existed between TXB$_2$ concentrations in right ventricle and in arteriolo-capillary vessels [75.49 ± 67.82 vs. 107.18 ± 74.38 pg/ml ($p < 0.01$)] (Fig. 1).

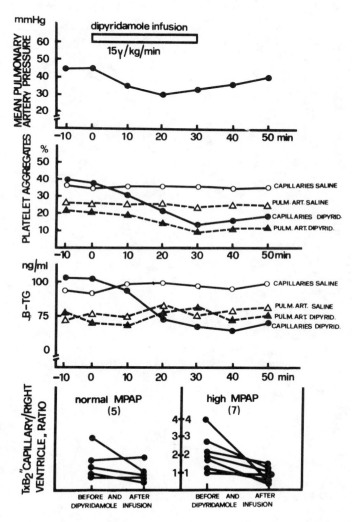

FIG. 2. Effects of dipyridamole infusion on mean pulmonary artery pressure, platelet aggregates, β-TG, and TXB$_2$ capillary/right ventricle ratio.

A good correlation existed between MPAP and TXB_2 levels in arteriolo-capillary blood ($r = 0.61$, $p < 0.001$).

Dipyridamole infusion lowered β-TG and platelet aggregate levels in arteriolo-capillary blood, whereas TXB_2 levels in arteriolo-capillary blood were slightly lowered. The high ratio between TXB_2 plasma levels in pulmonary capillaries and in the right ventricle was significantly reduced by dipyridamole (from 1.76–0.96, $p < 0.005$). Systolic and diastolic pulmonary pressure were transiently lowered by dipyridamole in H-MPAP patients. Saline infusion did not produce any change in platelet aggregation, β-TG, or pulmonary pressures (Fig. 2).

DISCUSSION

Our results indicate that platelet activation does occur in the arterial pulmonary bed in patients with pulmonary hypertension secondary to COPD but not in normotensive patients. Platelet aggregates, β-TG, and TXB_2 levels are significantly higher in arteriolo-capillary blood than in the right ventricle, indicating that local platelet activation occurs in pulmonary vessels. The increased TXB_2 levels in arteriolo-capillary blood show a good correlation with mean pulmonary artery pressure and pulmonary vascular resistance suggesting a possible role of TXA_2 in pulmonary hypertension in addition to the hypoxemic vasoconstriction. Experimental evidence in animals indicates that TXA_2 is responsible for acute pulmonary hypertension (2).

Acute diypridamole infusion proved to be effective in lowering the enhanced platelet aggregation and TXB_2 concentration in arteriolo-capillary blood in hypertensive patients. A parallel decrease in MPAP was shown with peak reduction of pulmonary pressure after 10 min infusion. The favorable effects of dipyridamole are probably related both to antiaggregating effects and to prostacyclin stimulation activity (6,8). Prostacyclin production by pulmonary vessels has been reported to contribute to decrease pulmonary vascular resistance (1). However, more extensive investigations on the efficacy of chronic treatment are needed to validate the value of dipyridamole in the chronic treatment of secondary pulmonary hypertension.

REFERENCES

1. Dusting, J. D., Moncada, S., and Vane, J. (1979): Prostaglandins, their intermediate and precursor: Cardiovascular actions and regulatory roles in normal and abnormal circulatory systems. *Prog. Cardiovasc. Dis.*, 21:405–430.
2. Frölich, J C., Ogletree, M., Peskar B. B., and Brigham, K. L. (1980): Pulmonary hypertension correlated to thromboxane synthesis. In: *Advances in Prostaglandin and Thromboxane Research* Vol. 7, edited by B. Samuelsson, P. W. Ramwell, and R. Paoletti, pp. 745–750. Raven Press, New York.
3. Granström, E., Kindhal, H, and Samuelsson, B. (1976): Radioimmunoassay for TXB_2. *Analyt. Lett.*, 9:611–627.
3a. Hyman et al. (1978): Prostaglandins and the lung. *Am. Rev. Resp. Dis.*, 117:111–135.
4. Ludlam, C. A., Moore, S., Bolton, A. E., Pepper, D. S., and Cash, J. D. (1975): The release of a human specific protein measure by radioimmunoassay. *Thromb. Res.*, 6:543–548.
5. Mitchell, R. S., Silvers, G. W., Dart, G. A., Petty, T. L., Vincent, T. M., Ryan, S. F., and Filly

(1968): Clinical and morphological correlations in chronic airway obstruction *Am. Rev. Resp. Dis.*, 97:54–62.

6. Moncada, S., and Korbut, R. (1978): Dipyridamole and other phosphodiesterase inhibitors act as antithrombotic agents by prostacyclin. *Lancet*, 1:1286–1289.

7. Nenci, G. G. (1980): Platelet, hypoxemia and pulmonary hypertension. *II European Symposium on Coagulation, Platelet Function, Fibrinolysis and Vascular Disease*, Palermo, Italy.

8. Neri Serneri, G. G., Masotti, G., Poggesi, L., Galanti G., and Morettini, A. (1981): Enhanced prostacyclin production by dipyridamole in man. *Eur. J. Clin. Pharmacol.*, 21:9–15.

9. Steele, P. P., Hellis, J. H., Weiley, H. S. Jr., and Genton, E. (1977): Platelet survival time in patients with hypoxemia and pulmonary hypertension. *Circulation*, 55:660–662.

10. Walcott, G., Burchell, H. B., and Brown, A. L. Jr., (1970): Primary pulmonary hypertension. *Am. J. Med.*, 49:70–79.

11. Wu, K. K., and Hoak, J. C. (1974): A new method for the quantitative detection of platelet aggregates in patients with arterial insufficiency. *Lancet*, 2:924–926.

Advances in Prostaglandin, Thromboxane, and Leukotriene Research, Vol. 13, edited by G. G. Neri Serneri, et al. Raven Press, New York © 1985.

Influence of Antiplatelet Drugs on βtg and PF4 Levels in Patients with Transient Ischemic Attacks

*F. Fabris, *M. L. Randi, *A. Casonato, *R. Dal Bo Zanon,
**S. Manzoni, **P. Tonin, **L. De Zanche, and *A. Girolami

*Institute of Medical Semiotics and **Clinical Neurology, University of Padua Medical School, Padua, Italy

Platelets play an important role in hemostasis and in the pathogenesis of thromboembolic episodes. In recent years it has been suggested that evaluation of platelet-specific proteins released in blood might provide a better index in vascular disease (4) and in monitoring the effectiveness of antiplatelet therapy. In this chapter we report the levels of β-thromboglobulin (βtg) and platelet factor 4 (PF4) in patients with transient ischemic attacks (TIA) and the influence of treatment with antiplatelet drugs.

MATERIAL AND METHODS

Forty-six patients with TIA were studied [29 males, 17 females, mean age 51.4 ± 9.5 (SD) years]. As controls, 33 healthy subjects with comparable sex and age were considered. At the time of the study, 22 of the patients were taking dipyridamole (225 mg/day): 20 of them presented TIA related to the carotid arterial system (CAS) and 2 TIA related to the vertebrobasilar arterial system (VBAS). Nine patients (8 with TIA related to CAS and 1 related to VBAS) were taking dipyridamole (225 mg/day) plus aspirin (ASA, 500 mg/day); the other 15 patients (11 TIA related to CAS and 4 related to VBAS) were not taking antiaggregating agents. No patient had had a TIA episode in the preceding 2 months.

The βtg and PF4 determinations were performed using commercially available radioimmunoassay kits supplied by Radiochemical Centre (Amersham, England) for βtg and by Abbott Labs (North Chicago, Illinois) for PF4. The reproducibility was tested by collecting two blood samples (24 hr apart) for each patient or control. The analysis of variance (ANOVA) test was used to compare the means for statistical significance using an Olivetti P 6040 computer. Bartlett's test was carried out to verify the variance's equivalence.

RESULTS

Results are summarized in Table 1. High values of βtg were obtained in patients not receiving antiplatelet drugs (85 ± 62 ng/ml) or taking ASA plus dipyridamole (69 ± 43.7 ng/ml, $p = 0.01$) in comparison to healthy controls (41 ± 23 ng/ml). Nevertheless, no statistical difference was observed between dipyridamole and ASA plus dipyridamole groups ($p = 0.09$). PF4 levels were significantly elevated only in untreated patients (17 ± 16 ng/ml, $p = 0.02$) (controls 9.6 ± 4.7 ng/ml).

DISCUSSION

The pathophysiology of TIA is not yet understood. Hemodynamic factors and thrombotic events are clearly important. Recently many studies have focused on the evaluation of βtg and PF4 released during platelet activation: increase of βtg and PF4 has been demonstrated in myocardial infarction, angina pectoris, prosthetic heart valvular disease, and other vascular diseases (2). In our study, βtg levels were statistically higher in patients with TIA in spite of a wide distribution of values. High values of βtg and PF4 have been frequently shown shortly after TIA or stroke (2,6,9). On the contrary, our results refer to patients evaluated almost 2 months after the onset of symptoms and therefore they suggest a continuous platelet activation as recently reported (9). No statistical difference was obtained, with regard to PF4, between patients taking or not taking antiplatelet therapy, despite the fact that the levels were higher than the controls in patients without therapy.

Several studies on the effectiveness of antiplatelet drugs in the prevention of cerebrovascular accidents have been performed. Treatment with ASA alone (3) or in combination with dipyridamole (7) has been shown to reduce the number of TIAs. The patients with dipyridamole showed significantly lower levels of plasma βtg as compared to patients not receiving therapy. Therapy with dipyridamole alone reduced the amount of plasma βtg of the patients with ischemic heart disease after isometric exercise (8), whereas no effect was reported in normal volunteers (5). On the other hand, treatment with ASA plus dipyridamole has no effect on the reduction of plasma βtg of the patients with coronary artery disease (1). The βtg

TABLE 1. *Mean βtg and PF4 levels in controls and in patients with transient ischemic attacks*

Treatment (no. of patients)	βtg (ng/ml)[a]	p[**b]	p[***b]	PF4 (ng/ml)[a]	p[**b]	p[***b]
Controls (33)	41 ± 22.9	—	—	9.6 ± 4.7	—	—
No therapy (15)	85.1 ± 62	0.001	—	17 ± 16.7	0.02	—
Dipyridamole (22)	45 ± 22	NS	0.008	12 ± 6	NS	NS
ASA + dipyridamole (9)	69 ± 43.7	0.01	NS	12 ± 5.5	NS	NS

[a]Mean $\pm$ SD.
[b]p** = Statistical difference from the controls; p*** = statistical difference from the patients without therapy.
NS = not significant.

levels of our patients not receiving therapy or treated with ASA plus dipyridamole were comparable.

In conclusion, our results show an increase of βtg levels in patients suffering from TIA, which confirms the participation of platelets in cerebrovascular diseases. The favorable effect of dipyridamole, as demonstrated by the improvement of βtg levels may be an incentive for the use of antiaggregating agents in cerebrovascular diseases.

We have evaluated the levels of βtg and PF4 in 46 patients with TIA. Patients not receiving therapy showed levels of βtg statistically higher than the controls, while we observed normal levels of βtg in patients taking dipyridamole and pathological amounts in those assuming aspirin plus dipyridamole. No statistical difference was observed with regard to PF4 among the three groups of patients.

REFERENCES

1. Boer, A. C., Han, P., Turpie, A. G. G., Butt, R., Gent, M., and Genton, E. (1981): The effect of antiplatelet drugs on platelet survival time and β-thromboglobulin in coronary artery disease. *Thromb. Haemostas.* (Abstr.), 46:192.
2. Cella, G., Zahavi, J., Haas, H. A., and Kakkar, V. V. (1979): β-Thromboglobulin, platelet production time and platelet function in vascular disease. *Br. J. Haematol.*, 43:127–136.
3. Fields, W. S., Lemak, N. A., Frankowski, R. F., Hardy, R. J., and Bigelow, R. H. (1977): Controlled trial of aspirin in cerebral ischemia. *Stroke*, 8:301–314.
4. Kaplan, K. L., Himie, L., Nossel, L., Drillings, M., and Lesznik, G. (1978): Radioimmunoassay of platelet factor 4 and β-thromboglobulin: Development and application studies of platelet release in relation to fibrinopeptide A generation. *Br. J. Haematol.*, 39:129–146.
5. Lensing, A. W. A., Sturk, A., and Cute, J. W. (1981): No effect of persantin on platelet aggregation and plasma βtg levels in healthy volunteers. *Thromb. Haemostas.*, 46:406 (abstract).
6. Levine, P. H., Fisher, M., Fullerton, A. L., Duffy, C. P., and Hoogasian, J. J. (1981): Human platelet factor 4: Preparation from outdated platelet concentrates and application in cerebrovascular disease. *Am. J. Haematol.*, 10:375–385.
7. Olsson, J. E., Brecher, C., Backlung, H., Krook, H., Muller, R., Nitelius, E., Olsson, O., and Tornberg, A. (1980): Anticoagulant as antiplatelet therapy as prophylactic against cerebral infarction in transient ischemic attacks. *Stroke*, 11:4–9.
8. Sano, T., Motomya, T., and Yamazaki, H. (1980): Platelet release reaction *in vivo* in patients with ischemic heart disease after isometric exercise and its prevention with dipyridamole. *Thromb. Haemostas.*, 42:1589–1597.
9. Stuart, M. E., Douglas, J. T., Lowe, G. D. O., Prentice, C. R. M., and Forbes, C. D. (1983): Prognostic value of beta-thromboglobulin in patients with transient cerebral ischemia. *Lancet*, ii:479–482.

*Advances in Prostaglandin, Thromboxane, and
Leukotriene Research, Vol. 13*, edited by G. G. Neri
Serneri, et al. Raven Press, New York © 1985.

Aspirin after Acute Myocardial Infarction: A Systematic Approach to Compare the Hemostatic Effects of Three Different Doses

*R. De Caterina, *D. Giannessi, *W. Bernini, *A. Boem,
**P. Patrignani, **P. Filabozzi, and **C. Patrono

*C.N.R. Institute of Clinical Physiology, University of Pisa, Pisa, Italy, and **Department
of Pharmacology, Catholic University School of Medicine, Rome, Italy

Clinical studies (5) generally support the concept that aspirin is an effective antithrombotic medication when given as a single daily dose ranging from 324 to 1,500 mg; however, no dose has ever been demonstrated superior to any other. On the other hand, pharmacological studies (6) have shown that doses of aspirin of 30 mg/day are capable of reducing the platelet-thromboxane B_2 (TXB_2) production by more than 90%. Because the pharmacologic effects of aspirin can be explained by a single mechanism, i.e., covalent acetylation of the active site of cyclooxygenase (7), we may wonder if it is possible to interfere significantly with platelet function using aspirin at low doses, close to those recommended by the pharmacological studies, in the clinical situation in which the drug has to be used. If so, it will be interesting to know to what extent a small change of platelet TXB_2 inhibition, such as passing from 30 mg/day to higher doses, will cause variation of platelet function.

The aim of this study was to compare the alterations of the hemostatic system induced by three different aspirin regimens: namely, 30, 50, and 324 mg daily. The three doses were given to patients recovering from myocardial infarction, since these patients represent the most common candidates for long-term therapy with aspirin in ischemic heart disease. The aspirin doses were chosen in the following manner: 30 mg/day is the dose proved to be capable of reducing TXB_2 more than 90% without reducing prostacyclin (PGI_2) renal production (6); 324 mg/day is the smallest dose of proved clinical usefulness in ischemic heart disease (3); and 50 mg/day is an arbitrary dose chosen because it probably increases TXB_2 inhibition with respect to the 30-mg/day dose, possibly at the expense of a reduced production of PGI_2.

METHODS

Twenty patients recovering after acute myocardial infarction within 2 weeks from admission in a coronary care unit were studied. Five patients were assigned randomly and in double-blind manner to each group of treatment with aspirin or placebo. Blood samples were obtained twice before, and on days 3, 7, 14, and 21 after beginning treatment. In all cases the following parameters were measured: bleeding time (BTI) (4), coagulation time, prothrombin time (PT), activated partial thromboplastin time (aPTT), circulating platelet aggregates (8), platelet aggregation induced by ADP, epinephrine, collagen, thrombin, and arachidonic acid (AA), TXB_2 generation (1) in platelet-rich plasma (PRP) after the same aggregation inducers, TXB_2 generation in serum (1), and platelet adhesiveness (2). The analysis of experimental data was performed by two-way analysis of variance with repeated measures to assess the time- and dose-dependence of the observed derangements after assessment of normality of distributions. Iterative single comparisons were made with the Student–Newman–Keuls test.

RESULTS AND CONCLUSIONS

A significant ($p < 0.01$) extension of BTI with aspirin dose with respect to basal level at all the doses employed was observed (Fig. 1). The increase is 40% at 30 mg, 75% at 50 mg, and 89% at 324 mg with respect to the basal, averaging the values at all times of sampling. The prolonging of BTI at the highest doses is significantly ($p < 0.05$) different from placebo. As far as platelet aggregation curves are concerned, we observed a slight and not significant tendency to decreasing for all the three doses employed of the ADP total curve and a complete abolition of the secondary wave. For the epinephrine total curve, we observed an inhibition of platelet aggregation of 82.8% ± 1.4 (SEM) at 30 mg/day, 64.5% ± 3.3 (SEM) at 50 mg/day, and 68.5% ± 3.2 (SEM) at 324 mg/day with respect to basal. The

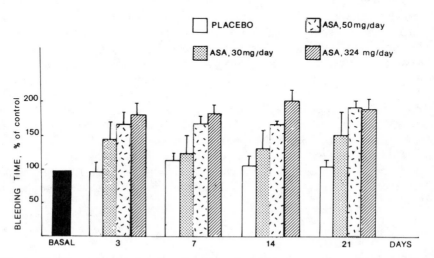

FIG. 1. Bleeding time variations (% of basal value) as a function of the time and of aspirin (ASA) dose or placebo. The mean ± SEM of each group of patients is reported.

observed variations are significant ($p<0.01$) with respect both to basal and to placebo for all the doses of aspirin employed. Similarly, when AA was used, a significant lowering of platelet aggregation was observed both with respect to basal ($p<0.01$) and to placebo ($p<0.05$), the percent of inhibition being 90.0 ± 1.3 (SEM) at 30 mg/day, 78.8 ± 7.3 (SEM) at 50 mg/day, and 89.0 ± 0.9 (SEM) at 324 mg/day. No significant differences among the three doses of aspirin were observed. When collagen and thrombin were used, only minor and not significant effects of inhibition could be observed. As far as TXB_2 is concerned, a significant inhibition with respect to basal and placebo in PRP was observed with all the examined aspirin doses and with all the aggregating agents. A close agreement is observed between the data of TXB_2 in PRP and the data of TXB_2 generation in serum, as can be seen in Fig. 2, where we report the values of TXB_2 in PRP after induction of platelet aggregation with AA and the TXB_2 levels in serum. In both cases the inhibition of the TXB_2 was about 93% using 30 mg/day, 96% using 50

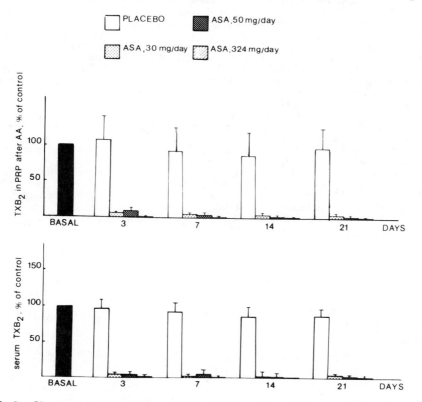

FIG. 2. Changes in platelet TXB_2 production as reflected by TXB_2 measured in platelet-rich plasma (PRP) after induction of platelet aggregation by arachidonic acid (AA) **(upper panel)** and by serum TXB_2 levels **(lower panel)** as a function of the time and of aspirin (ASA) dose or placebo. The mean $\pm$ SEM of each group of patients is reported.

mg/day, and 99% using 324 mg/day. No difference was observed in coagulation time, PT, aPTT, circulating platelet aggregates, and platelet adhesiveness.

The data so far gathered seem to indicate that low doses of aspirin are sufficient to inhibit, about maximally, the platelet aggregation without changes in prostacyclin production, at least for 30 mg/day, while in our experience, doses of 300 mg/day reduce by 20% the urinary 6-keto-PGF$_{1\alpha}$ in healthy subjects. Moreover, the improvement in TXB$_2$ inhibition when high doses of aspirin are used is not paralleled by a further impairment in platelet function, as evaluated by aggregation. We may conclude that in patients with acute myocardial infarction, daily aspirin doses of 324 mg/day do not yield significant advantages in antiplatelet effects with respect to low doses, which also minimize undesirable side effects. The results of our study clearly indicate the opportunity for using low doses of aspirin in clinical trials.

REFERENCES

1. Giannessi, D., De Caterina, R., Gazzetti, P., Bernini, W., Masini, S., and Zucchelli, G. C. (1982): Methodological assessment and applications of a radioimmunoassay for thromboxane (TX) B$_2$ to measurement of TXB$_2$ release by platelets. *J. Nucl. Med. All. Sci.*, 26:25–33.
2. Hellem, A. J. (1970): Platelet adhesiveness in von Willebrand's disease. A study with a new modification of the glass bead filter method. *Scand. J. Haematol.*, 7:374–382.
3. Lewis, D. L., Davis, J. W., Archibald, D. C., Stenike, W. E., Smitherman, T. C., Doherty, J. E. III, Schnaper, H. W., Le Winter, M. N., Linares, E., Pouget, J. M., Sabharwal, S. C., Chesler, E., and De Mots, H. (1983): Protective effects of aspirin against acute myocardial infarction and death in men with unstable angina. Results of a Veterans Administration cooperative study. *N. Engl. J. Med.*, 309:396–403.
4. Mielke, C. H. J. (1978): Template bleeding time: Technique. In: *Platelet Function Testing. Proceeding*, edited by H. J. Day, H. Holmsen, and M. D. Zucker, pp. 78–87. Department of Health, Education and Welfare, Bethesda, Md.
5. Passamani, E. R. (1980): Summary of ongoing clinical trials of platelet-active drugs in cardiovascular disease. *Circulation*, 62(suppl. V):106–110.
6. Patrignani, P., Filabozzi, P., and Patrono, C. (1982): Selective cumulative inhibition of platelet thromboxane production by low-dose aspirin in healthy subjects. *J. Clin. Invest.*, 69:1366–1372.
7. Roth, C. J., and Majerus, P. W. (1975): The mechanisms of the effect of aspirin on human platelets. I. Acetylation of a particular fraction protein. *J. Clin. Invest.*, 56:624–632.
8. Wu, K. K., and Hoak, J. C. (1974): A new method for the quantitative detection of platelet aggregates in patients with arterial insufficiency. *Lancet*, 2:924.

*Advances in Prostaglandin, Thromboxane, and
Leukotriene Research, Vol. 13*, edited by G. G. Neri
Serneri, et al. Raven Press, New York © 1985.

Dipyridamole and Aspirin in Arteriosclerosis Obliterans of the Lower Limbs

G. Davì, A. Pinto, M. G. Palumbo, V. Gallo, A. Mazza,
and A. Strano

*Istituto di Clinica Medica Generale e Terapia Medica I, University of Palermo,
Palermo, Italy*

Considerable evidence has been accumulated from clinical observations to establish an important role for blood platelets in thrombotic complications associated with atherosclerosis obliterans of the lower limbs (1,4,9,19,20); platelet survival time has been found to be decreased and plasma β-thromboglobulin (βTG) levels increased in arteriopathic patients compared with controls (19).

Because thrombosis *in situ* is frequently the final event in the occlusive process and because adhesion of platelets to an ulcerated atherosclerotic plaque may be the first step in thrombus formation, attempts to modify platelet behavior have theoretic support. The combination of dipyridamole (225 mg) and aspirin (ASA) (600 mg) seemed in a long-term study to show a positive effect on the free interval on the treadmill and venous occlusion plethysmography in patients with peripheral vascular disease (11); 300 mg dipyridamole alone, after 2 months continuous treatment, caused a significant increase in exercise muscle blood flow compared to placebo (18).

This study was therefore designed to determine, in patients with atherosclerosis obliterans of the lower limbs, the acute effects of dipyridamole alone or in combination with a low dose of aspirin that can largely inhibit platelet aggregation and thromboxane synthesis but that has much less effect on prostacyclin production in arterial and venous endothelium (21).

MATERIALS AND METHODS

Six patients (4 males and 2 females; mean age 58 ± 7.3 years) with arteriosclerosis obliterans of the lower limbs (II–III stage according to Fontaine) were treated with dipyridamole infusion at a dose of 8 μg/kg·min for 2 hr, which had previously been demonstrated to yield serum concentrations ranging from 1.5 to 2 μg/ml (16); 2 days later, the patients were treated with a low dose of aspirin (50 mg), and 2 hr later, dipyridamole infusion was repeated.

Rest flow (RF), peak flow (PF), basal vascular resistances (BVR), time to reach peak flow (tPF), time until 50% of reactive hyperemia ($t_{1/2}$) and total time of recovery (tT) were evaluated with strain-gauge plethysmography before and after the two treatments.

For the study of platelet aggregation, nine specimens of blood were drawn into a plastic syringe containing 1 volume of 0.126 M trisodium citrate. Platelet-rich plasma (PRP) was prepared centrifuging the citrated blood at 150 g for 8 min at room temperature.

Platelet counts were performed by phase-contrast microscopy. All aggregation was studied at 37°C with Born's method (3), using an Elvi 840 aggregometer (Elvi Logos, Milan, Italy); the threshold concentration of ADP required to produce a biphasic response was evaluated.

Inhibition of ADP- (2 μM) induced platelet aggregation by three different concentrations of prostacyclin (0.1, 0.5, and 2 ng/ml) was also studied. Platelet aggregates ratio (PAR) was estimated by the method of Wu and Hoak (22). For the estimation of plasma βTG, 2.5 ml blood was drawn into a plastic syringe; the samples were transferred immediately into plastic tubes containing EDTA (18 mM) and prostaglandin E_1 (2×10^{-7} M), placed in crushed ice.

The plasma was separated within 30 min of collection by centrifugation at 4°C. The middle third of platelet-poor plasma was removed and stored at -20°C until assayed. Specific radioimmunoassay (6) was performed for βTG (Amersham assay).

For the statistical analysis, Student's t-test was employed for comparison of paired data. Results are given as mean ± SD.

RESULTS

A slight increase of RF with a significant reduction of BVR and tPF, indicating an improvement of arterial wall reactivity, was observed after low-dose ASA pretreatment (Table 1). The threshold aggregating concentration of ADP was slightly increased after dipyridamole infusion but significantly augmented after ASA pretreatment (Table 2). A significant PAR reduction (Table 2) and synergism of the inhibition of ADP-induced platelet aggregation by prostacyclin (Fig. 1) was observed after dipyridamole infusion; no differences in these changes were observed

TABLE 1. Effects of low-dose aspirin pretreatment and dipyridamole infusion on parameters valued with strain-gauge plethysmography

	Baseline	DIP	DIP + ASA
RF (ml/min/100 g)	2.45 ± 0.38	2.58 ± 0.36	2.86 ± 0.39
PF (ml/min/100 g)	12.6 ± 4.8	12.75 ± 5.16	12.8 ± 5.06
BVR (AU)	67.3 ± 21.4	50.6 ± 17.2	37.5 ± 12.6[a]
tPF (sec)	8.9 ± 2.1	6.4 ± 2.0	5.8 ± 1.6[a]
$t_{1/2}$ (sec)	25.3 ± 12.1	23.3 ± 10.7	21.4 ± 13.4
tT (sec)	123.7 ± 58.7	110 ± 61.5	108 ± 59.6

[a]$p < 0.05$ versus baseline.

TABLE 2. *Effect of dipyridamole and aspirin on ADP-induced platelet aggregation and on circulating platelet aggregation*

	Baseline	DIP	DIP + ASA
PAR	0.82 ± 0.04	0.89 ± 0.04	0.90 ± 0.04[a]
Threshold aggregating concentration of ADP (μM)	0.48 ± 0.17	0.57 ± 0.17	0.80 ± 0.21[a]
βTG (ng/ml)	42 ± 9.6	40.5 ± 7.9	40.2 ± 6.6

[a]Significant difference from control at $p < 0.05$.

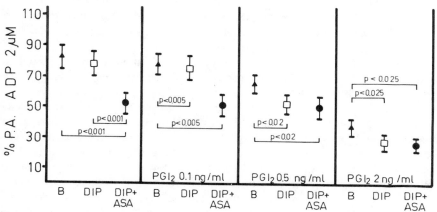

FIG. 1. Effect of dipyridamole (DIP) and aspirin (ASA) on ADP-induced platelet aggregation (P.A.) inhibited by varied levels of PGI_2. Mean $\pm$ SD shown.

after ASA pretreatment. Neither dipyridamole infusion nor ASA plus dipyridamole caused significant changes of plasma βTG levels (Table 2).

DISCUSSION

The mechanism of action of dipyridamole as an antithrombotic agent has not been completely clarified. Best et al. in 1979 demonstrated that dipyridamole not only may inhibit platelet function by increasing platelet cyclic AMP but may also exert a minor effect on platelet thromboxane synthesis (2). Di Minno et al. in 1980 observed that dipyridamole potentiates adenosine-induced inhibition of human platelet aggregation after oral dipyridamole administration (8). In 1981, Neri Serneri et al. demonstrated that dipyridamole increases PGI_2 production in healthy volunteers when given either by infusion or by oral administration (16). Preston et al. in 1982 observed that the *in vitro* stimulation of prostacyclin synthesis by dipyridamole is unrelated to the ability of the drug to block the high-affinity uptake of adenosine by endothelial cells and that the effect may also be independent of changes in the concentration of cAMP induced by the drug (10). Mehta et al. (13) suggested that the antithrombotic effect of dipyridamole in man is mediated mainly by potentiation of prostacyclin activity and to some extent by thromboxane A_2 suppression, as also observed previously (2,5,15).

In our study, threshold aggregating concentrations of ADP were slightly increased after dipyridamole, as also observed by Di Minno (8), but significantly augmented after ASA pretreatment.

Dipyridamole alone had no effects on ADP-induced platelet aggregation, but it potentiated the platelet aggregation inhibitory effects of low-dose ASA. Moreover, dipyridamole alone enhanced the platelet inhibitory effect of synthetic prostacyclin; similar results were recently obtained *in vitro* (12). PAR was significantly affected by dipyridamole infusion without further decrease after ASA pretreatment.

Treatment with dipyridamole or ASA/dipyridamole did not produce changes in plasma βTG concentration in our arteriopathic patients, as has also been observed in a trial in coronary artery disease patients (7).

Low-dose aspirin and dipyridamole infusion seemed, in our study, to ameliorate blood flow, improving arterial wall reactivity, and that could explain the positive effects found in chronic studies (11,14,18).

In conclusion, dipyridamole seems to have a positive effect on decreasing circulating platelet aggregates, enhancing prostacyclin-induced platelet aggregation inhibition; low-dose aspirin inhibits ADP-induced platelet aggregation and thromboxane synthesis (17), with no effect on prostacyclin generation (21) that could be potentiated by dipyridamole (16). Therefore the low-dose aspirin/dipyridamole combination seems useful in preventing platelet function in patients with atherosclerosis obliterans of the lower limbs that often present platelet hyperactivity (19).

REFERENCES

1. Baele, G., Bogaerts, H., Clement, D. L., Pannier, R., and Barbier, F. (1981): Platelet activation during treadmill exercise in patients with chronic peripheral arterial disease. *Thromb. Res.*, 23:215.
2. Best, L. C., McGuire, M. B., Jones, P. B. B., Holland, T. K., Martin, T. J., Preston, F. E., Segal, D. S., and Russell, R. G. G. (1979): Mode of action of dipyridamole on human platelets. *Thromb. Res.*, 16:367.
3. Born, G. V. R. (1962): Aggregation of blood platelets by adenosine diphosphate and its reversal. *Nature (Lond.)*, 194:927.
4. Cella, G., Zahavi, J., de Haas, H. A., and Kakkar, V. V. (1979): β-Thromboglobulin, platelet production time and platelet function in vascular disease. *Br. J. Haematol.*, 43:127.
5. Davì, G., Pinto, A., Palisi, F., Novo, S., Mendola, G., Mazzola, A., and Strano, A. (1982): Effetti dell'infusione di dipiridamolo sulla formazione di trombossano dalle piastrine e sul flusso arterioso in pazienti con arteriopatia obliterante degli arti inferiori. Estratto da *Il Progresso Medico, Vol. XXXVIII*, No. 5.
6. Davì, G., Rini, G. B., Averna, M., Novo, S., Di Fede, G., Mattina, A., Notarbartolo, A., and Strano, A. (1982): Enhanced platelet release reaction in insulin-dependent and insulin-independent diabetic patients. *Haemostasis*, 12:275.
7. De Boer, A. C., Han, P., Turpie, A. G. G., Butt, R., Gent, M., and Genton, E. (1983): Platelet tests and antiplatelet drugs in coronary artery disease. *Circulation*, 67:500.
8. Di Minno, G., Villa, S., Bertelè, V., and De Gaetano, G. (1980): Dipyridamole as an antithrombotic agent: An intricate mechanism of action. In: *Diet and Drugs in Atherosclerosis*, edited by G. Noseda, B. Lewis, and R. Paoletti, pp. 121–124. Raven Press, New York.
9. Gormsen, I., Dalsgaard-Nielsen, J., and Andersen, L. A. (1974): ADP-induced platelet aggregation *in vitro* in patients with ischaemic heart disease and peripheral thromboatherosclerosis. *Lancet*, 2:924.

10. Jackson, C. A., Greaves, M., and Preston, F. E. (1982): A study of stimulation of human venous prostacyclin synthesis by dipyridamole. *Thromb. Res.*, 27:563.
11. Libretti, A., and Catalano, M. (1983): Medical treatment of peripheral vascular diseases: Dipyridamole in combination with acetylsalicylic acid versus acetylsalicylic acid alone. *Thromb. Haemostas.*, 50:427.
12. Mehta, J., and Mehta, P. (1982): Dipyridamole and aspirin in relation to platelet aggregation and vessel wall prostaglandin generation. *J. Cardiovasc. Pharmacol.*, 4:688.
13. Mehta, J., Mehta, P., and Hay, D. (1982): Effect of dipyridamole on prostaglandin generation by human platelets and vessel walls. *Prostaglandins*, 24:751.
14. Morris-Jones, W., Preston, F. E., Greaney, M., and Chatterjee, D. K. (1981): Gangrene of the toes with palpable peripheral pulses: Response to platelet suppressive therapy. *Ann. Surg.*, 193:462.
15. Neri Serneri, G. G., Masotti, G., Abbate, R., Poggesi, L., Gensini, G., Favilla, S., Galanti, G., and Laureano, R. (1979): Enhanced prostacyclin production and decreased thromboxane formation by dipyridamole. *Proceedings of Florence International Meeting on Myocardial Infarction*, May 8–12, p. 489.
16. Neri Serneri, G. G., Masotti, G., Poggesi, L., Galanti, G., and Morettini, A. (1981): Enhanced prostacyclin production by dipyridamole in man. *Eur. J. Clin. Pharmacol.*, 21:9.
17. Patrono, C., Ciabattoni, G., Pinca, E., Pugliese, F., Castrucci, G., De Salvo, A., Satta, M. A., and Peskar, B. A. (1980): Low dose aspirin and inhibition of thromboxane B_2 production in healthy subjects. *Thromb. Res.*, 17:317.
18. Smith, R. S., and Warren, D. J. (1981): Effect of nicotinic acid and dipyridamole on tissue blood flow in peripheral vascular disease. *Pharmatherapeutica*, 2:616.
19. Strano, A., Davì, G., Avellone, G., Novo, S., and Pinto, A. (1983): Haemostatic alteration in peripheral artheriopathies. Proceedings of Ettore Majorana course *Advances in Haemostasis and Thrombosis*, Erice 20–26 April, pp. 217–226.
20. Ward, A. S., Porter, N., Preston, F. E., and Morris-Jones, W. (1978): Platelet aggregation in patients with peripheral vascular disease. *Atherosclerosis*, 29:63.
21. Weksler, B. B., Pett, S. B., Alonso, D., Richter, R. C., Stelzer, P., Subramanian, V., Tack-Goldman, K., and Gay, W. A. Jr. (1983): Differential inhibition by aspirin of vascular and platelet prostaglandin synthesis in atherosclerotic patients. *N. Engl. J. Med.*, 7:800.
22. Wu, K. K., and Hoak, J. C. (1974): A new method for the quantitative detection of platelet aggregates in patients with arterial insufficiency. *Lancet*, 2:924.

Advances in Prostaglandin, Thromboxane, and
Leukotriene Research, Vol. 13, edited by G. G. Neri
Serneri, et al. Raven Press, New York © 1985.

Effects of Ticlopidine on Platelet Function and on Coronary Insufficiency in Patients with Angina Pectoris

U. Berglund and L. Wallentin

Department of Internal Medicine, University Hospital, S-581 85 Linköping, Sweden

There is increasing evidence of platelet involvement in the different manifestations of coronary artery disease. A limited number of studies have been performed with antiplatelet drugs in angina pectoris. The results of these studies have been somewhat conflicting. In the present study we therefore investigated the possible effects of ticlopidine on platelet function and on myocardial ischemia in patients with stable angina pectoris.

MATERIAL

Thirty-eight men 41 to 65 years of age (median 58 years) referred for evaluation and treatment of incapacitating angina were studied. All patients had typical chest pain on exertion and some also had angina at rest. Only patients with a diagnostic exercise tolerance test interrupted because of chest pain and ST-T changes typical of myocardial ischemia were included. Coronary angiography was performed in 75% of the patients, all of whom had more than 50% stenosis or occlusion of at least one major coronary artery. No patient had heart failure or valvular disease, and none had earlier cardiac surgery. The pattern of anginal symptoms had been stable during the last 3 months in all patients. Beta-adrenoceptor blocking drugs were used by 37 patients, and 21 used calcium inhibitory drugs. This medication was kept unchanged during the study. All medication that could influence platelet function was excluded 1 week before and during the study.

METHODS

The design of the study was prospective, placebo-controlled, and double-blind. After a 2-week run-in period on placebo, the patients were randomized to oral treatment with either ticlopidine (T) at 250 mg twice daily ($n = 21$) or corresponding placebo (P) ($n = 17$). The treatment period was 8 weeks. All tests were performed after the run-in period, and after 4 and 8 weeks of treatment.

At each occasion, blood samples were drawn after an overnight fast. Platelet-rich plasma was isolated by centrifugation at 900 rpm for 15 min. Platelet aggregation was performed in a Payton aggregometer, mainly according to Born (2). Standardized amounts of ADP, collagen, and epinephrine were added to the platelet-rich plasma incubated at 37°C. The aggregation response was determined as the maximal percentage change of the light absorption compared to platelet-poor plasma. The platelet sensitivity to prostacyclin was tested by preincubation of platelet-rich plasma at 37°C for 4 min with different amounts of prostacyclin before the addition of ADP at 5 μM (5).

At each occasion, two exercise tolerance tests were performed: one at 21°C, and the other at 0°C. These tests were performed by sitting bicycle ergometry. The initial work load was low (in general 10 W). The load was increased continuously (in general by 10 W/min) until the patient experienced moderately severe angina. The electrocardiogram (ECG) was registered continuously, and the blood pressure was measured every minute. During the whole study the patients kept a diary recording the number of anginal attacks, the amount of nitroglycerin tablets consumed, and the possible side effects observed.

Statistical differences between the two groups were calculated by *t*-tests and Wilcoxon rank sum tests, and $p < 0.05$ was taken as significant.

RESULTS

Six patients were withdrawn from the study, 3 because of increasing angina necessitating urgent bypass surgery and 3 because of rash or diarrhea. All these patients turned out to belong to the T group. After 8 weeks of treatment with T there was a 48% mean reduction of maximal aggregation induced by ADP at 1 μM. Similar reductions of maximal aggregation were obtained with collagen and epinephrine in the T group. After the addition of prostacyclin in a concentration of 0.5 ng/ml and 1.0 ng/ml, the mean maximal aggregation was reduced by 65 and 78%, respectively, in the T group compared to the results obtained after the run-in period (Fig. 1). In the P group there were no significant changes of maximal aggregation in any of these aggregation tests.

After 8 weeks of treatment there was a nonsignificant mean reduction of maximal work load at 21°C by 4% in the T group and 2% in the P group, compared to the

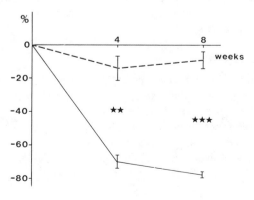

FIG. 1. Mean (± SEM) percentage change of maximal aggregation induced by ADP at 5 μM after preincubation with prostacyclin at 1.0 ng/ml during the treatment with ticlopidine *(continuous line)* or placebo *(dashed line)* compared to the results before treatment. Significances of differences between the groups during treatment were judged by unpaired *t*-tests and are symbolized by **$p < 0.01$; and ***$p < 0.001$.

findings after the run-in period. However, at 0°C there was a significant difference between the T group with a mean decrease of maximal work load by 3% and the P group with a mean rise of maximal work load by 10% (Fig. 2). The treatments did not induce any significant differences within or between the groups regarding ST-segment changes during exercise at 21°C or at 0°C.

Analysis of the patients' diaries showed no significant differences between the T group and the P group after 8 weeks of treatment concerning nitroglycerin consumption or the number of anginal attacks at rest or on exertion.

DISCUSSION

In the present study of patients with stable angina, there was a 50% reduction of ADP-induced aggregation during T treatment. This inhibition of ADP-induced aggregation is somewhat smaller than the results obtained in healthy volunteers (6), and less than what is obtained during aspirin (ASA) treatment. The T also reduced collagen-induced aggregation, an effect that is not obtained during ASA therapy. Furthermore, the present study demonstrated, for the first time in man, that T potentiated the platelet inhibitory effect of prostacyclin, indicating a synergistic effect between T and prostacyclin. Thus, in the dosage used (500 mg daily), T seemed to be an effective platelet inhibitor, which should influence the platelet–vessel wall interactions.

Despite the inhibitory effects on platelet function, T did not have any beneficial effects on anginal pain on exertion in our patients. It has been speculated that substances released from aggregating platelets might be involved in the spastic component of angina, which might be elicited by cold or occur spontaneously at rest. However, there was no effect on angina at rest, and T even seemed to reduce the maximal work load in the cold. Consequently, the transient episodes of myocardial ischemia in patients with stable angina do not seem to be influenced by platelet activation. This finding agrees with the previous results during ASA and dazoxiben treatment (3,4), but is at variance with the recent report from Fox et

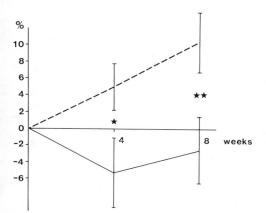

FIG. 2. Mean (± SEM) percentage change of maximal work load at sitting bicycle ergometry at 0°C during the treatment with ticlopidine *(continuous line)* or placebo *(dashed line).* $*p < 0.05$; $**p < 0.01$.

al. (1). However, even if platelet-inhibitory drugs do not influence anginal symptoms in patients with stable angina pectoris, this kind of treatment might play a role in preventing coronary thrombosis in these patients (4).

ACKNOWLEDGMENTS

This study was supported by the Swedish Medical Research Council (grant 19X-4529), by the King Gustafs and Queen Victorias Foundation, and by the Meda Pharmaceutical Company.

REFERENCES

1. Fox, K. M., Jonathan, A., and Selwyn, A. P. (1982): Effects of platelet inhibition on myocardial ischemia. *Lancet*, 2:727–730.
2. Gormsen, J., Dalsgaard Nielsen, J., and Agerskov Andersen, L. (1977): ADP-induced platelet aggregation *in vitro* in patients with ischemic heart disease and peripheral thromboatherosclerosis. *Acta Med. Scand.*, 201:509–513.
3. Hendra, T., Collins, P., Penny, W., and Sheridan, D. J. (1984): Failure of thromboxane synthetase inhibition to improve exercise tolerance in patients with stable angina pectoris. *Int. J. Cardiol.*, 5:382–385.
4. Lewis, H. D. Jr. et al. (1983): Protective effects of aspirin against acute myocardial infarction and death in men with unstable angina. *N. Engl. J. Med.*, 309:396–403.
5. Sinzinger, H., Kaliman, J., Widhalm, K., Pachinger, O., and Probst, P. (1981): Value of platelet sensitivity to antiaggregatory prostaglandins (PGI_2, PGE_1, PGD_2) in 50 patients with myocardial infarction at young age. *Prostaglandins Med.*, 7:125–132.
6. Thébault, J. J., Blatrix, C. E., Blanchard, J. F., and Panak, E. A. (1975): Effects of ticlopidine, a new platelet aggregation inhibitor in man. *Clin. Pharmacol. Ther.*, 18:485–490.

Advances in Prostaglandin, Thromboxane, and
Leukotriene Research, Vol. 13, edited by G. G. Neri
Serneri, et al. Raven Press, New York © 1985.

Metabolic Side Effects of the Platelet-Inhibitory Drug Ticlopidine

U. Berglund and L. Wallentin

Department of Internal Medicine, University Hospital, S-581 85 Linköping, Sweden

Platelet-inhibitory drugs are often suggested for use in patients with arteriosclerotic cardiovascular diseases in order to prevent thromboembolic events and to retard the arteriosclerotic process. Before starting long-term treatment with such a drug, it seems important to investigate its effects not only on platelet function but also on other cardiovascular risk factors. We therefore performed a study on the influence of ticlopidine on lipid metabolism in patients with coronary artery disease.

MATERIAL

Thirty-eight men 41 to 65 years of age (median 58 years) referred for evaluation and treatment of incapacitating angina were studied. All patients had typical chest pain on exertion and some also had angina at rest. Only patients with a diagnostic exercise tolerance test interrupted because of chest pain and ST-T changes typical of myocardial ischemia were included. Coronary angiography was performed in 75% of the patients, all of whom had more than 50% stenosis or occlusion of at least one major coronary artery. No patient had heart failure or valvular disease, and none had earlier cardiac surgery. The pattern of anginal symptoms had been stable during the last 3 months in all patients. Beta-adrenoceptor blocking drugs were used by 37 patients, and 21 subjects used calcium-inhibitory drugs. This medication was kept unchanged during the study. All medication that could influence the platelet function was excluded 1 week before and during the study.

METHODS

The design of the study was prospective, placebo-controlled, and double-blind. After a 2-week run-in period on placebo, the patients were randomized to oral treatment with either ticlopidine (T) at 250 mg twice daily ($n = 21$) or corresponding placebo (P) ($n = 17$). The treatment period was 8 weeks. All tests were performed after the run-in period, and after 4 and 8 weeks of treatment.

At each occasion, venous blood samples were obtained after an overnight fast for determination of lipid concentrations in plasma and in lipoprotein fractions. The plasma lipoprotein fractions were separated by ultracentrifugation at $d = 1.006$

and heparin–MnCl₂ precipitation (3). The determination of cholesterol and triglyceride concentrations were performed by enzymatic methods (3).

Statistical differences between the two groups were calculated by *t*-tests, and $p < 0.05$ was taken as significant.

RESULTS

In the T group, the cholesterol concentration showed a mean increase from 6.3 before treatment to 7.2 mmol/l after 8 weeks of treatment ($p < 0.001$). The elevation of the plasma cholesterol level was caused by an increase in the very low-density lipoprotein fraction from 0.71 to 1.04 mmol/l and in the low-density lipoprotein fraction from 4.6 to 5.3 mmol/l (Fig. 1). The mean level of cholesterol in the high-density lipoprotein fraction was unchanged during T treatment. Furthermore, there was a mean increase in the triglyceride concentration from 2.17 before treatment to 2.78 mmol/l after 8 weeks of treatment ($p < 0.01$) in the T group, mainly due to the increase of the very low-density lipoprotein fraction (Fig. 2). In the P group, there were no changes in lipoprotein levels during the study.

DISCUSSION

Ticlopidine has been shown to be an effective platelet inhibitor. The present study was the first that evaluated the effects of T on plasma lipids in coronary

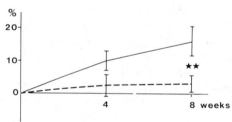

FIG. 1. Mean (± SEM) percentage change of the low-density lipoprotein cholesterol concentration during treatment with ticlopidine *(continuous line)* or placebo *(dashed line)*, compared to the results before treatment. Significances of differences between the groups during treatment were judged by unpaired *t*-tests and are symbolized by **$p < 0.01$.

FIG. 2. Mean (± SEM) percentage change of the triglyceride concentration during treatment with ticlopidine *(continuous line)* or placebo *(dashed line)*. Significances of differences between the groups during treatment were judged by unpaired *t*-tests and are symbolized by **$p < 0.01$.

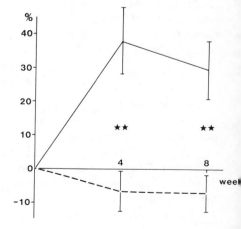

artery disease patients using a prospective double-blind placebo-controlled design. To our knowledge, no previous study has evaluated the effects of T on plasma lipoprotein fractions. The present findings of significant elevations of the cholesterol and triglyceride levels during T treatment agree with some animal studies and findings in healthy volunteers (Sanofi research data). These elevations of the cholesterol and triglyceride levels were confined to the "atherogenic" very low-density lipoprotein and low-density lipoprotein fractions, while there was no change of the "antiatherogenic" high-density lipoprotein fraction. The credibility of the present observations was supported by the unchanged lipoprotein levels in the placebo group.

It is well established that elevated levels of cholesterol in the very low-density lipoprotein and low-density lipoprotein fractions accelerate the development of atherosclerosis and increase the risk of ischemic cardiovascular events. Platelet activation seems to participate in the development of arteriosclerosis and to initiate thromboembolic events. Therefore, treatment with antiplatelet drugs might be beneficial in coronary artery disease, as suggested by some previous studies (1,2). The present study emphasizes the importance of monitoring several risk factors in the evaluation of drugs suggested to influence the cardiovascular morbidity by its beneficial effect on one of these factors. This study indicates that long-term treatment with T should be used with caution in coronary artery disease patients and that blood lipid levels should be monitored during the treatment.

ACKNOWLEDGMENTS

This study was supported by the Swedish Medical Research Council (grant 19X-4529), by the King Gustafs and Queen Victorias Foundation, and by the Meda Pharmaceutical Company.

REFERENCES

1. Lewis, H. D. Jr. (1983): Protective effects of aspirin against acute myocardial infarction and death in men with unstable angina. *N. Engl. J. Med.*, 309:396–403.
2. Persantine-Aspirin Reinfarction Study Group (1980): Persantine and aspirin in coronary heart disease. *Circulation*, 62:449–661.
3. Wallentin, L., and Fåhraeus, L. (1981): HDL₃ and HDL₂ determination by a combined ultracentrifugation and precipitation procedure. *Clin. Chim. Acta*, 116:199–208.

Advances in Prostaglandin, Thromboxane, and Leukotriene Research, Vol. 13, edited by G. G. Neri Serneri, et al. Raven Press, New York © 1985.

Coronary Artery Bypass Grafting. A Model for the Understanding of the Progression of Atherosclerotic Disease and the Role of Pharmacological Intervention

*Valentin Fuster and **James H. Chesebro

*Division of Cardiology, Mount Sinai Medical Center, New York, New York 10029; and
**Division of Cardiology, Mayo Clinic and Mayo Foundation, Rochester, Minnesota 55905

Evidence in experimental animals and humans suggests that atherosclerotic plaques may progress at two rates: (a) rapidly, by a gross mechanism of mural thrombus formation leading to its fibrotic organization and (b) slowly, by repeated platelet–arterial wall interaction leading to proliferation of smooth muscle cells and synthesis of fibrillar material. Our objective was to determine whether platelet-inhibitor drugs could prevent one or both mechanisms of progression. In dogs and humans, we have used the coronary artery bypass vein graft model because it tends to develop a rapid thromboatherosclerotic type of progression (within 2 weeks after operation) and a slow atherosclerotic type of progression (within 1 year postoperatively).

In dogs, platelet inhibition, based on the combination of dipyridamole plus aspirin significantly reduced the rapid thromboatherosclerotic type of progression within 2 weeks after operation, but only slightly reduced the slow atherosclerotic type of progression within 6 months. In a prospective, randomized, double-blind trial in 407 patients, the combination of dipyridamole plus aspirin significantly reduced the rapid thrombotic occlusion within 4 weeks of operation, but only slightly reduced the slow atherosclerotic type of late progressive occlusion within 1 year.

On the basis of this information, platelet inhibition seems more promising for the reduction of the rapid thrombotic type than of the slow type of progression of atherosclerosis. Indeed, for the slow type of progression of atherosclerosis, which tends to occur in a period of decades, prevention and modification of the risk factors for atherosclerotic disease should be the fundamental approach.

In part published in the *Proceedings of the International Symposium on Atheroma and Thrombosis*, edited by V. V. Kakkar, London, July 1983.

BACKGROUND

Over the last few years we have been particularly interested in the understanding, experimentally and clinically, of two vascular disease processes. The first relates to the coronary saphenous vein bypass graft, which has a high incidence of narrowing and occlusion. The second relates to the pathological process in the arteries, that is, the process of atherogenesis. We believe that the two processes are actually very similar, and their development is based on similar principles. In addition, both processes can progress under two completely different mechanisms. One is a thrombogenic mechanism of progression, which may be sensitive to platelet inhibition. The second is a much more complex mechanism of progression, based on an interaction of endothelial cells, platelets, smooth muscle cells, connective tissue, lipoproteins, and macrophages. This second mechanism is probably resistant to the use of platelet-inhibitor drugs.

We will summarize the experimental and clinical experience that we have gained, first in the saphenous vein bypass graft model, and second in the atherogenic model.

SAPHENOUS VEIN BYPASS GRAFT MODEL

Pathogenesis of Vein Graft Occlusion

This process is illustrated in Fig. 1. Damage to the endothelium occurs in all veins grafts. It appears to start with procurement of the saphenous vein and is probably enhanced by surgical handling and placing the vein in the arterial system. This is followed by platelet deposition to the subendothelial structures in areas of endothelial damage as soon as blood starts to flow through the graft (18). Thus, platelets initiate mural thrombus formation that starts during the operation. If this thrombus formation is severe, total occlusion of the vein graft may occur in the early days after operation (22). The mural or occlusive thrombus can organize with

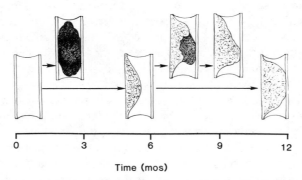

Time (mos)

FIG. 1. Scheme of gross processes leading to aortocoronary vein graft occlusion: early thrombotic occlusion **(high in panel, left)**, late occlusion as a result of an accelerated atherosclerotic process **(lower in panel)**, and late occlusion as a result of organization or complicating mural thrombus superimposed over a growing atherosclerotic plaque **(high in panel, right)**.

secondary ingrowth of smooth muscle cells and connective tissue (secondary proliferation) (26).

Whereas early occlusion is due to thrombosis, late occlusion, which tends to occur within 1 year, appears to be related to a more complex mechanism of disease progression (5). That is, intermittent platelet adhesion to a minimally injured endothelial surface, without thrombus formation, is associated with chronic smooth muscle cell and connective tissue proliferation (primary proliferation), which eventually may lead to the late occlusion of the graft with or without associated complicating thrombus. The pathogenesis of such primary proliferative process in the graft has most likely some similarities to the pathogenesis of the early atherosclerotic lesions in the arteries discussed later in the chapter.

Role of Platelet-Inhibiting Drugs

Since platelet deposition appears to initiate the pathophysiologic mechanism of vein graft occlusion starting during the operation, platelet-inhibitor therapy started before operation would be a logical choice for intervention. This is illustrated in Fig. 2. Thus, dipyridamole started 48 hr before operation and adding aspirin following operation greatly decreased platelet thrombus formation in the early hours to days after operation, as well as the secondary proliferation of smooth muscle cells and connective tissue (18,22,26) in the canine model; also importantly, there was no obvious perioperative bleeding, since aspirin was not started until after operation. The late progressive process of primary proliferation of smooth muscle cells and connective tissue was less affected by platelet inhibition.

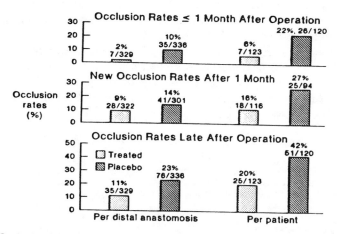

FIG. 2. Occlusion rates for all types of vein grafts per distal anastomosis and per patient (proportion with at least one occlusion). Occlusion is shown within 1 month, new beyond 1 month (in distal anastomoses and patients without occlusion within 1 month of operation) from angiography performed 1 year later, and at a median of 1 year after operation. These subjects include only patients who had angiography within 1 month of operation and again 1 year later. Below each percentage is shown the number of distal anastomoses or patients with occlusion/total number of distal anastomoses or patients. (From Chesebro et al., ref. 6.)

Using the rationale above, we designed and conducted a prospective, randomized, double-blind, placebo-controlled trial using dipyridamole (started 2 days before operation) plus aspirin (started 7 hr after operation; see Table 1 for schedule) in 407 patients (4). Vein graft angiography was performed early after operation (within 6 months) and again a median of 1 year after operation. Within 1 month of operation, vein graft distal anastomoses were occluded in 2% in the treated group and 10% in the placebo group; the proportion of patients with one or more distal anastomoses occluded was 6% in the treated group and 22% in the placebo group ($p = 0.0003$). At 4 to 6 months or less after operation, there were even greater differences in the occlusion rates per distal anastomosis and per patient ($p = 0.000001$). Perioperative dipyridamole and aspirin therapy is safe and did not cause perioperative bleeding. Therefore, the therapeutic benefit observed in the canine model was confirmed in humans.

At 1 year after operation, the beneficial effect of platelet inhibition in preventing graft occlusion was less striking than early after operation. Thus, of all grafts patent within 1 month after operation, the percentage developing late occlusion was reduced from 14% in the placebo group to 9% in the treated group; of patients with all grafts patent within 1 month after operation, the percentage developing late occlusion was reduced from 27% in the placebo group to 16% in the treated group ($p = 0.038$). This less striking beneficial effect of platelet inhibition late after operation is also in agreement with the results obtained in the canine model. As we will discuss later in the section on atherosclerosis, we cannot expect the primary proliferative process that affects late graft occlusion to be significantly prevented by platelet inhibitors. In fact, we believe that the slight therapeutic benefit of these agents late postoperatively is not related to the prevention of the primary occlusive proliferative process, but rather to the prevention of complicating superimposed thrombus, which in some cases may lead to the final occlusion.

As we discuss in the next section, our observations in the saphenous vein graft model compliment our present understanding of the process of atherosclerotic disease and its complications, as well as the possible role of platelet-inhibitor drugs in such arterial disease.

TABLE 1. *Platelet-inhibitor therapy for aortocoronary vein bypass operations*[a]

Starting 2 days before operation
Dipyridamole 100 mg orally, four times daily
Day of operation
6 a.m.: Dipyridamole 100 mg orally
1 hr After operation: dipyridamole 100 mg down nasogastric tube (clamp 1½ hr)
7 hr After operation: dipyridamole 75 mg and aspirin 325 mg, down nasogastric tube (clamp 1½ hr)
Day after operation and then daily for 1 year
Dipyridamole 75 mg and aspirin 325 mg orally three times daily

[a]No other aspirin or prostaglandin-inhibitor drugs.

ATHEROSCLEROTIC DISEASE

Natural Evolution of Atherosclerotic Lesions

A critical study for the understanding of the natural evolution of atherosclerotic lesions was the International Atherosclerosis Project (25), which involved 14 countries with 19 different racial groups. This study had the objective of describing the incidence and natural history of coronary and aortic atherosclerotic lesions found at autopsy in these different populations. In the study, 23,000 sets of coronary arteries and aortas were evaluated. The findings of the survey demonstrated that fatty streaks are a universal phenomenon in young persons in all geographic racial groups; however, their evolution into clinically relevant fibrous plaques and complicated lesions varies in incidence and extent among different geographic and ethnic groups.

In the natural history of the atherosclerotic lesions (Fig. 3), two facts are important: (a) that the progression of early atherosclerotic lesions (fatty streaks) to clinically relevant advanced atherosclerotic lesions (fibrous plaques, etc.) tends to occur in those individuals with the so-called risk factors of atherosclerotic disease, and (b) that the early and some of the advanced atherosclerotic lesions progress very slowly, probably by means of a complex biological step-by-step phenomenon, while some of the advanced atherosclerotic legions progress very rapidly, probably by means of a thrombogenic phenomenon.

Pathogenesis of Early Atherosclerotic Lesions

We will first review the major critical events in the development of the early atherosclerotic lesions (12): (a) hemodynamic stress, endothelial injury, and smooth

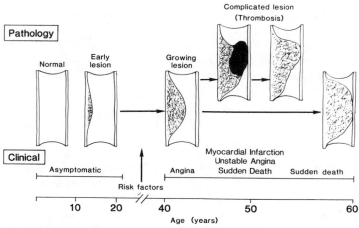

FIG. 3. Scheme of the gross evolution of coronary atherosclerosis. The growing fibrous plaque can progress to total occlusion of an artery, either through slow progression or rapidly by thrombus formation with subsequent fibrotic organization.

muscle cell proliferation; (b) interaction between arterial wall and blood cells; (c) lipoprotein entry and accumulation; and (d) fibrous tissue synthesis. As mentioned earlier in the chapter, this complex step-by-step phenomenon in the arteries appears to have some similarities to the progressive disease narrowing that affects the saphenous vein bypass graft, leading to late graft occlusion.

Endothelial Cell, Hemodynamic Stress, and Smooth Muscle Cell Proliferation

The aortic branch points and other areas where atherosclerotic plaques usually develop have been shown to be sites of endothelial injury (29). There is some evidence that hemodynamic factors are involved in causing such focal and chronic or continuous minimal endothelial injury. Thus, from experiments in which hydraulic models of various flow patterns were used, it was possible to predict from the site of maximal turbulence the areas of predilection for occurrence of atherosclerosis within the human arterial tree (34). In addition, in the experimental animal it has been found that some of the so-called risk factors of atherosclerotic disease may potentiate this process of endothelial injury (13).

The concept that atherosclerosis is a local response to chronic or continuous minimal endothelial injury has also received further support (33). Experimental endothelial injury reproduces the full spectrum of early atherosclerotic lesions. In such experiments one of the first structural changes, as in spontaneous atherosclerosis, is an intimal proliferation of smooth muscle cells that presumably derive from the medial of the artery. The fact that in these experiments the arterial injury was very superficial suggests the possibility that the migration and proliferation of smooth muscle cells are related to the interaction of plasma components. Furthermore, there have been a number of observations from *in vitro* systems to suggest that there may be components normally present in plasma that may act, at least *in vitro*, as stimulus for proliferation of smooth muscle cells. Thus, as discussed later, Ross et al. (31) have developed a method of studying the growth of these cells in culture and have shown that smooth muscle cells from the aortas of pigtail monkeys actively multiply in culture only when the medium in which they are grown contains macromolecules derived from serum.

Interaction Between Arterial Wall and Platelets

As already pointed out, hemodynamic factors plus endothelial injury and smooth muscle cell proliferation have been considered important in the development of atherosclerosis. There have been increasing indications that platelets, by interacting with the arterial wall, may be involved in these early stages of the disease.

Evidence that platelets and other formed blood elements can be involved in the primary minimal injury to the vascular endothelium in regions of blood turbulence has been obtained in a number of studies. Thus, examination of the endothelial surface of vessels from pigs, rabbits, mice, and pigeons, and from young humans who died suddenly, showed formed elements, mainly platelets, on the arterial surface near those sites where atherosclerosis develops (12).

Thus far, it appears that the observed attachment of platelets to damaged endothelial surfaces and particularly their activation mainly depends on a complex molecule related to factor VIII (27). This molecule, which is called Willebrand factor, is normally present in the circulating plasma and platelet, as well as in the endothelial and subendothelial regions—here probably attached to collagen fibrils—and there is increasing evidence that it favors the platelet–arterial wall interaction and platelet activation in the regions of endothelial damage.

Significant observations have raised the possibility that these platelets attached to the mildly injured arterial wall are one of the principal stimulating factors of the smooth muscle cell proliferation that occurs at the initial stages of atherosclerosis. In experimental atherosclerosis induced by endothelial injury, one of the first morphologic events is the appearance of platelets undergoing intracytoplasmic degranulation and adhering to the endothelial surface and subendothelial denuded areas. This precedes the migration and proliferation of smooth muscle cells (33). An important finding by Ross et al. (31) was that substance derived from platelets was necessary for the proliferation of smooth muscle cells and fibroblasts in culture, and it has been assumed that this substance is one of the main factors responsible for the smooth muscle cell proliferation of the atherosclerotic lesions. Such platelet-derived growth factor (PDGF) is a low molecular weight, heat-stable protein purified recently (1). PDGF, together with platelet factor 4 (PF-4), which is an anti-heparin factor, and β-thromboglobulin are all released from the platelet α-granules during platelet activation (16). The observation that PF-4 can penetrate the vessel wall intima during the process of platelet–arterial wall interaction (21) is of interest, particularly in view of the recent observation of its chemotactic properties (7). That is, it is conceivable that during platelet–arterial wall interaction, PF-4 and PDGF penetrate the vessel wall and, while PF-4 may play a role in attracting the smooth muscle cells from the media towards the intima, the PDGF, together with other growth factors, may play a role in the intimal smooth muscle cell proliferation.

Insight into the significance of platelets in initiating atherosclerosis has also been gained by investigating whether experimental animals with inhibited platelet function are resistant to the development of atherosclerosis. For several years, a breeding colony of pigs with severely impaired platelet function in the form of homozygous von Willebrand's disease has been maintained in Rochester, Minnesota. Fuster et al. have shown that such pigs with a lack of Willebrand factor have a marked impairment in platelet attachment to the vascular wall, and the pigs are resistant to the initiation and progression of both spontaneous atherosclerosis (19) and that induced by a mildly high cholesterol diet (15). However, pigs with less severely impaired platelet function in the form of heterozygous von Willebrand's disease are not resistant to atherosclerosis (2). This, again, indicates that the presence of normal or nearly normal functioning platelets may be important in the initial stages of atherosclerosis.

Lipoprotein Entry and Accumulation by Arterial Wall

The major class of lipids accumulating in the arterial wall during atherogenesis is cholesterol esters. The cholesterol is derived from plasma lipoproteins. Biochemical studies of atherosclerotic vessels at various stages of development have shown that whereas plasma and the normal arterial wall contain cholesterol linoleate, the development of atherosclerotic plaques is characterized by the accumulation of cholesterol oleate. This is also the case for most types of experimentally-induced atherosclerosis. As plaques become more advanced, free cholesterol and cholesterol linoleate from trapped plasma also accumulate.

We have recently reviewed (13) and now summarize the possible ultrastructural and biochemical role of lipids in atherosclerotic plaque formation.

1. It appears that high-serum low-density lipoproteins (LDL) contribute to the process of endothelial injury.

2. It appears that lipoproteins may be mitogenic, according to studies with smooth muscle cell cultures, probably by contributing to cell membrane formation.

3. The space occupying intracellular and extracellular accumulation of fat may also contribute to the growing of the atherosclerotic plaque.

4. It has been suggested that factors impairing the process of arterial wall removal of cholesterol may favor its accumulation and so the progression of the disease. Thus, epidemiologic data have established a consistent correlation between high concentrations of high-density lipoproteins (HDL) in plasma and a decreased incidence and progression of atherosclerotic disease. Since HDL molecules easily traverse the arterial wall and are able to transport cholesterol away from aortic smooth muscles in culture, it has been suggested that the observed protection against atherosclerosis is related to this removal of cholesterol from the arterial wall.

5. There is evidence that lipoproteins enhance platelet reactivity and may alter the prostaglandin production; as discussed later in this chapter with the pathogenesis of the advanced atherosclerotic lesions, this enhancement in platelet reactivity may well explain the thrombogenicity of an ulcerated atherosclerotic plaque in which the arterial wall fat may come in contact with the circulating platelet.

Fibrous Tissue Synthesis

The formation of fibrous tissue contributes significantly to the initiation of the atherosclerotic plaque and, most importantly, in its progression, as discussed later. The elements making up this fibrous tissue are collagen, proteoglycans, elastin, and glycoproteins (13), and all of them appear to be synthesized by the arterial smooth muscle cells (32).

Collagen formation is the major contributor to the growth of the atherosclerotic plaque. The glycosaminoglycans appear to be important in the binding of lipid into the arterial wall. Elastin fibers appear to be important in the binding of lipid into the arterial wall; in addition, they contribute significantly to the process of calcification of the atherosclerotic plaque. Glycoproteins appear to be important in certain interactions of collagen and elastin fibers.

This concept of fibrous tissue synthesis assumes that the endothelial injury and platelet deposition lead not only to the migration and proliferation of the smooth muscle cells but also to their synthesis of fibrous tissue components. In addition, it appears that the chronic pulsatile distention of the arteries also favors the synthesis of collagen by the smooth muscle cells and thus the slow progression of the atherosclerotic plaque.

Pathogenesis of Advanced Atherosclerotic Plaques

As already mentioned in this chapter, early atherosclerotic lesions, particularly in the form of fatty streaks, are a universal phenomenon in young persons; however, this evolution into advanced clinically relevant lesions tends to occur in those individuals with the so-called risk factors of atherosclerotic disease. Today there is increasing experimental, pathological, and clinical evidence that the early atherosclerotic lesions can progress into the advanced and clinically relevant atherosclerotic plaques by at least two completely different pathogenetic processes. The first is related to a continuation of the process responsible for the development of the early atherosclerotic lesions. That is, it is a chronic phenomenon leading to a slow progression of the atherosclerotic plaque over a period of decades.

The second mechanism by which atherosclerotic lesions can progress is a thrombogenic process. This process has some similarities to the thrombogenic process that affects the saphenous vein bypass graft leading to early graft occlusion. However, in patients with atherosclerotic disease, the thrombus is superimposed on an atherosclerotic plaque, while in the vein graft the thrombus formation occurs early, in areas of significant endothelial damage probably related to the surgical handling of the graft. In relation to the atherosclerotic process, indeed, the atherosclerotic plaques, particularly those of already moderate or significant degree, may progress rapidly by means of superimposed platelet and fibrin thrombus, which then tends to suffer a process of phagocytosis and fibrotic atherogenic transformation (12,16). It is likely that this fibrotic organization of thrombi is also dependent on the activation of the smooth muscle cells, not only by the platelet-derived growth factor but also probably by the fibrin itself, as well as by the thrombin and plasmin generated in the thrombus media.

An important question to be answered is why thrombus formation tends to occur over atherosclerotic plaques. In this context there are at least three important steps to consider: (a) hemodynamic factors, (b) arterial damage and thrombogenicity, and (c) hypercoagulable state.

Hemodynamic Factors

There is evidence that in regions of focal arterial narrowing there is a significant wall shear stress (force parallel to luminal surface and independent of turbulence) and/or wide variations in the direction of these forces (11). These observations are of particular significance in view of calculations that forces at or exceeding the yield stress of the endothelial lining probably explain the superficial arterial wall damage and thrombus formation characteristic of these regions. In addition, if the arterial narrowing caused by an atherosclerotic plaque is severe enough to cause stasis, this in itself may also potentiate thrombogenicity.

Arterial Damage and Thrombogenicity

There are two different types of arterial damage that probably lead to thrombus formation superimposed over the atherosclerotic plaques: (a) superficial damage mainly involving the endothelial and subendothelial layers and (b) deep damage mainly involving ulceration of the atherosclerotic plaque.

Superficial damage

In areas of arterial narrowing there is superficial damage mainly affecting the endothelial and subendothelial layer. Such damage is probably related to the hemodynamic factors already described. It is now evident experimentally that in such damaged areas there is a significant tendency for platelet aggregation and thrombus formation (9,20,24). Contrary to the minimal endothelial injury of the early atherosclerotic lesions—which, as discussed earlier in the chapter, appears to just lead to platelet adhesion—this type of superficial arterial damage in regions of arterial narrowing appears to be somewhat deeper, affecting the endothelial and subendothelial layers and leading to platelet aggregation and thrombogenicity. That is, in these constricted arterial regions, platelets become easily attached to the damaged surfaces: first, as a result of the same factors earlier described in the endothelial injury of the early atherosclerotic plaques (i.e., Willebrand factor, collagen fibrils), and second, in this type of deeper damage the thrombogenicity is, in addition, favored by the absence of two natural antithrombotic systems usually present in the intact endothelial and subendothelial arterial layers (9,16)—that is, the fibrinolytic system and the prostaglandin system [particularly prostacyclin (PGI_2)].

In this stenotic superficial region of arterial damage, the secondary superimposed deposition of thrombus (mural thrombus) may undergo atherogenesis with plaque growth; in addition, the thrombus may totally occlude the artery (occlusive thrombus), so contributing, for example, to the development of myocardial infarction (16). On some occasions, either mural or occlusive thrombus may also spontaneously disappear because of the blood lytic system or because of embolization (16). In fact, there is now increasing evidence that in these atherosclerotic damaged regions where thrombus tends to form there is a continuous dynamic formation and disappearance of platelet thrombi (9,16), as well as fluctuating vasotonicity (spasm) (24); both of these intermittent phenomena may explain some of the intermittent coronary syndromes.

Deep damage and ulceration

Arteries that have advanced atherosclerotic lesions show fragmentation of their elastic elements. This, together with the biochemical alteration of the elastic fibers in atherosclerotic disease, appears to promote conditions that lead to superficial ulceration with thrombus formation (3,13). Thus, it is not an infrequent finding at autopsy of patients with acute myocardial infarction to observe an acute ulcerated, ruptured, and hemorrhagic atherosclerotic plaque, at the site of the complicative occlusive thrombi that presumably contributed to the infarction (8,30). In addition, similar to the regions of superficial damage, in these ulcerated regions the complicating thrombi may just be partially occlusive or mural leading to atherogenesis and plaque growth (13).

In the genesis of thrombi as a complication of ulcerated atherosclerotic plaques, apart from the thrombogenic factors when the damage is superficial, there are three other important factors to be considered (12,16): (a) when the atherosclerotic plaque ruptures and there is hemorrhage into the plaque, there is adenosine diphosphate released from red blood cells which likely contributes to the process of platelet aggregation; (b) in the advanced atherosclerotic plaque the accumulated fat is usually underneath, but when the plaque ruptures such fat can come into contact with the circulating blood and so activate platelets and promote thrombogenicity; and (c) the acute damage site of the vascular wall can make available tissue thromboplastine, which also leads to the genesis of thrombi.

Hypercoagulable State

It is well known that focal thrombosis can lead to a secondary hypercoagulable or thrombotic state of the circulation, which may favor progression or recurrence of the thrombi (16). However, it is not entirely clear whether there really exists a primary hypercoagulable or thrombotic state of the circulation that can promote focal thrombosis and atherosclerosis. Thus, as we have reviewed (16), platelet aggregation and the subsequent generation of thrombin may be activated by circulating catecholamines. This interrelationship may be of major importance because it may be a link between conditions of stress and the development of arterial thrombosis. Of no less importance is the increasing evidence of an enhanced platelet reactivity in cigarette smokers, in patients with a strong family history of coronary disease, in patients with hyperlipidemia, and in patients with diabetes mellitus. However, in such high-risk conditions for atherosclerotic and thrombotic disease, the enhanced platelet and coagulable reactivity may be a secondary phenomenon rather than a primary cause of the disease.

Role of Platelet-Inhibiting Drugs

Our discussion will be focused in the two different mechanisms of atherosclerotic plaque progression (Table 2): (a) the slow progression of the early atherosclerotic lesions towards the advanced atherosclerotic plaques, and (b) the rapid thrombogenic progression of the advanced atherosclerotic plaques.

TABLE 2. *Coronary atherosclerotic disease: sequential events and the role of platelets and thrombosis*

Early lesions
    Rheologic factors—endothelial damage
    Platelet deposition
    Smooth muscle cell migration and proliferation
    Connective tissue synthesis
    Lipid transformation and deposition
Growing lesions
    Progression of above (slow process)
    Organization of thrombi (rapid process)[a]
Complications
    Myocardial infarction with *thrombotic occlusion[a]*

[a]Platelet-thrombotic events that perhaps may be reduced by the use of platelet-inhibitor drugs.
Italics = role of platelets and thrombosis.

Slow Process of Atherosclerotic Progression

As already discussed, there is evidence that platelet–arterial wall interaction is an important step in the pathogenesis of the early atherosclerotic lesions and of their slow progression towards the advanced atherosclerotic plaques. Indeed, it appears that minimal endothelial injury caused by chronic hemodynamic stress and by some of the so-called risk factors may lead to intermittent platelet–arterial wall interaction and the slow development of atherosclerotic lesions. We have been able to reproduce in the experimental pig such minimal endothelial injury (without descamation of the endothelial cells from the subendothelial layer) (14); a single layer of platelets interacting with the damaged endothelium appears to be sufficient to induce the intimal smooth muscle cell proliferation compatible with the athero-sclerotic lesion. The important point is that, at present, there is no platelet-inhibitor drug available that can totally prevent this single layer of adhering platelets. There-fore, we feel that by the use of platelet-inhibiting drugs the slow growth of the atherosclerotic process will not be totally prevented. In fact, the previously dis-cussed lesser beneficial effect of platelet inhibition in saphenous vein bypass grafts, late when compared with early postoperatively, is probably because late postoper-atively a similar type of atherosclerotic process develops in the graft and is resistant to platelet inhibition.

If a new platelet-inhibitor drug that can totally prevent the platelet adhesion to the vessel wall becomes available in the future, then a new threatening risk will emerge: the risk of bleeding. Thus, our pigs with homozygous von Willebrand's disease, which have a marked impairment in platelet attachment to the vascular wall (14), are resistant to the initiation and progression of atherosclerotic disease (15,19), but they have a very severe bleeding tendency; on the other hand, pigs having a less severely impaired platelet–arterial wall interaction in the form of heterozygous von Willebrand's disease develop atherosclerosis (2) and are free of significant bleeding. Also, Friedman and associates (10) produced marked thrombocytopenia (platelet count less than 7,000/mm³) in rabbits by administering anti-platelet serum. Injuring the endothelium in these rabbits with a polyethylene catheter was not followed by the development of atherosclerotic lesions, but the animals had a significant bleeding tendency; on the other hand, rabbits with less severe thrombocytopenia were not protected from atherosclerosis.

These findings emphasize that prevention of the initiation and progression of the slow atherosclerotic process in the arteries might be accomplished only if platelet function and counts are reduced to the point of causing significant bleeding. Therefore, it is not unreasonable to think that only those platelet-inhibitor agents leading to severe platelet dysfunction and bleeding might be of benefit in preventing the progression of the slow atherosclerotic process. Fortunately, such platelet-inhibitor agents are not yet available (17) and, of course, we feel they are undesirable.

Rapid Thrombogenic Process of Atherosclerotic Progression

As already discussed, in some patients with advanced atherosclerotic plaques, such plaques continue to progress rapidly, and a thrombogenic mechanism seems to be important. In addition, a sudden thrombotic occlusion superimposed on an atherosclerotic plaque can lead to a myocardial infarction. Since in these arterial thrombi platelet aggregation appears to be essential, it is reasonable to assume that platelet-inhibiting drugs may be beneficial in preventing this rapid progressive type of atherosclerotic process. Based on the striking antithrombotic effect obtained with platelet-inhibitor drugs in the saphenous vein grafts model early postoperatively, we believe that these agents may also turn out to be of benefit in the prevention of the rapid thrombogenic atherosclerotic process and thrombotic myocardial infarction. A most recent drug trial (23) and our studies in progress (28) may substantiate this belief. Nevertheless, at the present time, it is not known how frequently and in what specific patients with atherosclerotic disease this complicating thrombogenic process takes place.

REFERENCES

1. Antoniades, H. N., and Hunkapiller, M. W. (1983): Human platelet-derived growth factor (PDFG): Amino-terminal amino acid sequence. *Science*, 20:963.
2. Badimon, L, Rosemark, J. A., Badimon, J. J., Bowie, E. J. W. and Fuster, V. (1985): Diet induced atherosclerosis in pigs heterozygous for von Willebrand's disease. Comparison with homozygous von Willebrand pigs and normal pigs. (*submitted for publication*).
3. Chandler, A. B. Chapman, I. Erhardt, L. R., et al. (1974): Coronary thrombosis in myocardial infarction: Report of a workshop on the role of coronary thrombosis in the pathogenesis of acute myocardial infarction. *Am. J. Cardiol.*, 34:823.
4. Chesebro, J. H., Clements, I. P., Fuster, V., Elveback, L. R., Smith, H. C., Bardsley, W. T., Frye, R. L., Holmes, D. R., Vlietstra, R. E., Pluth, J. R., Wallace, R. B., Puga, F. J., Orszulak, T. A., Piehler, J. M., Schaff, H. V., and Danielson, G. K. (1982): A platelet-inhibitor-drug trial in coronary-artery bypass operations: Benefit of perioperative dipyridamole and aspirin therapy on early postoperative vein-graft patency. *N. Engl. J. Med.*, 307:73.
5. Chesebro, J. H., and Fuster, V. (1983): Platelets and platelet-inhibitor drugs in aortocoronary vein bypass operations. *Int. J. Cardiol.*, 2:511.
6. Chesebro, J. H., Fuster, V., Elveback, L. R., et al. (1984): Platelet-inhibitor-drug trial in coronary-

artery bypass operations: Benefit of perioperative dipyridamole and aspirin therapy on late-postoperative vein-graft patency. *N. Engl. J. Med.*, 310:209.

7. Deuel, T. F., Senior, R. M., Chang, D., et al. (1981): Platelet factor 4 is chemotactic for neutrophils and monocytes. *Proc. Natl. Acad. Sci. U.S.A.*, 78:4584.

8. DeWood, M. A., Spores, J., Notske, R., Mouser, L. T., Burroughs, R., Golden, M. S. and Lang, H. T. (1980): Prevalence of total coronary occlusion during the early hours of transmural myocardial infarction. *N. Engl. J. Med.*, 303:897.

9. Folts, J. D., Gallagher, K., and Rowe, G. G. (1982): Blood flow reductions in stenosed canine coronary arteries: Vasospasm or platelet aggregation? *Circulation*, 65:2.

10. Friedman, R. J., Stemerman, M. B., Wenz, B., Moore, S., Gauldie, J., Gent, M., Tiell, M. L., and Spaet, T. H. (1977): The effect of thrombocytopenia on experimental atherosclerotic lesion formation in rabbits. *J. Clin. Invest.*, 60:1191.

11. Fry, D. L. (1968): Acute vascular endothelial changes associated with increased blood velocity gradients. *Circ. Res.*, 22:165.

12. Fuster, V. (1981): Coronary atherosclerotic disease. The role of platelets and platelet inhibitor drugs. *Scand. J. Haematol.*, 38 (suppl. 27):1.

13. Fuster, V. (1981): Pathogenesis of atherosclerosis and the role of risk factors. *Coeur*, 12:65.

14. Fuster, V., Badimon, L., Rosemark, J. A., and Bowie, E. J. W. (1983): Platelet-arterial wall interaction: Quantitative and qualitative study following selective carotid endothelial injury in normal and von Willebrand pigs. *Clin. Res.*, 31:2, 459A.

15. Fuster, V., Bowie, E. J. W., Lewis, J. C., et al. (1978): Resistance to arteriosclerosis in pigs with von Willebrand's disease: Spontaneous and high cholesterol diet-induced arteriosclerosis. *J. Clin. Invest.*, 61:722.

16. Fuster, V., and Chesebro, J. H. (1981): Current concepts of thrombogenesis. Role of platelets. *Mayo Clin. Proc.*, 56:102.

17. Fuster, V., and Chesebro, J. H. (1981): Pharmacologic effects of platelet inhibitor drugs. *Mayo Clin. Proc.*, 56:185.

18. Fuster, V., Dewanjee, M. K., Kaye, M. P., Josa, M., Metke, M. P., and Chesebro, J. H. (1979): Noninvasive radioisotopic technique for detection of platelet deposition coronary artery bypass grafts in dogs and its reduction with platelet inhibitors. *Circulation*, 60:1508.

19. Fuster, V., Fass, D. N., Kaye, M. P., Josa, M., Zinsmeister, A. R., and Bowie, E. J. W. (1982): Arteriosclerosis in normal and von Willebrand pigs: Long-term prospective study and aortic transplantation study. *Circ. Res.*, 51:587.

20. Gertz, S. D., Uretsky, G., Wainberg, R. S., et al. (1981): Endothelial cell damage and thrombus formation after partial arterial constriction: Relevance to the role of coronary artery spasm in the pathogenesis of myocardial infarction. *Circulation*, 63:3.

21. Goldberg, J. D., Stemerman, M. B., and Handin, R. I. (1980): Vascular permeation of platelet factor 4 after endothelial injury. *Science*, 209:611.

22. Josa, M., Lie, J. T., Bianco, R. L., and Kaye, M. P. (1981): Reduction of thrombosis in canine coronary bypass vein grafts with dipyridamole and aspirin. *Am. J. Cardiol.*, 47:1248.

23. Lewis, H. D. Jr., Davis, J. W., Archibald, D. G., et al. (1983): Protective effects of aspirin against acute myocardial infarction and death in men with unstable angina. *N. Engl. J. Med.*, 309:7, 396.

24. Maseri, A., L'Abbate, A., Baroldi, G., Chierchia, S., Marzilli, M., Ballestra, A. M., Severi, S., Parodi, O., Biagini, A., Distante, A., and Pesola, A. (1978): Coronary vasospasm as a possible cause of myocardial infarction. *N. Engl. J. Med.*, 299:1271.

25. McGill, H. C., Jr. (editor) (1968): *The Geographic Pathology of Artherosclerosis*. Williams & Wilkins, Baltimore.

26. Metke, M. P., Lie, J. T., Fuster, V., Josa, M., and Kaye, M. P. (1979): Reduction of intimal thickening in canine coronary bypass vein grafts with dipyridamole and aspirin. *Am. J. Cardiol.*, 43:1144.

27. Meyer, D., and Baumgartner, H. P. (1983): Annotation: Role of von Willebrand factor in platelet adhesion to the subendothelium. *Br. J. Haematol.*, 54:109.

28. Passamani, E. R. (1980): Summary of ongoing clinical trials of platelet-active drugs in cardiovascular disease (Discussion). *Circulation*, 62 (suppl. 5):106.

29. Reidy, M. A., and Bowyer, D. E. (1977): Scanning electron microscopy of arteries: The morphology of aortic endothelium in haemodynamically stressed areas associated with branches. *Atherosclerosis*, 26:281.

30. Rentrop, K. P., Blanke, H., Karsch, K. R., and Kreuzer, H. (1979): Initial experience with

transluminal recanulization of the recently occluded infarct-related coronary artery in acute myocardial infarction—comparison with conventionally treated patients. *Clin. Cardiol.*, 2:92.

31. Ross, R., Glomset, J., Kariya, B., et al. (1974): A platelet-dependent serum factor that stimulates the proliferation of arterial smooth muscle cells *in vitro*. *Proc. Natl. Acad. Sci. U.S.A.*, 71:1207.
32. Ross, R., and Klebanoff, S. J. (1971): The smooth muscle cell: I. *In vivo* synthesis of connective tissue proteins. *J. Cell. Biol.*, 50:159.
33. Spaet, T. H., Stemerman, M. B., Veith, F. J., et al. (1975): Intimal injury and regrowth in the rabbit aorta: Medial smooth muscle cells as a source of neointima. *Circ. Res.*, 36:58.
34. Wesolowski, S. A., Fries, C. C., Sabini, A. M., et al. (1965): The significance of turbulence in hemic systems and in the distribution of the atherosclerotic lesion. *Surgery*, 57:155.

Advances in Prostaglandin, Thromboxane, and
Leukotriene Research, Vol. 13, edited by G. G. Neri
Serneri, et al. Raven Press, New York © 1985.

Platelet-Inhibitory Therapy in Reconstructive Arterial Surgery

Charles N. McCollum and Mark Goldman

Department of Surgery, Charing Cross Hospital, London W6 8RF, England

Vascular surgery developed rapidly following the introduction of various prosthetic materials for arterial replacement over 20 years ago. As a result, blood could
be diverted past areas of occlusion to relieve symptoms of ischemia. Furthermore,
the strength and durability of materials such as Dacron were such that they could
be implanted to replace aneurysms or occlusions of large arteries such as the aorta
and iliacs. In this high-flow location, these relatively unsophisticated materials
perform well with few thrombotic complications. However, when prosthetic materials of any type are used to bypass medium-sized or small arteries, such as the
superficial femoral, then graft thrombosis becomes an important problem. In femoropopliteal bypass, the overwhelming majority of vascular surgeons cannot
achieve patency rates with prosthetic materials equivalent to the results using
autologous saphenous vein (1,2). As the long saphenous vein is often inadequate
or not available for reconstruction, there remains the need to find approaches to
improve patency rate in prosthetic grafts. This is particularly true as aortocoronary
bypass is now one of the most frequent forms of reconstruction, where the results
with prosthetic grafts are poor.

If we are to improve patency rates in prosthetic graft bypass it seems important
to consider the possible reasons for their early failure. Whereas a great deal of
research has been directed to physical characteristics of the graft such as durability,
elasticity, and compliance, the most obvious difference relates to the luminal surface.
Whenever circulating blood comes in contact with a foreign surface, or possibly
any surface that does not secrete inhibitors, then platelets will adhere and potentially
initiate laminated thrombus deposition. The current view is that vascular endothelium secretes the inhibitor prostacyclin, which is a direct antagonist to the action
of the platelet aggregating substance thromboxane. It may well be, however, that
this is a gross oversimplification of the complicated interaction of the various
pathways involved in stimulating and inhibiting thrombus formation.

NATURE AND DURATION OF GRAFT THROMBOGENICITY

When various grafts are placed in an artificial circulation containing human
blood, platelets rapidly adhere to the luminal surface at a rate that varies according

to the graft material (7,15). This process is not entirely confined to platelets, as fibrinogen consumption is also increased in the months following the implantation of Dacron aortobifemoral grafts in patients (18). The precise role of platelets and the coagulation cascade in the formation of luminal thrombus is poorly understood. However, it appears that platelet adherence may initially be reversible but becomes stabilized by fibrin deposition. If platelet-inhibitory therapy is to be prescribed, it is important to consider the duration of these processes.

Initially the flow surface of recently implanted Dacron grafts is highly thrombogenic (15,23). It was thought that, with time, pseudointima forms, and that this pseudointima was relatively nonthrombogenic (22). Sauvage et al. (22) also produced evidence, predominantly from animal models, that a high porosity in the construction of Dacron allows living tissue to grow through the interstices to produce more rapid and complete luminal healing. Until recently the only methods by which this could be measured in patients was by estimating platelet survival. Using ^{51}Cr-labeled platelets, it was found that survival was shortened for between 6 and 9 months following implantation of Dacron aortoiliac grafts, but subsequently platelet survival was normal and the graft said to be nonthrombogenic (16,18). More recently, however, the development of ^{111}In labeling has permitted the direct measurement of platelet adherence to grafts in man, and it has clearly been shown that Dacron grafts continue to accumulate platelets for many years (11,21). Furthermore, it appears that the increased porosity and the incorporation of a double velour, which are features of the modern Dacron prostheses, do not influence either initial thrombogenicity or the rate that this thrombogenicity is reduced by healing and graft maturation (10).

It therefore seems logical that, where platelet-inhibitory drug therapy is indicated, it should be continued indefinitely. However, it should not be forgotten that the risk of treatment must not outweigh the risk of graft thrombosis and that platelet-inhibitory regimes containing aspirin produce a range of gastrointestinal side effects, the most ominous being hemorrhage.

INFLUENCE OF PLATELET-INHIBITORY DRUGS ON GRAFT THROMBOGENICITY

As the luminal surface of prosthetic grafts in patients rarely, if ever, heals to a confluent endothelial lining, it seems that further manipulations in graft construction are unlikely to produce substantial improvements (2). The logical approach therefore is to investigate whether the administration of drugs, either anticoagulants or platelet inhibitors, may reduce the rate of thrombus accumulation. Anticoagulants have never been adequately studied, but where they have been used there has been no evidence of benefit (5). In recent years, interest has centered on the potential of platelet-inhibitory drugs, and several studies have been performed in animals and then in clinical practice. The effect of aspirin, dypyridamole, sulfinpyrazone, and a combination of aspirin and dypyridamole was compared in Dacron grafts perfused in an experimental model with human blood (17). In these experiments, it seemed that aspirin was the most effective single agent, but the dosage of aspirin employed may be reduced by combination with dipyridamole. This combination of aspirin and dipyridamole has been studied further in animal models using a variety of species and graft materials: patency was enhanced and there was evidence that pseudointimal hyperplasia was prevented (6,14,20). In patients the same drug combination was initially studied for its effect on platelet survival, and Harker et al. found that the shortening of platelet survival encountered following Dacron graft implantation could be "normalized" (16).

In our own studies we have investigated the influence of this drug combination on ^{111}In-labeled platelet accumulation on various grafts both in dogs and in clinical practice. In our *in vivo* experiments in dogs, the combination of aspirin and dipyridamole was more effective than a specific thromboxane synthetase inhibitor (dazoxiben; Pfizer Ltd.), although the difference in terms of graft patency failed to achieve statistical significance. The clinical study consisted entirely of patients awaiting femoropopliteal bypass from September 1979 to February 1981 who were allocated at random and double-blind to receive either a combination of aspirin (300 mg) with dipyridamole (75 mg) or identical placebo capsules three times daily. Whenever possible, reversed saphenous vein was used for bypass, with double-velour knitted Dacron (Meadox, Microvel) or PTFE (Gore-Tex) used only as an alternative when the vein was absent or inadequate. Medication was started 48 hr before surgery in all patients, but only patients with prosthetic grafts contin-ued to take the trial drug beyond hospital discharge at 2 weeks. The methods we used to measure graft thrombogenicity in patients have been described previously (12). Briefly, autologous platelets labeled with 150 mCi ^{111}In oxine were injected on postoperative day 7. At 1 hr later, radioactivity was counted over three sites along the graft to include both anastamoses and a midpoint with equivalent sites marked on the contralateral thigh. The measurements were made daily for 7 days. Gamma images of both thighs were obtained on days 1, 3, and 5 using a large field of view gamma camera. Graft thrombogenicity was calculated as previously de-scribed using the ratio of counts over the graft to those over the reference leg on each day of study (12). The rate of platelet accumulation in a graft was then obtained by computing the slope of the line of best fit placed through the daily ratios by linear regression analysis. It is the rise in this ratio of radioactivity graft over a reference per day that we have called the thrombogenicity index (TI).

Platelet accumulation on autologous vein was found to be consistently low, with a mean TI ($\pm$ SEM) of 0.03 ± 0.010 unaffected by aspirin and dipyridamole (Table 1). This being the case, we ceased to enter patients with vein grafts to the study after 14 had been evaluated. In all, 67 patients were entered, and of these 53 had prosthetic femoropopliteal bypasses (37 PTFE, 16 Dacron) (19). Six of these (4 placebo, 2 aspirin plus dipyridamole) failed during the first week before platelet studies could be completed. For this reason, thrombogenicity index measurements were available in 61 patients, and the results are shown in Table 1. Aspirin and dipyridamole had no influence on the thrombogenicity of vein grafts but reduced the thrombogenicity of prosthetic grafts from a mean of 0.17 ± 0.02 on placebo to

TABLE 1. *Influence of aspirin and dipyridamole on thrombogenicity index*

| | Thrombogenicity index[a] for material | | |
Treatment	Dacron ($n = 12$)	PTFE ($n = 35$)	Vein ($n = 14$)
Placebo	0.25 ± 0.09	0.14 ± 0.01	0.03 ± 0.01
Aspirin plus dipyridamole	0.16[b] ± 0.05	0.09[c] ± 0.01	0.03 ± 0.01

[a]Mean ± SEM.
[b]Significant difference at $p < 0.05$ compared with placebo.
[c]Significant difference at $p < 0.02$ compared with placebo.

0.11 ± 0.01 on platelet inhibitory therapy ($p<0.02$). This influence of the drug combination on radiolabeled platelet uptake in the grafts is illustrated by the gamma images in Fig. 1, which demonstrates the often impressive differences between patients on aspirin and dipyridamole compared to placebo.

RELATIONSHIP BETWEEN THROMBOGENICITY AND GRAFT PATENCY

In both our animal studies and the femoropopliteal study just described, we examined the influence of thrombogenicity measured 1 week following graft implantation on subsequent graft patency (8). In both, subsequent patency appeared to depend strongly on the rate of platelet accumulation shortly following graft implantation. Of the 67 patients randomized to aspirin and dipyridamole or placebo, 57 were able to complete radiolabeled platelet studies and follow-up to 1 year. The mean thrombogenicity index in the 21 grafts that subsequently occluded, 0.19 ± 0.018, was considerably greater than that of 0.07 ± 0.009, that found in the 36 bypasses that remained patent ($p<0.001$) (Fig. 2). Calculated by the life table method, the cumulative 12-month patency rate of all grafts entered was 58%. When the patients were divided into two groups around the median TI of 0.094, those patients with a TI below the median had a 1-year cumulative patency of 90%, compared with 39% where the TI fell in the upper half of the range ($p<0.001$) (Fig. 3). Femoropopliteal patency is obviously determined by several other factors, of which indications for surgery, placement of the graft above or below the knee, and the number of patent calf arteries are thought to be the most important. The influence of these risk factors was also determined by life table. Neither the indications for surgery comparing rest pain and gangrene to claudication nor the placement of the distal anastomosis below the knee significantly influenced subsequent graft patency rates. This relationship between thrombogenicity index and subsequent patency was equally strong even if the vein grafts were excluded; the mean TI in the 20 prosthetic grafts which occluded, 0.20 ± 0.081, was more than double that (0.09 ± 0.046) in the 23 that remained patent to 1 year ($p<0.01$). This relationship was tested for a single graft material; the mean TI, 0.08 ± 0.042, in the 20 PTFE grafts patent at 1 year was significantly less than that (0.18 ± 0.060) found in the 11 that occluded

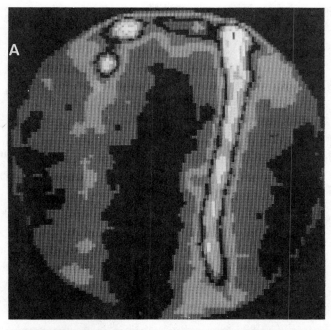

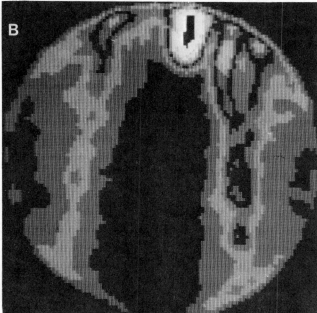

FIG. 1. Images on day 5 from two patients with left PTFE grafts. **A:** The patient on placebo had a more radioactive graft, with a TI of 0.15, which thrombosed between 2 and 3 months later. **B:** On aspirin plus dipyridamole, TI was 0.08 and the graft was still patent at 12 months.

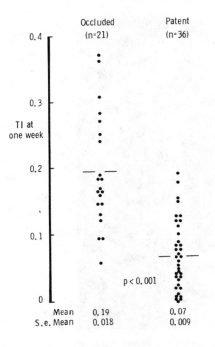

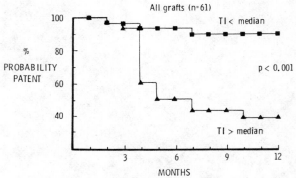

FIG. 2. Thrombogenicity index (TI) for each femoropopliteal graft plotted to compare those that subsequently occluded or remained patent for 12 months. Clearly, grafts with a high TI were more likely to fail, and those with a low TI were more likely to remain patent.

FIG. 3. Subsequent patency of femoropopliteal bypass grafts with a thrombogenicity index (TI) in the upper half of the range, compared by life table with that of patients with TI below the median ($n = 28$ in each group). Those with a TI less than 0.094 had a cumulative patency of 90%, compared with 39% in those with higher TI values.

($p < 0.01$). It is interesting to note that throughout this study we found that patients with rapid platelet accumulation on prosthetic grafts suffered early occlusion.

It remains possible that TI is itself influenced by other risk factors, such as blood flow and physical and chemical composition of the flow surface. Assessed individually, the small effect of each on graft patency may be difficult to demonstrate, but their combined influence with the platelet acting as the common pathway may be what is measured by thrombogenicity index. Although TI is a sensitive predictor during the early high-risk period, failure of the more thrombogenic prostheses will result in the remaining grafts predominently being those of low thrombogenicity. It therefore seems likely that patency beyond 1 year will increasingly be dicatated by other factors, such as smoking habits and progression of arterial disease in proximal or distal vessels. Obviously, sporadic graft failures will also occur for reasons unrelated to thrombogenicity, such as mechanical deterioration of the materials.

CLINICAL STUDIES

Clearly, the final decision on the widespread application of platelet inhibitory drug therapy will be based on the results of clinical studies. We are aware of only three double-blind and randomized studies on the effect of platelet-inhibitory drug therapy on graft patency in peripheral vascular surgery. Donaldson et al. studied the influence of aspirin and dipyridamole on the patency of Dacron femoropopliteal grafts (4). DeWeese and colleagues undertook a similar study in patients with PTFE grafts (13). In both these studies, the results were similar to those in our own clinical study using both Dacron and PTFE grafts, we will briefly describe our results (9). Fifty-three patients undergoing femoropopliteal bypass with prosthetic grafts were randomized, giving 31 on placebo and 22 on the combination of aspirin and dipyridamole. The various risk factors were equally distributed between the two groups, and only 3 patients failed to complete follow-up to 12 months; 2 died with patent grafts at 6 and 7 months, respectively, while a third required reoperation for a false aneurysm. Analysis was on the "intention to treat" basis. Overall, there were 26 occlusions during the first year, all but one of which occurred during the first 6 months. Among those patients that completed follow-up to 1 year, 19 grafts occluded in the 28 patients on placebo, compared to only 7 in the 21 patients receiving aspirin and dipyridamole ($\chi^2 = 4.44$, $p<0.05$). Cumulative patency by life table is shown in Fig. 4. Placebo grafts performed badly, with a

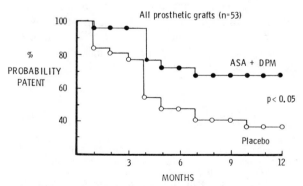

FIG. 4. Prosthetic graft patency by life table plotted for patients randomized to aspirin plus pyridamole or placebo. The cumulative patency rates at 12 months are 67% and 36%, respectively.

36% patency by 12 months compared to 67% in the aspirin and dipyridamole group ($p < 0.05$). In the 37 patients with reconstruction with PTFE grafts, our results were very similar to those of De Weese's group (13) with cumulative patency of 50% and 80% for placebo and for aspirin plus dipyridamole, respectively. Gastrointestinal side effects were volunteered by only 2 patients on aspirin and dipyridamole, compared to 1 receiving placebo.

In general, the results for femoropopliteal graft patency using various prosthetic materials vary widely between the different series. Many surgeons report these results without describing their policy on the use of platelet-inhibitory drugs. We feel that reexamination of the various retrospective studies with respect to anti-thrombotic policy may help to explain some of the discrepancies that have been reported.

Based on the results that we have discussed, our current policy for prosthetic bypasses placed below the groin is to prescribe aspirin and dipyridamole and continue therapy indefinitely. As graft thrombosis is relatively rare in the aortoiliac segment, we feel that the risk of long-term aspirin therapy cannot be justified in these patients. For patients undergoing femoro–femoral and other extraanatomic bypass, the decision is more difficult as the relative risks are more finely balanced. However, wherever there is cause for concern that thrombosis may occur, for example as a result of severe distal disease, then our policy is to prescribe platelet-inhibitory therapy. There is currently no adequate information to guide the surgeon on appropriate therapy following saphenous vein femoropopliteal bypass. The risk of thrombosis is high enough to justify therapy if such therapy were effective. Our only guide at present is the effect of aspirin and dipyridamole on coronary artery bypass (3). In this large study with patency assessed objectively, this drug combination was effective even on autologous vein bypasses. We are pleased to indicate that a multicenter study is now being started among vascular surgeons in England to evaluate further whether platelet-inhibitory therapy is required when saphenous vein is used in femoropopliteal bypass. We look forward to the development of new platelet-inhibitory drugs that will hopefully have less gastrointestinal side effects. Our hopes are currently pinned on specific inhibitors or antagonists to thromboxane; ultimately, efficacy will require to be proven against the existing and effective combination of aspirin and dipyridamole. With the radiolabeled platelet techniques, we now also have adequate methods to assess the influence of new drugs on the rate of platelet accumulation in a developing thrombus in man.

REFERENCES

1. Bergan, J. J., Yao, S. T., Flinn, W. R., and Graham, L. M. (1982): Prosthetic grafts for the treatment of lower limb ischaemia. *Br. J. Surg.*, 69:S34–S37.
2. Callow, A. D. (1982): Current status of vascular grafts. *Surg. Clin. North Am.*, 62:501–513.
3. Chesebro, J. H., Clements, I. P., Fuster, V., et al. (1982): A platelet inhibitor drug trial on coronary artery bypass operations. Benefit of peroperative dipyridamole and aspirin therapy on early post operative vein graft patency. *N. Engl. J. Med.*, 307:73–78.
4. Donaldson, D. R., Kester, R. C., Hall, T. J., Rajah, S. M., Crow, M. J., and Salter, M. C. P. (1982): Do platelet-modifying agents influence the patency of femoropopliteal Dacron bypass grafts? *Br. J. Surg.* (Abstr.), 60:284.

5. Evans, G., and Irvine, W. T. (1966): Long term arterial graft patency in relation to platelet adhesiveness, biochemical factors and anticoagulant therapy. *Lancet*, ii:353–355.
6. Feins, R. H., Roedersheimer, R. L., Green, R. M., and DeWeese, J. A. (1979): Platelet aggregation inhibition in human umbilical vein grafts and negatively charged bovine heterografts. *Surgery*, 85:395–399.
7. Goldman, M., Gunson, B., Hawker, R. J., et al. (1983): Human umbilical vein and polytetrafluorethylene compared in an artifical circulation. *Br. J. Surg.*, 70:4–6.
8. Goldman, M., Hall, C., Dykes, J., Hawker, R. J., and McCollum, C. N. (1983): Does ¹¹¹indium-platelet deposition predict patency in prosthetic arterial grafts? *Br. J. Surg.*, 70:635–638.
9. Goldman, M., and McCollum, C. N. (1984): A prospective randomised study to examine the effect of aspirin plus dipyridamole on the patency of prosthetic femoro-popliteal grafts. *Vasc. Surg.*, 18:217–221.
10. Goldman, M., McCollum, C. N., Hawker, R. J., Drolc, Z., and Slaney, G. (1982): Dacron arterial grafts: The influence of porosity, velour, and maturity on thrombogenicity. *Surgery*, 92:947–952.
11. Goldman, M., Norcott, H. C., Hawker, R. J., et al. (1982): Platelet accumulation on mature Dacron grafts in man. *Br. J. Surg.*, 69:S38–40.
12. Goldman, M., Simpson, D., Hawker, R. J., Norcott, H. C., and McCollum, C. N. (1983): Aspirin and dipyridamole reduce platelet deposition on prosthetic femoro-popliteal grafts in man. *Ann. Surg.*, 198:713–717.
13. Green, R. M., Roedesheimer, L. R., and DeWeese, J. A. (1982): Effects of aspirin and dipyridamole on expanded polytetrafluoroethylene graft patency. *Surgery*, 92:1016–1026.
14. Hagen, P.-O., Wang, Z.-G., Mikat, E. M., and Hackel, D. B. (1982): Antiplatelet therapy reduces aortic intimal hyperplasia distal to small diameter vascular prostheses (PTFE) in non-human primates. *Ann. Surg.*, 195:328–339.
15. Hamlin, G. W., Rajah, S. M., Crow, M. J., and Kester, R. C. (1978): Evaluation of the thrombogenic potential of three types of arterial graft studied in an artificial circulation. *Br. J. Surg.*, 65:272–276.
16. Harker, L. A., Slichter, S. J., and Sauvage, L. R. (1977): Platelet consumption by arterial prostheses. The effects of endothelialisation and pharmacological inhibition of platelet function. *Ann. Surg.*, 186:594–601.
17. McCollum, C. N., Crow, M. J., Rajah, S. M., and Kester, R. C. (1980): Antithrombotic therapy for vascular prosthesis; An experimental model testing platelet inhibitory drugs. *Surgery*, 87:668–676.
18. McCollum, C. N., Kester, R., Rajah, S. M., Learoyd, P., and Pepper, M. (1981): Arterial graft maturation: The duration of thrombotic activity in Dacron aortobifemoral grafts measured by platelet and fibrinogen kinetics. *Br. J. Surg.*, 68:61–64.
19. Norcott, H. C., Goldman, M., Hawker, R. J., et al. (1982): Platelet arterial grafts. *Thromb. Haemostas.*, 48:307–310.
20. Oblath, R. W., Buckley, F. O., Green, R. M., Schwartz, S. I., and DeWeese, J. A. (1978): Prevention of platelet aggregation and adherence to prosthetic vascular grafts by aspirin and dipyridamole. *Surgery*, 84:37–43.
21. Ritchie, J. L., Stratton, J. R., Hamilton, G. W., et al. (1981): Indium¹¹¹ platelet imaging for detection of platelet deposition in abdominal aneurysms and prosthetic arterial grafts. *Am. J. Cardiol.*, 47:882–889.
22. Sauvage, L. R., Berger, K., Barros D'Sa, A. A. B., Yates, S. G., Walter, M. W., Robel, S. B., Lischko, M. M., Wood, S. J., Davis, C. C., and Rittenhouse, E. A. (1978): Graft materials in vascular surgery. *Miami*, 153–165.
23. Yates, S. G., Nakagawa, Y., Berger, K., and Sauvage, L. R. (1973): Surface thrombogenicity of arterial prostheses. *Surg. Gynaecol. Obstet.*, 136:12–16.

*Advances in Prostaglandin, Thromboxane, and
Leukotriene Research, Vol. 13*, edited by G. G. Neri
Serneri, et al. Raven Press, New York © 1985.

Patency of Saphenous Veins Used for Aortocoronary Bypass Grafting: Effects of Platelet-Derived Mediators

*M. Chiavarelli, **F. Fabi, *R. Chiavarelli, *M. Toscano,
**A. Carpi, and *B. Marino

*Department of Cardiac Surgery, University of Rome; and **Department of
Pathophysiology, Istituto Superiore di Sanità, 00199 Rome, Italy

After coronary artery surgery, perioperative vasospasm may produce a marked hemodynamic compromise, leading to circulatory collapse and death (2). Recently, a new potentially lethal expression of vascular spasm has been described: aorto-coronary vein graft spasm. Spasm involving a saphenous vein graft may explain the recurrence of angina after successful surgery with patent grafts (4), may cause early closure of the vein (1), or may produce late occlusion with myocardial infarction (3,5).

Platelet hyperactivity is present in most patients with coronary heart disease, and platelet-derived products have been implicated as a potential factor in the genesis of coronary arterial spasm. Vasoactive substances released during platelet activation include 5-hydroxytryptamine (5-HT) and thromboxane A_2 (TXA_2), which may contribute to saphenous vein spasm. In order to investigate the putative role played by these autacoids, their effect on human saphenous veins was studied *in vitro*.

MATERIALS AND METHODS

Rings of the greater saphenous vein (3 mm wide, obtained at surgery) were suspended in organ chambers by placing two L-shaped metal holders in the lumen of the vessel. They were equilibrated for 90 min under a 2-g isometric tension in Krebs solution at 37°C, aerated with 95% oxygen and 5% carbon dioxide. Concentration–response curves to U46619 (10^{-9}–10^{-6} M), considered to be a thromboxane mimetic, and to 5-HT (10^{-8}–10^{-4} M) were constructed by increasing organ chamber concentrations cumulatively by fourfold to fivefold. In a different set of experiments, phenoxybenzamine (0.1 mg/liter) was added for 60 min and then washed out to study the pretreatment effect on the 5-HT dose–response curve.

Male guinea pigs 3 to 4 weeks old (200–250 g) were sacrificed by cervical dislocation. The pulmonary artery was cannulated, and the lungs were removed and perfused at 10 ml/min with Krebs solution at 37°C. The effluent from the lungs superfused over human saphenous vein spiral strips, mounted auxotonically in cascade. To analyze the effect of authentic TXA_2, arachidonic acid (0.1–10 μg) was given by intrapulmonary arterial injection, and thromboxane release was confirmed by the inhibition with 1-benzylimidazole (10–100 mg/liter).

Circulating rat platelets were used as a source of platelet mediators. Male rats (300–400 g) were anesthetized with ethyl urethane (1 g/kg i.p.). After i.v. heparin (2,000 u/kg), blood was continuously withdrawn (2.5 ml/min) by a peristaltic pump from a catheter inserted into the left common carotid artery, used to bath saphenous vein strips, and returned to the animal by a roller pump via the right jugular vein. Arachidonic acid was injected (0.03–0.09 mg) or infused (2.5–10 mg/liter) into the extracorporeal circuit so that it mixed with blood for 1 min before reaching saphenous veins. Aspirin (1–10 mg/kg) was given to block platelet activation by arachidonic acid.

RESULTS

Dose–response curves are shown in Fig. 1. U46619 ($pD_2 = 7.75$) was more potent than 5-HT ($pD_2 = 6.46$), with lower intrinsic activity (84.55%). Phenoxybenzamine pretreatment reduced noncompetitively the 5-HT-evoked contraction ($pD'_2 = 6.56$).

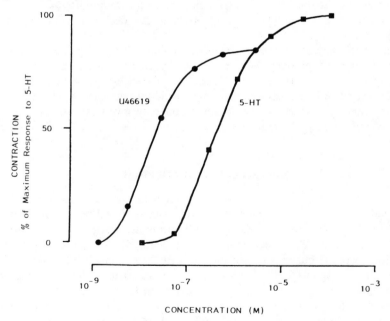

FIG. 1. Effect of increasing concentration of 5-HT and U46619 (TXA_2 mimetic) in human saphenous veins. Data are expressed as percent of the maximal response to 5-HT and shown as means of 10 experiments.

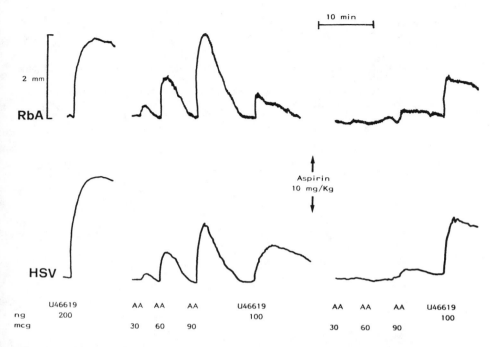

FIG. 2. Responses of superfused rabbit aorta (RbA) and human saphenous vein (HSV) to substances released from circulating rat platelets after 1 min incubation with arachidonic acid (AA). The administration of aspirin prevented the vascular contraction to subsequent injection of AA, while the response to U46619 was retained.

Thromboxane A_2 released by guinea pig lungs strongly contracted saphenous veins, which were almost insensitive to other prostaglandins.

Arachidonic acid-activated, circulating rat platelets produced a powerful saphenous vein vasoconstriction, which was antagonized by low-dose aspirin pretreatment (Fig. 2). Phenoxybenzamine pretreatment did not influence the response, while it markedly reduced 5-HT contraction.

CONCLUSIONS

Platelet-derived mediators are powerful vasoconstrictors of human saphenous veins, TXA_2 being more active than 5-HT. They may start or at least favor venous graft spasm, with further platelet aggregation and release of potent vasoconstrictors, leading ultimately to thrombosis of the venous graft.

Low-dose aspirin, by preventing platelet aggregation, could also reduce the incidence of dynamic venous graft stenoses and favor early graft patency.

REFERENCES

1. Baduini, G., Marra, S., and Angelino, P. F. (1981): Sudden occlusion of a saphenous vein bypass graft relieved by direct injection of nitroglycerin. *Cathet. Cardiovasc. Diagnosis*, 7:87–95.

2. Buxton, A. E., Goldberg, S., Harken, A., Hirshfeld, J., and Kastor, J. A. (1981): Coronary artery spasm immediately after myocardial revascularization. *N. Engl. J. Med.*, 304:1249–1253.
3. Heijman, J., El Gamal, M., and Michels, L. (1983): Catheter induced spasm in aortocoronary vein grafts. *Br. Heart J.*, 49:30–32.
4. Victor, M. F., Kimbiris, D., Iskandrian, A. S., et al. (1981): Spasm of a saphenous vein bypass graft. *Chest*, 80:413–415.
5. Walinsky, P. (1982): Angiographic documentation of spontaneous spasm of saphenous vein coronary artery bypass graft. *Am. Heart J.*, 103:290–292.

Advances in Prostaglandin, Thromboxane, and Leukotriene Research, Vol. 13, edited by G. G. Neri Serneri, et al. Raven Press, New York © 1985.

Aspirin and Dipyridamole Reduce Lipid Accumulation in Vein Bypass Grafts: Combination Versus Single Drug Therapy

*Lawrence E. Boerboom, *Gordon N. Olinger,
*Lawrence I. Bonchek, and **Ahmed H. Kissebah

*Departments of *Cardiothoracic Surgery and **Medicine, Medical College of Wisconsin, Milwaukee, Wisconsin 53226*

It is now well established that saphenous vein aortocoronary bypass grafts undergo progressive changes that result in a cumulative occlusion rate of approximately 44% within 10 to 12 years of operation (3). The association of classic atherosclerotic lesions with late graft failure invokes the hypothesis that endothelial injury and platelet involvement play a role in graft degeneration.

Histologic studies, studies of platelet survival, and imaging with radiolabeled platelets confirm platelet aggregation in grafts and its attenuation with platelet inhibition. We have demonstrated that platelet inhibition with a combination of aspirin and dipyridamole therapy reduces cholesterol and apolipoprotein-B accumulation by vein grafts in both normolipemic and hyperlipemic monkeys (2). This combination therapy has also been demonstrated by Chesebro et al. (4) to improve vein graft patency in patients.

The latter trial of the effect of platelet inhibition on graft patency has provoked widespread acceptance of the postoperative prescription for platelet inhibition with both aspirin and dipyridamole. While a positive effect of treatment was noted as late as 12 months postoperatively in this study, many practitioners seem prone to continue dipyridamole no longer than 3 months because of this drug's expense, its numerous annoying side effects, and poor patient compliance when such an agent must be taken several times daily.

Our most recent study therefore assessed whether aspirin or dipyridamole given separately mitigates the cholesterol and apolipoprotein-B uptake by vein grafts (1). Cephalic vein grafts were interposed in the femoral arteries of stump-tailed macaque monkeys as described previously (2) and were removed for analysis 3 months later. Biochemical results are shown in Table 1. In all groups receiving medication, both cholesterol and apolipoprotein-B concentrations in grafts were similar to the concentrations found in respective ungrafted veins, and in each of the treated groups cholesterol ($p < 0.001$) and apolipoprotein-B ($p < 0.001$) concentrations in grafts were significantly reduced compared with grafts from control monkeys.

TABLE 1. *Tissue cholesterol and apolipoprotein-B concentration*

Treatment	Cholesterol (mg/100 mg)		Apolipoprotein-B (μg/100 mg)	
	Vein	Graft	Vein	Graft
Control	0.08 ± 0.02	0.20 ± 0.02[a]	2.0 ± 0.3	18.5 ± 2.5[a]
Aspirin + dipyridamole	0.06 ± 0.02	0.07 ± 0.03[b]	1.6 ± 0.6	1.9 ± 0.4[b]
Aspirin	0.06 ± 0.02	0.09 ± 0.02[b]	1.8 ± 0.4	1.6 ± 0.3[b]
Dipyridamole	0.06 ± 0.02	0.09 ± 0.04[b]	1.8 ± 0.5	1.8 ± 0.5[b]

Data are mean ± SD.
[a]Significant at $p < 0.001$ compared to vein.
[b]Significant at $p < 0.001$ compared to control.

There were no significant differences in cholesterol or in apolipoprotein-B concentrations among the three treated groups. In striking contrast, in grafts from control monkeys, cholesterol concentration was 250% ($p<0.001$) and apolipoprotein-B concentration was 925% ($p<0.001$) of that observed in ungrafted vein. These data demonstrate that, in monkeys, platelet inhibition with either aspirin or dipyridamole given individually reduces the uptake of cholesterol and apolipoprotein-B by experimental vein bypass grafts to the same degree as therapy with these drugs combined.

The mechanism by which aspirin or dipyridamole diminished lipid accumulation in our monkey vein grafts remains speculative. It is possible that platelet inhibition prevents the secondary endothelial injury and increased endothelial permeability postulated to result from interaction between the vessel wall and the contents released from platelet storage granules. It is also possible that platelet inhibition prevents platelet-derived growth factor from stimulating cholesterol and phospholipid biosynthesis in smooth muscle cells, or that platelet inhibition prevents platelet-derived growth factor from stimulating proliferation of low-density lipoprotein receptors on smooth muscle cells.

With the population of coronary bypass patients increasing by approximately 150,000 yearly in the United States alone, a recommendation of "prophylactic" platelet inhibition with combination therapy for life translates to annual patients' cost of tens of millions of dollars. The data we have developed short-term from our normocholesterolemic monkey vein graft preparation suggest there is no additional benefit to combined therapy. For the time being, we are comfortable based on this information to discontinue dipyridamole or aspirin earlier postoperatively as patient tolerance dictates, but we eagerly await results from long-term studies that should have more bearing on the late fate of vein grafts in patients. Should long-term platelet inhibition prove to be of continued benefit, and the results extrapolated to the human condition, the issue of combined versus single drug therapy could have enormous implications.

REFERENCES

1. Boerboom, L. E., Olinger, G. N., Bonchek, L. I., Gunay, I. I., and Kissebah, A. H. (1984): Veingraft atherogenesis: Effect of different platelet inhibitors. *J. Am. Coll. Cardiol.*, 3:510.

2. Bonchek, L. I., Boerboom, L. E., Olinger, G. N., Pepper, J. R., Munns, J., Hutchinson, L., and Kissebah, A. H. (1982): Prevention of lipid accumulation in experimental vein bypass grafts by antiplatelet therapy. *Circulation*, 66:338–341.
3. Campeau, L., Enjalbert, M., Lesperance, J., Vaislic, C., Grondin, C. M., and Bourassa, M. G. (1983): Atherosclerosis and late closure of aortocoronary saphenous vein grafts: Sequential angiographic studies at 2 weeks, 1 year, 5 to 7 years, and 10 to 12 years after surgery. *Circulation*, 68(suppl. II):1–7.
4. Chesebro, J. H., Fuster, V., Elveback, L. R., Clements, I. P., Smith, H. C., Holmes, D. R., Bardsley, W. T., Pluth, J. R., Wallace, R. B., Puga, F. J., Orszulak, T. A., Piehler, J. M., Danielson, G. K., Schaff, H., and Frye, R. L. (1984): Effect of dipyridamole and aspirin on late vein-graft patency after coronary bypass operations. *N. Engl. J. Med.*, 310:209–214.

Advances in Prostaglandin, Thromboxane, and
Leukotriene Research, Vol. 13, edited by G.G. Neri
Serneri, et al. Raven Press, New York © 1985.

Role of Prostaglandins in the Activity of Some Cardiovascular Drugs

Giulio Masotti

Clinica Medica I, University of Florence, 50134 Florence, Italy

The effects of cardiovascular drugs on prostaglandin (PG) synthesis are reported in a continuously increasing number of papers, but these effects do not always seem important from a clinical point of view. In this chapter, only those drugs whose activity on prostaglandins is of clinical relevance will be examined.

Among the antianginal drugs, nitroglycerin has been reported to stimulate the synthesis of vasodilating prostaglandins, not only in animals (27,38) and *ex vivo* human cells (Fig. 1) and vessels (15,24) but also in patients (39,48). However, the relevance of the released prostaglandins to the vasodilating activity of nitroglycerin is less certain. In experiments by Morcillio et al. (27), the fall in dog coronary resistance caused by nitroglycerin is blunted by indomethacin. Subsequent authors, both in dog experiments (33,45) and in humans (39,41), using indomethacin and other cyclooxygenase inhibitors, found conflicting results, so that the possible contribution of the stimulated prostaglandins to the vasodilating activity of nitroglycerin has been negated by some of them (33,41). However, the use of indomethacin and related drugs is not the ideal approach to demonstrate that prostaglandins

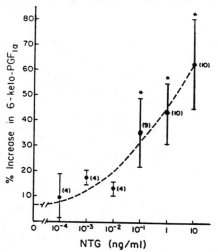

FIG. 1. 6-Keto-PGF$_{1\alpha}$ production by cultured human endothelial cells incubated with increasing concentrations of nitroglycerin (NTG). (From Levin et al., ref. 15, with permission.)

participate in the activity of nitroglycerin. These drugs not only block prostaglandin synthesis by the coronary vasculature but also increase nitroglycerin plasma levels (50), probably by interfering with hepatic drug clearance (10). Therefore, the participation of prostaglandins in the vasodilating activity of nitroglycerin cannot be excluded and could explain its ineffectiveness in some types of myocardial ischemia if we recall the different impairment of prostacyclin (PGI_2) synthetic capacity in the various forms of ischemic heart disease (30).

Among antihypertensive drugs, it has been reported that propranolol and bendrofluazide owe part of their antihypertensive activity to the stimulation of prostaglandin synthesis (49). The mediation of prostaglandins also takes part in and is particularly relevant to the antihypertensive activity of captopril. This drug is an inhibitor of the converting enzyme that is responsible for the conversion of angiotensin I to angiotensin II (32) and for the breakdown of bradykinin (11,31) (Fig. 2). Therefore, the inhibition of converting enzyme leads to a decrease in the level of angiotensin II and an increase in the plasma kinin levels (20,52). The antihypertensive activity of captopril occurs in patients with high and normal or with low levels of plasma renin activity (4). Therefore the inhibition of angiotensin II production alone cannot account for the antihypertensive activity. Potentiation of the vasodilating effect of bradykinin may be a second possible mechanism. Further hypotensive actions could be connected with a stimulation of the prostaglandin system, since both bradykinin (21) and, to a lesser extent, angiotensin I (9) have been shown to stimulate prostaglandin synthesis. Indeed, captopril is able to increase blood levels of PGE_2, a vasodilating prostaglandin that modulates the effects of adrenergic stimulation by decreasing the discharge of the neuroeffector (28) and whose production is significantly lower in patients with essential hypertension (44). The increase in plasma PGE_2 after captopril has been observed in patients with essential hypertension, not only in resting conditions (1) but also, in experiments carried out by our group, during sympathetic stimulation induced by cold appli-

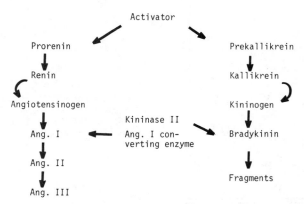

FIG. 2. Activity of converting enzyme on the kinin and angiotensin (Ang.) system. *Downward arrow*, converts to or yields a product; *curving arrow*, acts on.

cation. In such a condition, the impairment of this modulating mechanism, typical of the hypertensive state, is particularly evident when compared with normotensive subjects (Fig. 3). The stimulation of PGE_2 and vasodilating prostaglandins is an essential part of the antihypertensive activity of captopril, since the suppression of this mechanism by cyclooxygenase-inhibiting drugs significantly reduces its hypotensive effect (40,43).

In recent years the interest in antiaggregating agents has greatly increased for their potential importance in prevention of thrombosis. Two antiaggregating agents have been, until now, more extensively studied—aspirin and dipyridamole. The antiaggregating activity of aspirin is due to the inhibition of platelet cyclooxygenase and therefore to the blockade of thromboxane formation. But after the discovery of prostacyclin (PGI_2) in 1976 (25), it became clear that the favorable effect of blocking platelet thromboxane was inevitably coupled with the deleterious inhibition of a potent vasodilating and antiaggregating substance such as PGI_2. From this premise, many studies have been designed in order to find the ideal dosage of aspirin capable of a maximum inhibition of platelet thromboxane with a minimum effect on vascular PGI_2. In 1979, our group (18) demonstrated that the inhibition of thromboxane can be dissociated from that of PGI_2. An aspirin dose of 3.5 mg/kg (about 250 mg as a single dose), while inducing a nearly maximal inhibition of platelet aggregation, gives only a 20% inhibition of PGI_2 production (Fig. 4). The inhibition of platelet aggregation lasts for 72 hr, while PGI_2 production is completely restored after 24 hr (Fig. 5).

More recently, Weksler et al. (51) demonstrated that a single dose of 80 mg was able to suppress platelet thromboxane production by 95%, whereas PGI_2 production

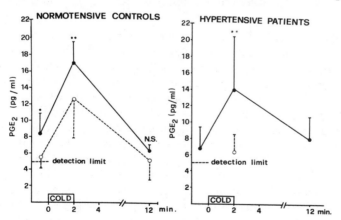

FIG. 3. Effects of captopril treatment (300 mg/day for 7 days) in 6 normotensive controls and 6 patients with low-renin essential hypertension (*dashed line,* before captopril; *solid line,* after captopril). In controls, captopril significantly enhances both baseline plasma PGE_2 concentration and its increase induced by sympathetic stimulation [cold application (23)]. In low-renin hypertensives, plasma PGE_2 concentration, undetectable in baseline conditions and very low after sympathetic stimulation, is increased after captopril to levels comparable to normotensive controls. Statistical significance is shown by *$p<0.05$; **$p<0.001$.

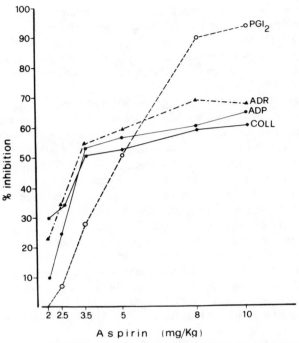

FIG. 4. Effect of different single doses of aspirin on prostacyclin production and platelet aggregation induced by different agents [ADP, 2 umol/liter; adrenaline (ADR), 10 umol/liter and collagen (COLL), 5 ug/ml], 2 hr after administration. (From Masotti et al., ref. 18, with permission.)

was inhibited only by 38% in aortic tissue and unchanged in veins. Patrono's group (35), on the other hand, could demonstrate that a daily dose of 0.45 mg/kg given for 7 days produces a virtually complete inhibition of platelet thromboxane (TX) B_2 production, while PGI_2 production, as expressed by urinary excretion of 6-keto-$PGF_{1\alpha}$, is unaffected. Despite these pharmacological data, the use of low doses of aspirin in the prevention of thrombosis did not enter the clinical practice because it seemed unfair to abandon doses of 1 g aspirin whose usefulness was substantiated by large clinical trials. The recent double-blind trial (16) showing that 324 mg aspirin has a protective effect against myocardial infarction and death in patients with unstable angina is the demonstration that protection of thrombosis is not peculiar to high doses. Dipyridamole, as demonstrated by Moncada et al. in 1978 (26), acts as a phosphodiesterase inhibitor, thus potentiating the effect of endogenous PGI_2 on platelets. Besides this activity, dipyridamole is also capable of stimulating prostacyclin production. In studies by our group (19,29), dipyridamole in humans increased PGI_2 production both after acute i.v. infusion and after a 7-day oral treatment with 375 mg daily. Subsequently, several authors confirmed our data (3,7,14,22,36,46). Therefore the mechanism of the antiaggregating activity of

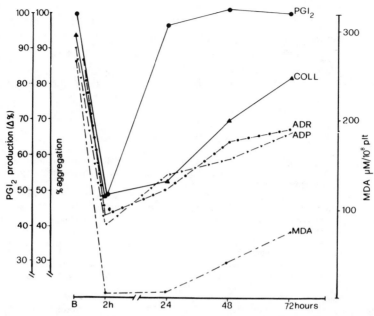

FIG. 5. Duration of effect of one dose of aspirin (5 mg/kg) on platelet aggregation induced by different agents [ADP, 2 umol/liter; adrenaline (ADR), 10 umol/liter, and collagen (COLL), 5 ug/ml] and on production of prostacyclin and malondialdehide (MDA) in healthy volunteers. (From Masotti et al., ref. 18, with permission.)

dipyridamole must be interpreted as due to inhibition of phosphodiesterase and to stimulation of PGI$_2$ production.

More recently, the problem of antithrombotic therapy was faced by attempting to develop drugs able to produce a selective inhibition of thromboxane synthesis. These agents could have greater potential as antithrombotic agents, since in addition to reducing TXA$_2$ formation, they would leave PGI$_2$ synthesis unaffected or even increased as a consequence of redirection of platelet cyclic endoperoxides to vascular PGI$_2$ synthetase (8,47). Toward this aim, various selective thromboxane inhibitors such as Dazoxiben (6,12,34,37), OKY (23,42), CGS-13080 (5), and RO-22-4679 (13) have been tested. Although each of these drugs was shown, from *in vitro* studies, to be a potent thromboxane synthetase inhibitor, data available so far from *in vivo* studies raise some doubt on whether they represent a real progress in prevention of thrombosis. The effects of thromboxane synthetase inhibitors on platelet aggregation is weaker than aspirin, probably because endoperoxide formation is not prevented (2,6). The increase in PGI$_2$ production, on the other hand, has been observed only in particular experimental conditions (6,12,17,23), and the antithrombotic potential of this increase remains to be demonstrated. Finally, the increase in PGI_2, production is also associated with the stimulation of other prostaglandins, such as PGE_2 and $PGF_{2\alpha}$ (6), which could promote platelet aggregation.

These data represent the most impressive examples of the interactions between cardiovascular drugs and prostaglandins. From these data, the mediation of prostaglandins appears as a crucial mechanism that the cardiologist must be well aware of, since it strongly affects both the clinical effects and the adverse reactions of these drugs.

REFERENCES

1. Abe, K., Ito, T., Sato, M., Haruyama, T., Sato, K., Omata, K., Hiwatari, M., Sakurai, Y., Imai, Y., and Yoshinaga, K. (1980): Role of prostaglandin in the antihypertensive mechanism of capropril in low renin hypertension. *Clin. Sci.*, 59:141s–144s.
2. Bertele, V., Tomasiak, M., Falanga, A., Cerletti, C., and De Gaetano, G. (1982): Aspirin inhibits platelet aggregation but not because it prevents thromboxane synthesis. *Lancet*, 2:775.
3. Blass, K. E., Block, H. U., Forster, W., and Ponicke, K. (1980): Dipyridamole: A potent stimulator of prostacyclin (PGI_2) biosynthesis. *Br. J. Pharmacol.*, 68:71–73.
4. Bravo, E. L., and Tarazi, R. C. (1979): Converting enzyme inhibition with an orally active compound in hypertensive man. *Hypertension*, 1:39–46.
5. Burke, S. E., Di Cola, G., and Lefer, A. M. (1983): Protection of ischemic cat myocardium by CGS-13080, a selective potent thromboxane A_2 synthesis inhibitor. *J. Cardiovasc. Pharmacol.*, 5:842–874.
6. Dale, J., Thaulow, E., Myhre, E., and Parry, J. (1983): The effect of a thromboxane synthetase inhibitor, dazoxiben, and acetylsalicylic acid on platelet function and prostaglandin metabolism. *Thromb. Haemostas.*, 50:703–706.
7. Davì, G., Pinto, A., Palisi, F., Novo, S., Mendola, G., Mazzola, A., and Strano, A. (1981): Livelli plasmatici di 6-keto $PGF_{1\alpha}$ e formazione di trombossano dalle piastrine, prima e dopo infusione di dipiridamolo, in pazienti con arteriopatia obliterante degli arti inferiori. *III Congr. Naz. Soc. Ital. Patol. Vascol.*, Palermo, p. 84 (Abstr.).
8. Defreyn, G., Deckmin, H., and Vermylen, J. (1982): A thromboxane synthetase inhibitor reorients endoperoxide metabolism in whole blood towards prostacyclin and prostaglandin E_2. *Thromb. Res.*, 26:389.
9. Dusting, G. J., Mullins, E. M., and Doyle, A. E. (1980): Angiotensin-induced prostacyclin release may contribute to the hypotensive action of converting enzyme inhibitors. In: *Advances in Prostaglandin and Thromboxane Research, Vol. 7*, edited by B. Samuelsson, P. W. Ramwell, and R. Paoletti, pp. 815–819. Raven Press, New York.
10. Feely, J., and Wood, A. J. J. (1983): Effect of inhibitors of prostaglandin synthesis on hepatic drug clearance. *Br. J. Clin. Pharmacol.*, 15:109–111.
11. Ferreira, S. H., Greene, L. J., and Alabaster, V. A. (1970): Activity of various fractions of bradykinin-potentiating factor against angiotensin I-converting enzyme. *Nature*, 225:379–380.
12. Fitzgerald, G. A., Brash, A. R., Oates, J. A., and Pedersen, A. K. (1983): Endogenous prostacyclin biosynthesis and platelet function during selective inhibition of thromboxane synthase in man. *J. Clin. Invest.*, 71:1336–1343.
13. Huddleston, C. B., Lupinetti, F. M., Laws, K. H., Collins, L. C., Clanton, J. A., Hawiger, J. J., Oates, J. A., and Hammon, J. W. (1983): The effects of RO-22-4679, a thromboxane synthetase inhibitor, on ventricular fibrillation induced by coronary artery occlusion in conscious dogs. *Circ. Res.*, 52:608–613.
14. Jackson, C. A., Greaves, M., and Preston, F. E. (1982): A study of the stimulation of human venous prostacyclin synthesis by dipyridamole. *Thromb. Res.*, 27:563–573.
15. Levin, R. E., Jaffe, E. A., Weksler, B. B., and Tack-Goldman, K. (1981): Nitroglycerin stimulates synthesis of prostacyclin by cultured human endothelial cells. *J. Clin. Invest.*, 67:762–769.
16. Lewis, H. D., Davis, J. W., Archibald, D. G. et al. (1983): Protective effect of aspirin against acute myocardial infarction and death in man with unstable angina: Results of a Veterans Administration Cooperative Study. *N. Engl. J. Med.*, 309:396–403.
17. Maguire, E. D. and Wallis, R. B. (1983): *In vivo* redirection of prostaglandin endoperoxides into

6-keto PGF$_{1\alpha}$ formation by thromboxane synthetase inhibitors in the rat. *Thromb. Res.*, 32:15–27.

18. Masotti, G., Galanti, G., Poggesi, L., Abbate, R., and Neri Serneri, G. G. (1979): Differential inhibition of prostacyclin production and platelet aggregation by aspirin. *Lancet*, 2:1213–1216.

19. Masotti, G., Poggesi, L., Galanti, G., and Neri Serneri, G. G. (1979): Stimulation of prostacyclin by dipyridamole (letter). *Lancet*, 1:1412.

20. McCaa, R. E., Hall, J. E., and McCaa, C. S. (1978): The effects of angiotensin I converting enzyme inhibitors on arterial blood pressure and urinary sodium excretion. Role of the renal renin-angiotensin and kallikrein-kinin systems. *Circ. Res.*, 43(suppl.I):32–39.

21. McGiff, J. C., Terragno, N. A., Malik, K. U., and Lonigro, A. J. (1972): Release of a prostaglandin E-like substance from canine kidney by bradykinin. *Circ. Res.*, 31:36–43.

22. Mehta, J., Mehta, P., and Hay, D. (1982): Effect of dipyridamole on prostaglandin generation by human platelets and vessel walls. *Prostaglandins*, 24:751–761.

23. Mehta, J., Mehta, P., and Ostrowski, N. (1983): Stimulation of vessel wall prostacyclin by selective thromboxane inhibitor OKY 1581. *Prostaglandins Leukotrienes Med.*, 12:49–52.

24. Mehta, J., Mehta, P., Roberts, A., Faro, R., Ostrowski, N., and Brigmon, L. (1983): Comparative effects of nytroglycerin and nitroprusside on prostacyclin generation in adult human vessel wall. *J. Am. Coll. Cardiol.*, 2:625–630.

25. Moncada, S., Gryglewski, R. J., Bunting, S., and Vane, J. R. (1976): An enzyme isolated from arteries transforms prostaglandin endoperoxides to an unstable substance that inhibits platelet aggregation. *Nature*, 263:663–665.

26. Moncada, S., and Korbut, R. (1978): Dipyridamole and other phosphodiesterase inhibitors act as antithrombotic agents by potentiating endogenous prostacyclin. *Lancet*, 1:1286–1289.

27. Morcillio, E., Reid, P. R., Dubin, H., Ghadgaonkar, R., and Pitt, B. (1980): Myocardial prostaglandin E release by nitroglycerin and modification by indomethacin. *Am. J. Cardiol.*, 45:53–57.

28. Neri Serneri, G. G., Masotti, G., Castellani, S., Scarti, L., Trotta, F., and Mannelli, M. (1983): Role of PGE$_2$ in the modulation of the adrenergic response in man. *Cardiovasc. Res.*, 17:662–670.

29. Neri Serneri, G. G., Masotti, G., Poggesi, L., Galanti, G., and Morettini, A. (1981): Enhanced prostacyclin production by dipyridamole in man. *Eur. J. Clin. Pharmacol.*, 21:9–15.

30. Neri Serneri, G. G., Masotti, G., Poggesi, L., Galanti, G., Morettini, A., and Scarti, L. (1982): Reduced prostacyclin production in patients with different manifestations of ischemic heart disease. *Am. J. Cardiol.*, 49:1146–1151.

31. Ng, K. K., and Vane, J. R. (1968): Fate of angiotensin I in the circulation. *Nature*, 218:144–150.

32. Ondetti, M. A., Rubin, B., and Cushman, D. W. (1977): Design of specific inhibitors of angiotensin-converting enzyme: A new class of orally active antihypertensive agents. *Science*, 196:441–444.

33. Panzenbeck, M. J., Baez, A., and Kaley, G. (1984): Nitroglycerin and nitroprusside increase coronary blood flow in dogs by a mechanism independent of prostaglandin release. *Am. J. Cardiol.*, 53:936–940.

34. Parry, M. J., Randall, M. J., Tyler, H. M., Myhre, E., Daler, J., and Thaulow, E. (1982): Selective inhibition of thromboxane synthetase by dazoxiben increase prostacyclin production by leucocytes in angina patients and healthy volunteers. *Lancet*, 2:164.

35. Patrignani, P., Filabozzi, P., and Patrono, C. (1982): Selective cumulative inhibition of platelet thromboxane production by low-dose aspirin in healthy subjects. *J. Clin. Invest.*, 69:1366–1372.

36. Puustinen, T., and Uotila, P. (1983): Dipyridamole interferes with the incorporation of arachidonic acid and stimulates prostacyclin production in rat lungs. *Prostaglandins*, 26:265–274.

37. Randall, M. J., Parry, M. J., Hawkeswood, E., Cross, P. E., and Dichinson, R. P. (1981): UK-37, 248, a novel, selective thromboxane synthetase inhibitor with anti-aggregatory and antithrombotic activity. *Thromb. Res.*, 23:145–162.

38. Schrör, K., Grodzinska, L., and Darius, H. (1981): Stimulation of coronary vascular prostacyclin and inhibition of human platelet thromboxane A$_2$ after low-dose nitroglycerin. *Thromb. Res.*, 23:59–67.

39. Silberbauer, K., Sinzinger, H., Punzengruber, C., and Kefalides, A. (1982): Effect of nitroglycerin on prostaglandin I$_2$ synthesis modified by aspirin. *Circulation (Abstr.)*, 66(suppl. II):263.

40. Silberbauer, K., Stanek, B., and Templ, H. (1982): Acute hypotensive effect of captopril in man modified by prostaglandin synthesis inhibition. *Br. J. Clin. Pharmacol.*, 14(suppl. 2):87s–93s.

41. Simonetti, I., De Caterina, R., Marzilli, M., and L'Abbate, A. (1984): Coronary vasodilatation

by nitrates: Any role for prostaglandins? Int. Meeting on Platelets, Prostaglandins and the Cardiovascular System (Florence, February 8–11, 1984), page 125 (Abstr.).

42. Smith, J. B., and Jubiz, W. (1981): OKY-1581: A selective inhibitor of thromboxane synthesis *in vivo* and *in vitro*. *Prostaglandins*, 22:353–363.

43. Swartz, S. L., Williams, G. H., Hollenberg, N. K., Levin, L., Dluhy, R. G., and Moore, T. J. (1980): Captopril-induced changes in prostaglandin production. *J. Clin. Invest.*, 65:1257–1264.

44. Tan, S. Y., Sweet, P., and Mulrow, P. J. (1978): Impaired production of renal prostaglandin E_2: A newly identified lesion in human essential hypertension. *Prostaglandins*, 15:139–149.

45. Trimarco, B., Patrono, C., Ricciardelli, B., Volpe, M., Cuocolo, A., De Simone, A., and Condorelli, M. (1984): Indomethacin blunts the late phase of nitroglycerin-induced coronary vasodilatation in dogs. Int. Meeting on Platelets, Prostaglandins and the Cardiovascular System (Florence, February 8–11, 1984), page 126 (Abstr.).

46. Van de Velde, V. J., Bult, H., Weisenberger, H., and Herman, A.G. (1982): Dipyridamole stimulates prostacyclin production in isolated rat aortic tissue. *Arch. Int. Pharmacodyn. Ther.*, 256:327–328.

47. Vermylen, J., Carreras, L.O., Van Schaeren, J., Defreyn, G., Machin, S. J., and Verstraete, M. (1981): Thromboxane synthetase inhibition as antithrombotic strategy. *Lancet*, 1:1073–1075.

48. Wallis, J., Moses, J. W., Borer, J.S., Goldberg, H. L., Fisher, J., Kase, M., Weksler, B. B., and Tack-Goldman, H. L. (1982): Nitroglycerin increases coronary blood prostacyclin levels in coronary artery disease. *Circulation (Abstr.)*. 66(suppl. II):II:264.

49. Watkins, J., Abbot, E. C., Hensby, C. N., Webster, J., and Dollery, C. T. (1980): Attenuation of hypotensive effect of propranolol and thiazide diuretics by indomethacin. *Br. Med. J.*, 281:702–705.

50. Weber, S., Rey, E., Pipeau, C., Lutfalla, G., Richard, M. O., Daoud-El-Assaf, H., Olive, G., and Degeorges, M. (1983): Influence of aspirin on the hemodynamic effects of sublingual nitroglycerin. *J. Cardiovasc. Pharmacol.*, 5:874–877.

51. Weksler, B. B., Pett, S. B., Alonso, D., Richter, R. C., Stelzer, P., Subramanian, V., Tack-Goldman, K., and Gay, W. A. (1983): Differential inhibition by aspirin of vascular and platelet prostaglandin synthesis in atherosclerotic patients. *N. Engl. J. Med.*, 308:800–805.

52. Williams, G. H., and Hollenberg, N. K. (1977): Attenuated vascular and endocrine response to SQ20, 881 in hypertension. *N. Engl. J. Med.*, 297:184–188.

Advances in Prostaglandin, Thromboxane, and
Leukotriene Research, Vol. 13, edited by G. G. Neri
Serneri, et al. Raven Press, New York © 1985.

Coronary Vasodilation by Nitrates: Any Role for Prostaglandins?

I. Simonetti, R. De Caterina, C. Michelassi, M. Marzilli,
M. De Nes, and A. L'Abbate

*C.N.R. Clinical Physiology Institute and Istituto di Patologia Medica I,
University of Pisa, Pisa, Italy*

Since their introduction in cardiovascular therapy in the last century (1), nitrates represent the most widely used drugs for prophylactic and symptomatic management of myocardial ischemia.

In vitro studies have shown that nitrates are able to evoke prostacyclin production in human endothelial cell culture (5) and in isolated coronary arteries (8). These findings led some investigators to hypothesize that vasodilating properties of nitrates could be mediated by the prostaglandin (PG) system, and in particular by PGI_2 (6). The aim of this study was to determine *in vivo* in humans whether coronary vasodilation by nitrates is mediated by the PG system. For this purpose the effect of isosorbide dinitrate (ISDN) on coronary artery diameter and coronary flow, before and after acute administration of aspirin (ASA), was investigated.

METHODS

The study was carried out in 13 patients undergoing routine coronary angiography for suspected coronary heart disease (CHD). No patient had evidence of heart failure or other form of heart disease. All gave their consent to the study. Pharmacological therapy was discontinued 2 days before the study, and fast-acting nitrates were not allowed in the 8-hr period preceding the angiographic examination. No patient had taken ASA or other drugs known to interfere with prostaglandin synthesis in the 2-week period preceding the study. Coronary angiography was performed by the Judkins technique (4); coronary sinus flow (CSF) was measured according to the method of Ganz et al. (3). In 9 patients—group 1—coronary angiography and, in 4 of the 9, CSF measurements were performed in basal condition and 2 min after intracoronary administration of 3 mg ISDN. ASA, at 1 g i.v. and 100 mg intracoronary (2,7), was then injected and, following a time interval of 15 min, intended to be long enough to allow systemic and coronary endothelial inhibition of prostacyclin synthesis, coronary angiography and CSF measurement were repeated. A second intracoronary administration of 3 mg ISDN was then performed, and a last set of measurements was obtained 2 min later.

Thus, in this group, a first "control" ISDN vasodilation and a second vasodilation after ASA were obtained and compared.

In 4 patients—group 2—after control angiography, only the second step of the procedure was performed, i.e., ASA (1 g i.v. + 100 mg intracoronary); coronary angiography 15 min later; ISDN 3 mg intracoronary; coronary angiography 2 min later. This was performed in order to assess either the effect of ASA on resting coronary tone or the capability of ASA in preventing ISDN-induced vasodilation as in group 1, but without the interference of previous ISDN injection.

In each patient, end-systolic and end-diastolic frames were selected from the 35-mm angiographic film in the control condition and after each pharmacological intervention. The selected frames were projected by a photographic enlarger at a constant magnification onto a horizontal screen, where vascular and catheter profiles were accurately traced. The diameters of large and medium-sized coronary vessels were measured by means of a magnifying glass fitted with a scale of 0.1-mm divisions. Measurements were then normalized using the actual dimensions of the catheter (2 cm from the tip) as reference.

The error of this method had been assessed in a previous study on a population of 668 coronary artery segments. Each segment was traced and measured twice by the same operator. The analysis of measurement reproducibility revealed a variability around the identity line of 6.7%. The diameters of the analyzed segments were then distributed into classes of 1-mm stepwise increments, and the intraobserver percent error in each class was obtained, including 95% of the differences between the two measurements (i.e., all values within the confidence limits). This error was inversely related to the vascular diameter, being larger in the smallest classes (Fig. 1). In the evaluation of the results of the present study, the percentage variations in vascular diameter relative to control observed after each pharmacological administration were matched with the error of the method in the class of the control diameter.

RESULTS

Percentage diameter changes of each vascular segment relative to control in group 1 are shown in Fig. 2 (A). After the first ISDN administration there was a significant increase (20.7 ± 8%); vasodilation was less but still present 15 min after ASA (14.8 ± 7.2%) and was further enhanced by the second ISDN (24.9 ± 11.4%), indicating that ASA was not able to prevent ISDN-induced vasodilation. The lower degree of vasodilation observed after ASA could be related either to a time-dependent decrease of ISDN effect or to a vasoconstricting effect of ASA.

To elucidate whether ASA might induce such vasoconstriction, in group 2 it was injected first. Figure 2 (B) illustrates the results. No significant differences in coronary artery diameter relative to control were observed after ASA (1.1 ± 4.6%), whereas a significant increase was obtained after ISDN (21 ± 7%).

Independent of ASA administration, a comparable vasodilation was observed after each ISDN administration, with the smallest vessels exhibiting the greater

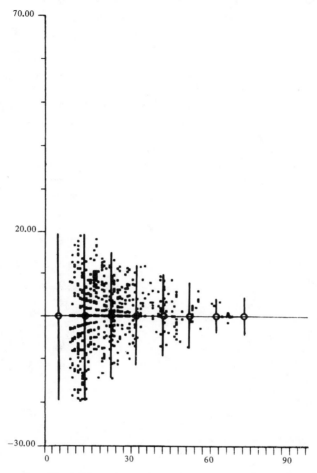

FIG. 1. Distribution of percentage difference between the two measurements of 668 coronary artery segments performed by the same operator (*y* axis), plotted against values of the first measurement (*x* axis, mm × 10⁻¹). The horizontal line parallel to the abscissa represents the zero or identity line; vertical bars represent the percentage error in the various diameter classes, of 1 mm each. Each class includes 95% of values. Values are symmetrically distributed around the identity line. Note that the smaller the vascular diameter, the larger is the percentage error of the measurement.

response. Coronary sinus flow measurements performed in 4 patients of group 1, all with normal coronary vessels, showed no significant changes in coronary flow and resistance, in spite of a significant decrease of pressure–rate product, which, from the control value of $9.5 \pm 1.9 \times 10^{-3}$ beats·mm Hg, dropped to 8.6 ± 1.6 ($p < 0.05$) and to 7.6 ± 2.0 ($p < 0.01$) after the first and the second ISDN administration, respectively. These findings indicate that ISDN induced a "relative" vasodilation that ASA was not able to prevent.

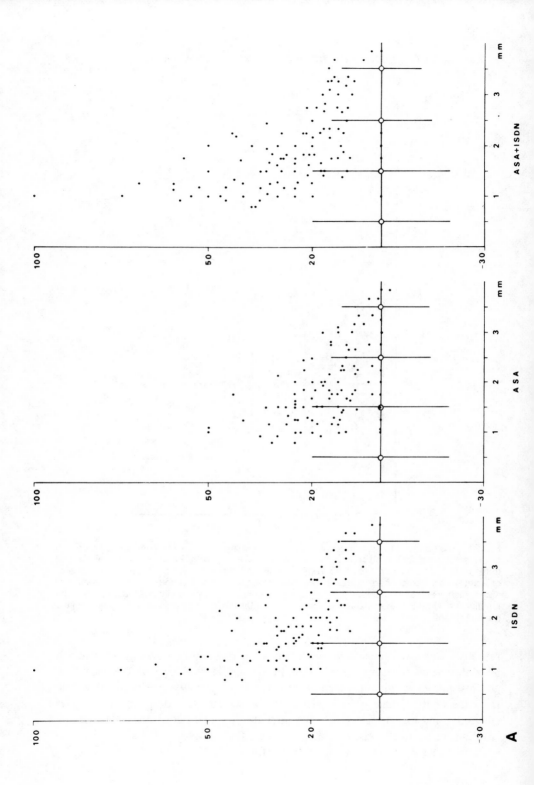

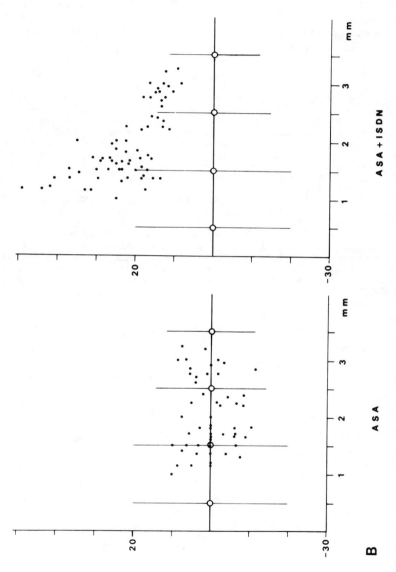

FIG. 2. Percentage variation of each vascular diameter (*y* axis) relative to control (*x* axis), observed after each pharmacological intervention in groups 1 (**A**) and 2 (**B**). The horizontal lines parallel to the abscissa represent the zero or identity line; vertical bars represent the percentage error in each diameter class. See text for description. ASA, aspirin; ISDN, isosorbide dinitrate.

CONCLUSIONS

Aspirin, at the dosage used, was not able to prevent coronary vasodilation by isosorbide dinitrate, at the level of both conductance and resistance vessels. Our data do not support the hypothesis that coronary vasodilation by nitrates is mediated by the prostaglandin system.

REFERENCES

1. Brunton, T. L. (1867): On the use of nitrite of amyl in angina pectoris. *Lancet*, 2:97.
2. FitzGerald, G. A., Oates, J. A., Hawiger, J., Maas, R. L., Jackson Roberts, L., II, Lawson, J. A., and Brash, A. R. (1981): Endogenous biosynthesis of prostacyclin and thromboxane and platelet function during chronic administration of aspirin in man. *J. Clin. Invest.*, 71:676–688.
3. Ganz, W., Tamura, K., Marcus, H., Donoso, R., Yoshida, S., and Swan, H. J. C. (1971): Measurement of coronary sinus blood flow by continuous thermodilution. *Circulation*, 44:181–195.
4. Judkins, M. P. (1967): Selective coronary arteriography. I. A percutaneous transfemoral technique. *Radiology*, 89:815–824.
5. Levin, R. I., Jaffe, E. A., Weksler, B. B., and Tack-Goldman, K. (1981): Nitroglycerin stimulates synthesis of prostacyclin by human endothelial cells. *J. Clin. Invest.*, 67:762–769.
6. Moncada, S., Higgs, E. A., and Vane, J. R. (1977): Human arterial and venous tissues generate prostacyclin (prostaglandin X), a potent inhibitor of platelet aggregation. *Lancet*, I(8001):18–20.
7. Petrignani, P., Filarozzi, P., and Patrono, C. (1982): Selective cumulative inhibition of platelet thromboxane production by low dose aspirin in healthy subjects. *J. Clin. Invest.*, 69:1366–1372.
8. Shror, K., Grodzinska, L., and Darius, H. (1981): Stimulation of coronary vascular prostacyclin and inhibition of human platelet thromboxane A_2 after low dose nitroglycerin. *Thromb. Res.*, 23:59–67.

Advances in Prostaglandin, Thromboxane, and Leukotriene Research, Vol. 13, edited by G.G. Neri Serneri, et al. Raven Press, New York © 1985.

Indomethacin Blunts the Late Phase of Nitroglycerin-Induced Coronary Vasodilatation in Dogs

*Bruno Trimarco, **Carlo Patrono, *Bruno Ricciardelli, *Massimo Volpe, *Alberto Cuocolo, *Antonio De Simone, and *Mario Condorelli

*Istituto di Clinica Medica I, II Facoltà di Medicina e Chirurgia, University of Naples, 80131 Naples, Italy; and **Istituto di Farmacologia, Facoltà di Medicina, Catholic University, Rome, Italy*

The present study was undertaken to further investigate the possibility that prostaglandins participate in the coronary hemodynamic response to nitroglycerin (NTG) intracoronary administration. For this purpose we assessed in the dog the effects of different doses of indomethacin (I) and naproxen (N) on the hemodynamic response induced by NTG intracoronary (i.c.) administration, in an attempt to demonstrate a relationship between these two phenomena that may confirm the hypothesis that the prostaglandin system is involved in the genesis of NTG-induced coronary vasodilatation.

METHODS

Mongrel dogs of both sexes weighing 10 to 20 kg were anaesthetized and instrumented as previously described (3).

Preparation of Animals

The surgical procedure has been previously described (3). The lumen of the left circumflex coronary artery was cannulated with a polyethylene catheter introduced through the right carotid artery and positioned under fluoroscopy. The wall of the left circumflex coronary artery was ligated around the catheter positioned into the lumen of the vessel. The coronary artery was then perfused at constant flow with a Sigmamotor T8S peristaltic pump with blood of the same animal obtained through a polyethylene catheter introduced through the external iliac artery in the abdominal aorta. Under such conditions, changes in vascular tone of the perfused district were reflected by proportional changes in perfusion pressure. Blood flow rate was adjusted to give perfusion pressure close to systemic blood pressure. This perfusion pressure was maintained slightly higher than systemic blood pressure in order to

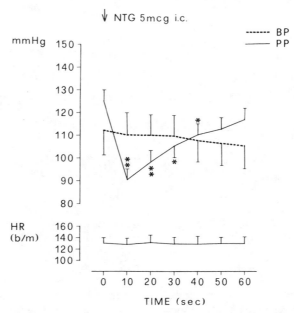

FIG. 1. Effects of nitroglycerin (NTG) intracoronary (i.c.) administration on coronary perfusion pressure (PP), systemic blood pressure (BP), and heart rate (HR) in control condition ($n = 5$). Each point represents mean ± SE. Each point is compared with the basal value by the paired t-test. Significant difference is shown by *$p < 0.05$; **$p < 0.01$.

TABLE 1. *Percentage of cyclooxygenase activity inhibition induced by increasing doses of indomethacin and naproxen*

Indomethacin		Naproxen	
Dose	% Inhibition	Dose	% Inhibition
0.1 mg kg	90	1 mg/kg	83
0.3 mg/kg	94	3 mg/kg	90
0.5 mg/kg	96	5 mg/kg	96
1.5 mg/kg	100	7 mg/kg	100
3 mg/kg	100	10 mg/kg	100
4 mg/kg	100	12 mg/kg	100
5 mg/kg	100	15 mg/kg	100

compensate the resistances of the tubing system, and was left unchanged throughout the experiment. The intraarterial administration of drugs was made in the perfused circuit after the pump and immediately before the perfused district. All drugs were injected into the coronary circulation in a volume of saline not exceeding 0.1 ml.

Analyses

The extent of systemic cyclooxygenase inhibition induced by different pharmacologic treatments was assessed through radioimmunoassay measurements of serum

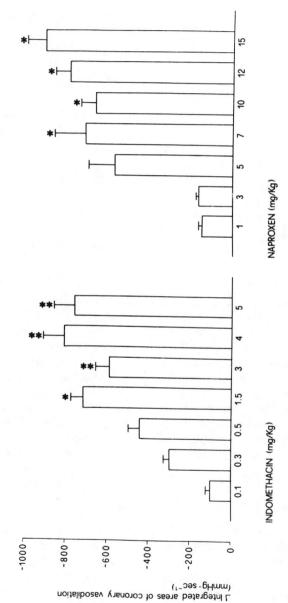

FIG. 2. Changes of the integrated areas of coronary vasodilatation after administration of increasing amounts of indomethacin and naproxen ($n = 5$). Each bar represents mean ± SE. Statistical analysis was performed by comparing the values obtained in control conditions and after each pharmacological treatment using the paired t-test. Symbols are as in Fig. 1.

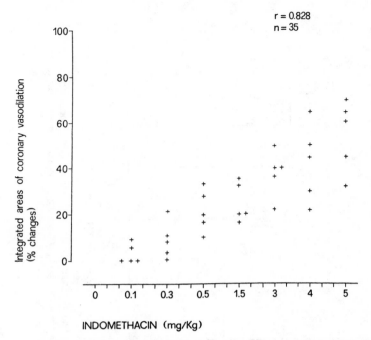

FIG. 3. Relationship between changes of integrated areas of coronary vasodilatation and the dose of indomethacin administered.

thromboxane (TX) B_2, which reflects thrombin-induced activation of platelet TXA_2 production during whole blood clotting (2).

Statistical analysis was performed by comparing the values of systemic and perfusion pressure recorded after i.c. drug injection with the basal value using a paired t-test. Furthermore, in order to assess the effect of different pharmacological treatment on the coronary response to NTG and hystamine i.c. injection, the integrated areas of coronary vasodilatation were measured by planimetry and the values obtained before and after each pharmacological treatment were compared by a paired t-test.

Experimental Protocol

Two series of experiments were performed. In the first group ($n = 20$), the effects of seven different doses of I (0.1, 0.3, 0.5, 1.5, 3, 4, and 5 mg/kg body weight i.v.) on the hemodynamic response to i.c. injection of NTG (5 μg) were evaluated. In the second group studied ($n = 19$), N substituted for I as the agent inhibiting prostaglandin synthesis. With this drug, seven dosage schedules were also given (1, 3, 5, 7, 10, 12, and 15 mg/kg body weight i.v.). In both groups, no more than two individual dosages were given per dog. The dosage schedules of each dog were determined by a computer-based randomization scheme, and they

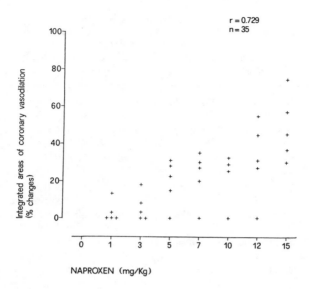

FIG. 4. Relationship between changes of integrated areas of coronary vasodilatation and the dose of naproxen administered.

were not necessarily in a step-progressive fashion. The dosages were cumulative, with the second dose being obtained adding the appropriate amount of drug to the first dose.

At the beginning of the study in each dog, a venous blood sample was withdrawn from the right atrium through a catheter introduced via the external iliac femoral vein, to measure TXB_2. Then, after a hemodynamic response to hystamine i.c. injection was recorded, the effects of NTG i.c. administration were evaluated. Subsequently, I or N was administered i.v. At 30 min following the administration of the specific prostaglandin-synthesis inhibiting agent, a second blood sample was withdrawn for assaying the level of systemic inhibition. Then, after the vascular responsiveness had again been evaluated by i.c. injection of hystamine, a second response to NTG i.c. administration was elicited. The higher dosage of I or N was then administered and its effects on cyclooxygenase activity, vascular responsiveness, and NTG-induced hemodynamic response were assessed as indicated above.

RESULTS

The i.c. injection of NTG elicited a consistent vasodilatation of the coronary bed (Fig. 1), while systemic blood pressure and heart rate were not significantly modified.

Effect of Indomethacin and Naproxen Treatment

Systemic cyclooxygenase activity was significantly reduced after I and N administration, with 100% inhibition reached after I at 1.5 mg/kg and N at 7 mg/kg

TABLE 2. *Maximum fall in coronary perfusion pressure after each dose of indomethacin and naproxen administered*

Indomethacin		Naproxen	
Basal value	31 mm Hg	Basal value	33 mm Hg
0.1 mg/kg	27 mm Hg	1 mg/kg	36 mm Hg
Basal value	29 mm Hg	Basal value	32 mm Hg
0.3 mg/kg	29 mm Hg	3 mg/kg	31 mm Hg
Basal value	28 mm Hg	Basal value	33 mm Hg
0.5 mg/kg	28 mm Hg	5 mg/kg	23 mm Hg
Basal value	23 mm Hg	Basal value	38 mm Hg
1.5 mg/kg	30 mm Hg	7 mg/kg	33 mm Hg
Basal value	26 mm Hg	Basal value	30 mm Hg
3 mg/kg	20 mm Hg	10 mg/kg	31 mm Hg
Basal value	21 mm Hg	Basal value	33 mm Hg
4 mg/kg	17 mm Hg	12 mg/kg	23 mm Hg
Basal value	20 mm Hg	Basal value	24 mm Hg
5 mg/kg	20 mm Hg	15 mg/kg	18 mm Hg

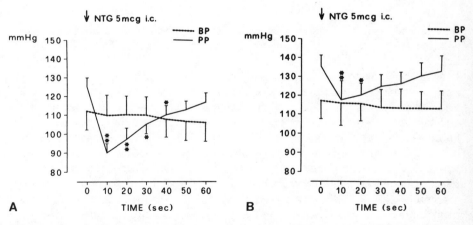

FIG. 5. Effects of nitroglycerin (NTG) intracoronary (i.c.) administration on coronary perfusion pressure and systemic blood pressure **(A)** in control condition and **(B)** after indomethacin (1.5 mg/kg i.v.) administration ($n = 5$). Each point represents mean ± SE. Statistical analysis and symbols are as in Fig. 1.

(Table 1). With both drugs there was an increase in the basal value of systemic and perfusion pressure that was statistically correlated with the percentage of systemic cyclooxygenase activity inhibition induced (I: $p<0.001$ for both blood and perfusion pressure; N: $p<0.01$ for both blood and perfusion pressure). Furthermore, after I or N i.v. treatment, we observed a reduction in the integrated areas of NTG-induced coronary vasodilatation that was increased by augmenting the

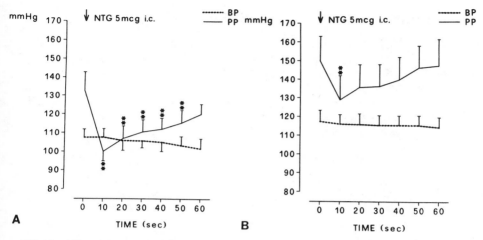

FIG. 6. Effects of nitroglycerin intracoronary administration on coronary perfusion pressure and systemic blood pressure **(A)** in control condition and **(B)** after naproxen (7 mg/kg i.v.) administration ($n = 5$). Each point represents mean ± SE. Statistical analysis and symbols as in Fig. 1.

amount of both drugs, until the dose of I at 1.5 mg/kg and N at 7 mg/kg, when the significance level was reached (Fig. 2). No further reduction in the integrated areas of coronary vasodilatation was detectable with the higher dosages of I or N. A statistically significant correlation was found when the decreases in the integrated areas observed were plotted against the dose of I or N administered ($p < 0.001$) (Figs. 3 and 4). After the complete blockade of prostaglandin synthesis induced by I or N, the NTG-induced coronary vasodilatation was not accompanied by a reduction in the maximum fall in perfusion pressure (Table 2) but was characterized by a faster return of the perfusion pressure to the basal value (Figs. 5 and 6). Finally, no significant change in the systemic blood pressure response was observed after the two pharmacological treatments (Figs. 5 and 6).

Specificity of Pharmacological Treatments

In no instance was the hemodynamic response induced by hystamine i.c. injection modified by the various pharmacological treatments (data not shown). Furthermore, in pilot experiments in which four NTG-induced coronary responses were evoked at 30-min intervals without any pharmacological treatment, no statistically significant change in coronary vasodilatation occurred (data not shown).

DISCUSSION

These results suggest that prostaglandins are involved in the mediation of the late phase of NTG-induced coronary vasodilatation. They represent a confirmation in an *in vivo* study of the data obtained *in vitro* by Levin and co-workers (1), who showed that NTG at clinically attainable concentrations causes a dose-dependent increase in prostacyclin (PGI_2) synthesis by endothelial cells.

REFERENCES

1. Levin, R. I., Jaffe, E. A., Weksler, B. B., and Tack-Goldman, K. (1981): Nitroglycerin stimulates synthesis of prostacyclin by cultured human endothelial cells. *J. Clin. Invest.*, 67:762.
2. Patrono, C., Ciabattoni, G., Pinca, E., Pugliese, F., Castrucci, G., DeSalvo, A., Satta, M. A., and Peskar, B. A. (1980): Low dose aspirin and inhibition of TxB_2 production in healthy subjects. *Thromb. Res.*, 17:317.
3. Trimarco, B., Chierchia, S., Ricciardelli, B., Cuocolo, A., Volpe, M., Saccà, L., and Condorelli, M. (1984): Ouabain-induced reflex coronary vasodilatation mediated by cardiac receptors with vagal afferents. *Am. J. Physiol.*, 15:H664.

*Advances in Prostaglandin, Thromboxane, and
Leukotriene Research, Vol. 13*, edited by G. G. Neri
Serneri, et al. Raven Press, New York © 1985.

Dilation of Large Coronary Arteries in Conscious Dogs by Prostacyclin

T. H. Hintze, M. R. Kichuk, H. Stern, and G. Kaley

Department of Physiology, New York Medical College, Valhalla, New York 10595

Prostacyclin (PGI_2) relaxes large coronary artery rings (7) and strips *in vitro*, a property that led to its discovery (6), and increases coronary blood flow in anesthetized dogs (3,8). PGI_2 has also been shown to reduce perfusion pressure in isolated perfused cat coronary artery segments (9) and to increase large coronary vessel dimensions in *in situ* perfused dog coronary arteries (2). The purpose of the present study was to determine the effects of PGI_2 on large coronary arteries in conscious dogs in the absence of the trauma of recent surgery and anesthetics that are known to influence cardiovascular regulation (10) and vascular smooth muscle tone directly (1).

METHODS

Dogs ($n = 6$) were instrumented using sterile surgical techniques under pentobarbital anesthesia through an incision in the left fifth intercostal space. A Konigsberg solid-state pressure gauge was placed in the apex of the left ventricle, and Tygon catheters were placed in the left atrial appendage and descending thoracic aorta. Piezoelectric transducers, 7-MHz crystals attached to a Dacron backing, were sutured to opposing surfaces of the left circumflex coronary artery for the instantaneous and continuous measurement of large coronary artery diameters. A Doppler flow probe was placed proximal to the coronary dimension crystals. The chest was closed in layers and the pneumothorax was reduced. When the animals had fully recovered, experiments were begun. Since the dose 2.0 μg/kg of PGI_2 caused a maximal change in coronary dimensions, the effects of this dose were compared to those of nitroglycerin, at 25 μg/kg, a drug known to dilate large coronary arteries in this model (4) and in man. Arterial pressure, heart rate, left ventricular (LV) pressure, change in LV pressure with time ($LVdP/dt$), and coronary diameter and blood flow were continuously recorded. In addition, internal coronary cross-sectional area (CSA) and late diastolic coronary vascular resistance (LDCR) were calculated and used as indices of large and small coronary dilation. These methods have been previously described in detail (4,5,11).

RESULTS

An actual record from a dog is shown in Fig. 1.

Effects of Prostacyclin at 2.0 μg/kg

The maximum changes in coronary diameter occurred 120 sec after injection; therefore, all data will be reported for this time period. At this dose of PGI_2, LV systolic pressure decreased 16 ± 5.4 mm Hg, arterial pressure decreased 48 ± 5.0 mm Hg, LV$dP/dt$ did not change from control, while heart rate increased slightly, 23 ± 8 b/min. PGI_2 increased large coronary vessel diameter (0.09 ± 0.02 mm from 3.70 ± 0.60 mm), coronary blood flow, and calculated coronary CSA, and decreased LDCR (Fig. 2).

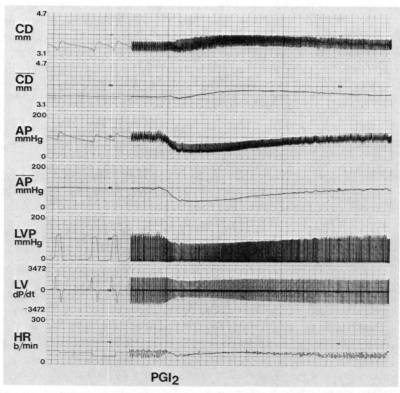

FIG. 1. Injection of PGI_2 (2 μg/kg) caused a reduction in left ventricular systolic pressure (LVP), LV *dP/dt*, phasic and mean arterial pressure (AP), and an increase in phasic and mean coronary diameter (CD) and heart rate (HR). The maximum effects of PGI_2 occurred 120 sec after injection. Notice the initial fall in heart rate, at the time of maximum fall in AP, which increases slightly at the time of maximum increase in CD. Overbars indicate mean values.

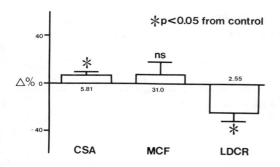

FIG. 2. Percent changes (Δ%) in large coronary cross-sectional area (CSA), mean coronary blood flow (MCF), and late diastolic coronary resistance (LDCR) during the maximum increase in CSA following injection of PGI₂ (2 μg/kg) are shown. PGI₂ increased CSA and reduced LDCR significantly but did not increase MCF. The dilation of large coronary artery by PGI₂ was relatively small when compared to the effects of nitroglycerin. Control values are shown beneath the bars.

Effects of a Thromboxane A₂-Like Substance (U46619) and Prostacyclin (2 μg/kg)

The maximum effects of this drug also occurred 120 sec after injection. At 5 μg/kg, U46619 increased LV systolic pressure 12 ± 5 mm Hg, mean arterial pressure 26 ± 3.1 mm Hg, and heart rate 17 ± 5 b/min, but did not change LV$dP/dt$. Coronary diameter decreased 0.15 ± 0.02 mm. CSA fell 0.95 ± 0.22 mm², and LDCR increased 2.07 ± 0.27 mm Hg·ml·min. Injection of PGI₂ reversed the constriction caused by U46619. In contracted vessels, PGI₂ increased coronary diameter 0.11 ± 0.03 mm and increased CSA $0.48 \pm .09$ mm².

Comparative Effects of Prostacyclin and Nitroglycerin

While PGI₂ (2 μg/kg) caused a small increase in CSA (Fig. 2), nitroglycerin had substantially larger effects. Nitroglycerin increased CSA $34 \pm 7.3\%$ from 5.90 ± 0.61 mm², significantly more ($p < 0.01$) than PGI₂ ($13 \pm 3.0\%$).

DISCUSSION

This is the first study of the effects of PGI₂ on large coronary vessels in conscious dogs. Results of a recent study by Dusting and Angus (3) in a perfused *in situ* dog coronary vessel are similar to our results. However, in their model, regulatory functions—especially changes in cardiac function and heart rate, which may contribute indirectly to the effects of PGI₂—could not be taken into consideration. In another previous study, Ogletree et al. (9) reported that PGI₂ reduced perfusion pressure in an isolated cat coronary artery perfused at constant flow. In our study the dilation of large coronary vessels was sufficient to reverse the coronary constriction caused by a thromboxane-like substance (U46619) but was much smaller than the dilation caused by nitroglycerin alone or nitroglycerin administered during the injection of U46619.

In our study, indomethacin had no significant effect on large coronary vessels, nor did it significantly potentiate the large coronary dilation resulting from PGI₂ administration. This indicates that little or no PGI₂ is formed in the large coronary vessels in the basal state. In conclusion, PGI₂ dilates large coronary vessels in the conscious dog, despite large reductions in arterial pressure. The dilation is sufficient to reverse coronary vasoconstriction induced by a thromboxane-like substance but is smaller than dilation of large coronary arteries to nitroglycerin.

ACKNOWLEDGMENTS

This study was supported by U.S. Public Health Service grant 30274 from the National Heart, Lung, and Blood Institute and an intramural grant from New York Medical College. M. R. Kichuk and H. Stern were summer medical student fellows in the Department of Physiology.

REFERENCES

1. Altura, B. T., and Altura, B. M. (1975): Pentobarbital and contraction of vascular smooth muscle. *Am. J. Physiol.*, 229:1635–1640.
2. Dusting, G. J., and Angus, J. A. (1984): Interaction of epoprostenol (PGI₂) with vasoconstrictors on diameters of large coronary arteries of the dog. *J. Cardiovasc. Pharmacol.*, 6:20–27.
3. Dusting, G. J., Moncada, S., and Vane, J. R. (1979): Prostaglandins, their intermediates and precursors: Cardiovascular actions and regulatory roles in normal and abnormal circulatory systems. *Prog. Cardiovasc. Dis.*, 21:405–430.
4. Hintze, T. H., and Vatner, S. F. (1983): Comparison of effects of nifedipine and nitroglycerin on large and small coronary arteries and cardiac function in conscious dogs. *Circ. Res.*, 52(suppl. I):139–146.
5. Hintze, T. H., and Vatner, S. F. (1983): Dipyridamole dilates large coronary arteries in conscious dogs. *Circulation*, 68:1321–1327.
6. Kulkarni, P. S., Roberts, R., and Needleman, P. (1976): Paradoxical endogenous synthesis of a coronary dilating substance from arachidonate. *Prostaglandins*, 12:337–352.
7. Mullane, K. M., Bradley, G., and Moncada, S. (1982): The interactions of platelet-derived mediators on isolated canine coronary arteries. *Eur. J. Pharmacol.*, 84:115–118.
8. Needleman, P., and Kaley, G. (1978): Cardiac and coronary prostaglandin synthesis and function. *N. Engl. J. Med.*, 298:1120–1128.
9. Ogletree, M. L., Smith, J. B., and Lefer, A. M. (1978): Actions of prostaglandins on isolated cat coronary arteries. *Am. J. Physiol.*, 235:H400–H406.
10. Vatner, S. F., and Braunwald, E. (1975): Cardiovascular control mechanisms in the conscious state. *N. Engl. J. Med.*, 293:970–976.
11. Vatner, S. F., and Hintze, T. H. (1983): Mechanism of constriction of large coronary arteries by β-adrenergic receptor blockade. *Circ. Res.*, 53:389–400.

*Advances in Prostaglandin, Thromboxane, and
Leukotriene Research, Vol. 13*, edited by G.G. Neri
Serneri, et al. Raven Press, New York © 1985.

Prostaglandins in Therapy of Cardiovascular Disease

*Andrzej Szczeklik and **Ryszard J. Gryglewski

*Department of Medicine and **Department of Pharmacology, Copernicus Academy of
Medicine, 31-066 Cracow, Poland

Prostaglandin (PG) E_1 was the first prostanoid to be tried in therapy of cardio-vascular disease (5). However, the discovery of prostacyclin (PGI_2) in 1976 (13,25) and demonstration of its powerful actions in man has shifted the clinical interest away from PGE_1. Recently, PGI_2, but not PGE_1, has been tried in numerous clinical situations. First came the open observations, to be followed by controlled clinical trials. Here we concentrate on the latter, moving through different clinical conditions in which PGI_2 has been used. Recent results obtained with PGE_1 are mentioned, but a reader interested in comprehensive PGE_1 coverage is referred to previous reviews (29,37).

ACTIONS OF PROSTACYCLIN IN MAN FORMING THE BASIS OF THERAPY

PGI_2 exerts multiple actions in man. Those that most probably account for its therapeutic values are (a) vasodilatation, (b) antiplatelet properties, (c) stimulation of fibrinolysis, and (d) cytoprotection.

The first two are relatively well-known. Vasodilatation reflects the action of PGI_2 on the resistance, rather than the capacitance, vessels (46). Relief by PGI_2 of ischemia-induced vasoconstriction of resistance vessels was suggested as a mechanism explaining clinical improvement in peripheral vascular disease (17). The profound antiplatelet properties of PGI_2 can be divided into antiaggregatory and disaggregatory. The former are reflected by inhibition of platelet aggregation, and the latter by dispersion of both circulating platelet aggregates and platelet thrombi formed on the collagen surface (39).

Infusion of PGI_2 in man at a dose of 2 to 5 ng/kg·min stimulates fibrinolysis (8,40). The activation reaches its peak 3 to 5 hr from the start of infusion, but disappears over the following hours if the infusion is continued. The distinct stimulation of fibrinolysis produced by PGI_2 might be of special clinical interest, because it does not result in systemic degradation of fibrinogen and is thus deprived of frequent side effects of streptokinase therapy. The effect is, furthermore, of long duration, extending at least up to 24 hr after cessation of 5-hr infusion of PGI_2 (40). Its therapeutic importance, however, remains to be established.

PGI_2 can exert protective action against experimental damage to gastric mucosa, myocardium, and liver. This mysterious property has been termed cytoprotection. Whereas this effect may reflect the PGI_2 potent vasodilatory and antiaggregating activities, a more distinct mechanism can also play an important role. Thus, PGI_2 directly preserves integrity of platelets and that of their internal structures, protects myocardial mitochondria against functional depression and disruption produced by endotoxemia or reduction in blood flow, and guards liver cell organelles against ischemia-induced injury (see refs. 48 and 51). Although the exact cytoprotective mechanisms of PGI_2 at the cellular level are still unclear, it has been linked to elevated ATP and cyclic nucleotide levels (35).

EXTRACORPOREAL CIRCULATION

Extracorporeal circulation of blood, with heparin as the only anticoagulant, activates and exhausts platelets, causing a bleeding diasthesis and also thrombosis. Bleeding sometimes suffered after cardiopulmonary bypass and after cerebral microembolization are examples of dreaded complications familiar to clinicians. PGI_2 has been shown to prevent platelet damage, formation of microemboli, and thrombocytopenia frequently associated with these procedures. These effects were demonstrated in hemodialysis, cardiopulmonary bypass, and charcoal hemoperfusion. PGI_2 can safely replace heparin as the sole antithrombotic agent during hemodialysis, but in cardiopulmonary bypass heparin has to be added to prevent consumption of fibrinogen. For a detailed discussion of this subject the reader is referred to recent comprehensive reviews (48,50).

PERIPHERAL ARTERIAL DISEASE

Arteriosclerosis Obliterans and Thromboangiitis Obliterans

When PGI_2 (13,25) was first given (41) to patients with advanced peripheral arterial disease (PAD), a sustained relief of rest pain and healing of ischemic ulcers were noticed. These early observations were confirmed by several (1,19,28,31) but not all (23) investigators, who, with one exception (19), carried out open clinical studies. A recent double-blind trial from Prentice's group (3) has pointed to long-term benefit from intravenous PGI_2 in patients with ischemic rest pain. Rest pain was reduced in all patients 1 day after the infusion; in some patients the effect lasted for over 1 month.

We have recently concluded a random-assignment, placebo-controlled study on treatment of ischemic ulcers with PGI_2 (27). The drug was given in a continuous 72-hr infusion into femoral artery. Thirty nondiabetic patients participating in the study were well-matched for age, sex, type, and localization of disease, rest pain, number and area of ulcers, calf blood flow, and previous sympathectomies. At 6 weeks after the infusion, there was a significant difference in ulcer area between the two groups ($p < 0.02$, unpaired t-test). By this time, mean ulcer area decreased significantly ($p < 0.02$, paired t-test) in the PGI_2-treated group but not in the placebo group. Thus, intraarterial infusion of PGI_2 promoted healing of ischemic ulcers in patients with peripheral arterial disease and without gangrene. If our results could be reproduced in a controlled study using an intravenous route, then more patients with ischemic ulcers refractory to conventional treatment might be expected to profit from the PGI_2 therapy.

The route of administration of PGI_2 might have an effect on the selection of patients. Thus, administration of the drug to femoral artery through a catheter introduced transcutaneously, as in our study, practically eliminates patients with aortoiliac disease, because of lack of feasibility of arterial catheterization. If intravenous infusion of PGI_2 is used, patients with proximal lesions respond more poorly to the therapy than those with distal localization of the disease, affecting vessels below the knee. Such has been our impression based on over 100 patients treated with i.v. PGI_2. No response should be expected in patients with deep black gangrene of the foot or in patients with grossly infected ulcers. Diabetes, in our material, seemed to affect unfavorably the results of the ulcer treatment. Similar experience was reported by Gruss et al. (12), who used 34-day-long intraarterial infusions of PGE_1. On the other hand, Eklund et al. (11), in a study showing significant short- but not long-term effects of PGE_1 on healing of ischemic ulcers, observed good responses in 2 diabetic patients.

High doses of prostaglandins used in treatment of ischemic ulcers may have detrimental effects. This conclusion was reached by Rhodes and Heard (33), who infused PGE_1 at a dose of 21 ng/kg·min. They also pointed to the fact that the worst results with PGI_2 were those of Machin et al. (23), who used the highest dosing regimen.

Raynaud's Disease

Prentice's group (2) has recently confirmed in a controlled study results of previous open observations on the utility of PGI_2 in Raynaud's disease. PGI_2 given as a 5-hr intravenous infusion at weekly intervals for 3 weeks reduced the frequency and duration of ischemic attacks and improved hand temperature measurements. This improvement lasted 6 to 10 weeks. Open clinical trials suggested that PGE_1 can also produce symptomatic improvement by increasing digital perfusion (6,30).

CORONARY HEART DISEASE

Angina Pectoris

Attacks of angina pectoris might occur during an effort or at rest. Accordingly, two forms of angina can be distinguished, with differing mechanisms. Effort angina is precipitated by increased oxygen demand of myocardium. Angina at rest (also referred to as spontaneous angina) is evoked by transient impairment of coronary blood flow, the causes of which are still largely speculative, including vasoconstriction and fluctuating intraluminal obstruction by plugging blood constituents. Spontaneous angina is a syndrome with various etiologies. Their clinical differentiation is difficult, sometimes not feasible. Equivocal results achieved with PGI_2 in angina might be explained by variations in patient selection criteria and in the importance of different mechanisms operating at various stages of the disease (21).

The effects of PGI_2 on effort-induced anginal attacks were studied in patients with coronary arteriosclerosis submitted to atrial pacing. PGI_2 induced distinct changes in hemodynamic parameters and indices of myocardial metabolism (4,43,44). In our patients (44), contrary to those studied by Bergman et al. (4), PGI_2 infusions offered no protection against ischemia, which was precipitated at the same pacing rate. This was in contrast to premedication with nitroglycerin, which prevented anginal pain in all patients. Why is there such a difference between the two drugs? Nitroglycerin reduces hemodynamic effects of angina by dilating capacitance vessels and lowering preload, while PGI_2 acts predominantly on resistance rather than capacitance vessels (46). Nitroglycerin also decreased oxygen demand of myocardium more effectively than PGI_2, as evidenced by its effects on left ventricular filling pressure and cardiac index. We therefore do not expect PGI_2 to be of therapeutic value in effort angina. This view is supported by lack of effects of long-term administration of PGI_2 on tolerance of exercise by patients with effort angina (43).

Spontaneous angina creates more problems. Because of its lack of homogeneity, we chose an approach in which each patient served as self-control. We then studied the effects of PGI_2 on the frequency, duration, and severity of ischemic attacks (42). Twenty-five patients with spontaneous angina who did not respond to 48-hr infusion of placebo received, after a 2-day observation period, 48-hr infusion of PGI_2 at an average rate of 4.0 ng/kg·min. PGI_2 decreased transiently the number of ischemic attacks in only 1 of 4 patients with Prinzmetal angina and was without any effect in 5 other patients whose attacks were associated with increase in heart rate and blood pressure. However, in 11 of 16 patients with coronary atherosclerosis, whose attacks were characterized by ST-segment depression without increase in heart rate or blood pressure and often occurred at night, PGI_2 consistently diminished the frequency of the ischemic episodes. This improvement lasted from 10 days to 3 months.

Thus, in spontaneous angina, selection of patients determines results of the therapy. Angiography in our hands was of no help in differentiating responders from nonresponders. Rarely, a positive effect can be obtained in Prinzmetal angina, as noted already by Chierchia et al. (7), who looked at the effects of PGI_2 only in this particular type of angina. Most of our responders just described had myocardial infarction in the past. Platelets of such subjects are known to display often augmented aggregatory tendency and increased release of thromboxane A_2 during aggregation (26,38). Activation of platelets at the site of endothelial damage could be responsible for symptoms of spontaneous angina in a subset of patients responding favorably to PGI_2.

Myocardial Infarction

There is an experimental evidence that exogenous PGI_2 has a beneficial effect in the acute myocardial infarction; it limits the infarct size and decreases mortality (48). PGI_2 appears to be well tolerated by humans when infused into coronary arteries (15) and by patients with acute myocardial infarction when given intravenously (10,37). These observations led to first controlled clinical trial on PGI_2 in myocardial infarction by Wennmalm's group (18).

Thirty patients with acute myocardial infarction of less than 16 hr duration were randomly allocated to infusion of either PGI_2 or inactive vehicle. The drug was infused at a rate of 4 to 5 ng/kg·min during 72 hr. The mean peak plasma levels of the enzymes did not differ between the patients receiving PGI_2 and the controls. Nonetheless, patients treated with PGI_2 within 10 hr after the onset of symptoms tended to display a lower rise in creatine phosphokinase myocardial isoenzyme MB (CPK-MB) during the first 24 hr of infusion as compared to controls. Furthermore, none of the PGI_2 patients, but 4 in the control group, displayed an extension of the infarct during the course of the infusion. However, follow-up disclosed that 2 patients in the PGI_2 group reinfarcted, compared to none in the control group.

Thus, results of the Swedish study suggest that PGI_2 might have a protective action on myocardium. This protection is limited to the period of infusion. It would therefore be necessary to offer the patient some conceptually related therapy after cessation of PGI_2 administration.

Another approach that merits further investigation is a direct infusion of PGI_2 into coronary vessels. Uchida et al. (47) reported on a successful coronary recanalization induced by intracoronary administration of PGI_2 to 9 patients with acute myocardial infarction.

ISCHEMIC STROKE

Stimulated by favorable results obtained in an open study (14), two controlled clinical trials on use of PGI_2 in ischemic stroke were recently completed (20,24). The trials were carried out in Sheffield and Cracow, according to a similar protocol, and included 24 and 26 patients with acute completed stroke, respectively. Following randomization, PGI_2 or its solvent were given by intravenous infusion at a dose of 2.5 to 5 ng/kg·min over 6 hr, followed by an equal volume of saline for a further 6 hr. This regimen was repeated until five 6-hr courses of PGI_2 (or its solvent) had been given. In Cracow, but not in Sheffield, in patients to whom PGI_2 was administered, a significant alleviation of aphasia and hemiparesis occurred at the end of the PGI_2 infusion period, i.e., 54 hr from the beginning of the treatment. By the end of 2 weeks observation, an improvement in neurological deficit could be detected, although it was not statistically significant in either of the trials.

Thus, two controlled trials did not reveal such a dramatic therapeutic effect of PGI_2 infusions as that reported in the open study (14). Apart from a tendency to spontaneous improvement in the placebo group, another reason could be age difference, since the controlled patients were significantly older than those partic-

TABLE 1. *Miscellaneous cardiovascular conditions in which prostacyclin has been used*

Clinical condition	No. of patients	Route and duration of treatment	Results	Investigators (ref.)
Pulmonary hypertension				
Idiopathic (child)	1	Right atrium, minutes	Pulmonary vasodilatation	Watkins et al. (49)
Persistent fetal circulation	1	Pulmonary artery, hours	Correction of hypoxia	Lock et al. (22)
Mitral stenosis	7	I.V., minutes	Pulmonary vasodilatation	Szczeklik et al. (45)
Pulmonary vascular disease	4	Right atrium, minutes	Fall in pulmonary and systemic pressure	Duadagni et al. (9)
Primary	7	I.V., hours	Pulmonary vasodilatation	Rubin et al. (34)
Central retinal vein occlusion	17	I.V., days	Improvement in visual acuity, regression of lesion in optic fundus in 12 patients	Zygulska-Mach et al. (53)
Congestive heart failure	9	I.V., 1 hr	Improvement in hemodynamic state	Yui et al. (52)
Vascular prosthetic grafting	11	I.V., hours	Decrease in platelet deposition on prosthetic graft surface	Sinzinger et al. (36)

ipating in the open study. Because in one of the trials a significant therapeutic effect of PGI_2 was seen as long as the treatment was continued—i.e., up to 54 hr—the most obvious approach would be to extend courses of PGI_2 infusions for a longer period of time, e.g., up to 2 weeks. Other options would be to use a long-lasting continuous infusion of PGI_2 or to combine it with heparin and indomethacin, as suggested by the results of experimental studies (16). Future controlled studies should bring answers to those problems and should establish the value of PGI_2 therapy in ischemic stroke.

MISCELLANEOUS CARDIOVASCULAR DISORDERS

PGI_2 and its stable analogs have a potential for use in certain clinical situations. These are listed in Table 1 and represent results of open observations, limited to a few patients.

SIDE EFFECTS

Headache is the most common adverse effect, besides facial flushing, experienced by patients receiving PGI_2 infusions. It disappears with reduction in infusion rate. Other side effects include tachycardia, decrease in blood pressure, and articular pains. Less common are restlessness, nausea, and drowsiness. Side effects can be avoided or their intensity reduced if the infusions of PGI_2 are started with a small dose of 1 ng/kg·min, to be increased gradually up to 5 ng/kg·min over a period of a few hours. A detailed review of side effects accompanying PGI_2 has appeared (32).

CONCLUDING REMARKS

Discovery of PGI_2 led to an explosion of scientific investigation, which enormously increased our understanding of the basis of cardiovascular disease. It also helped to bring some new therapeutic approaches a step closer. Several controlled clinical trials with PGI_2 gave encouraging results and defined the value of this therapy in selected diagnostic categories. One of the main problems is to sustain beneficial effects obtained with PGI_2 treatment. This might be achieved in the future by use of optimal regimens of PGI_2 infusion, stable PGI_2 analogs, releasers and potentiators of endogenous PGI_2, thromboxane A_2 (TXA_2) antagonists and TXA_2 synthetase inhibitors, and by combination of PGI_2 therapy with other drugs.

REFERENCES

1. Assal, J. P., Helg, C., Vonder Weld, N., et al. (1980): Prostacyclin perfusions in diabetic peripheral arterial insufficiency. *Diabetologia*, 19:254.
2. Belch, J. J. F., Drury, J. K., Capell, H., Forbes, C. D., Newman, P., McKenzie, F., Leiberman, P., and Prentice, C. R. M. (1983): Intermittent Epoprostenol (prostacyclin) infusion in patients with Raynaud's syndrome. *Lancet*, 1:313–315.
3. Belch, J. J. F., McArdle, B., Pollock, J. G., Forbes, C. D., McKay, A., Leiberman, P., Lowe, G. D. O., and Prentice, C. R. M. (1983): Epoprostenol (prostacyclin) and severe arterial disease. *Lancet*, 1:315–317.

4. Bergman, G., Daly, K., Atkinson, L., Rothman, M., Richardson, P. J., Jackson, G., and Jewitt, D. E. (1981): Prostacyclin: Haemodynamic and metabolic effects in patients with coronary artery disease. *Lancet*, 1:596–598.
5. Carlson, L. A., and Eriksson, I. (1973): Femoral artery infusion of prostaglandin E_1 in severe peripheral vascular disease. *Lancet*, 1:155.
6. Clifford, P. C., Martin, M. F. R., Sheldon, E. J., Kirby, J. D., Baird, R. N., and Dieppe, P. A. (1980): Treatment of vasospastic disease with prostaglandin E_1. *Br. Med. J.*, 281:1031–1034.
7. Chierchia, S., Patrono, C., Ciabattoni, G., De Caterina, R., Cinotti, G. A., Distante, A., and Maseri, A. (1982): Effect of intravenous prostacyclin in variant angina. *Circulation*, 65:470–477.
8. Dembińska-Kieć, A., Kostka-Trąbka, E., and Gryglewski, R. J. (1982): Effect of prostacyclin on fibrinolytic activity in patients with arteriosclerosis obliterans. *Thromb. Haemostas.*, 47:190.
9. Duadagni, D. N., Ikram, H., and Maslowski, R. (1981): Haemodynamic effects of prostacyclin (PGI_2) in pulmonary hypertension. *Br. Heart J.*, 45:385–388.
10. Edhog, O., Henriksson, P., and Wennmalm, A. (1983): Prostacyclin infusion in patients with acute myocardial infarction (preliminary report). *N. Engl. J. Med.*, 308:1032–1033.
11. Eklund, A. E., Eriksson, G., and Olsson, A. G. (1982): A controlled study showing significant short term effect of prostaglandin E_1 in healing of ischemic ulcers of the lower limb in man. *Prostaglandin Leukotriene Med.*, 8:265–271.
12. Gruss, J. D., Bartels, D., Ohta, T., Machado, J. L., and Schlechtweg, B. (1982): Conservative treatment of inoperable arterial occlusions of the lower extremities with intraarterial prostaglandin E_1. *Br. J. Surg.*, 69:S11–S13.
13. Gryglewski, R. J., Bunting, S., Moncada, S., Flower, R. J., and Vane, J. R. (1976): Arterial walls are protected against deposition of platelet thrombi by a substance (prostaglandin X) which they make from prostaglandin endoperoxides. *Prostaglandins*, 12:685–713.
14. Gryglewski, R. J., Nowak, S., Kostka-Trąbka, E., Kuśmiderski, J., Dembińska-Kieć, A., Bieroń, K., Basista, M., and Błaszczyk, B. (1983): Treatment of ischemic stroke with prostacyclin. *Stroke*, 14:197–202.
15. Hall, R. J., and Dewar, H. A. (1981): Safety of coronary arterial prostacyclin infusion (letter). *Lancet*, 1:949.
16. Hallenbeck, J. M., Leith, D. R., Dutka, A. J., and Greenbaum, L. J. Jr. (1982): PGI_2, indomethacin and heparin promote post-ischemic neuronal recovery in dogs administered therapeutically. In: *Prostaglandins in Clinical Medicine*, edited by K. K. Wu and E. C. Rossi, pp. 335–341. Year Book Medical, Chicago.
17. Hellström, H. R. (1983): Epoprostenol and severe arterial disease. *Lancet*, 1:712.
18. Henriksson, P., Edhog, O., and Wennmalm, A. (1984): Limitation of myocardial infarction with prostacyclin—A double-blind study. In: *Prostacyclin. Clinical Trials*, edited by R. J. Gryglewski, J. McGiff, and A. Szczeklik. Raven Press, New York.
19. Hossman, V., Heinen, A., Auel, H., et al. (1981): A randomized placebo-controlled trial of prostacyclin (PGI_2) in peripheral arterial disease. *Thromb. Res.*, 22:481–490.
20. Huczyński, J., Kostka-Trąbka, E., Sołowska, W., Bieroń, K., Grodzińska, L., Dembińska-Kieć, A., Pykosz-Mazur, E., Pęczek, E., and Gryglewski, R. J. (1984): Prostacyclin in patients with completed ischemic stroke—A controlled trial. In: *Prostacyclin. Clinical Trials*, edited by R. J. Gryglewski, A. Szczeklik, and J. McGiff. Raven Press, New York.
21. Linet, O. (1982): Prostacyclin. A review of clinical experience. *Postgrad. Med.*, 72:105–120.
22. Lock, J. E., Olley, P. M., Coceani, F., et al. (1979): Use of prostacyclin in persistent fetal circulation (Letter). *Lancet*, 1:1343.
23. Machin, S. J., Defreyn, G., Chamone, D. A., and Vermylen, J. (1981): Clinical infusions of prostacyclin in advanced arterial disease. In: *Clinical Pharmacology of Prostacyclin*, edited by P. J. Lewis and J. M. O'Grady, p. 173. Raven Press, New York.
24. Martin, J. F., Hamdy, N. A. T., Nicholl, J., Lewatas, N., Bergvall, U., Owen, P., Whittington, D., and Holryhod, M. (1984): Interim results from a double-blind controlled trial of prostacyclin in cerebral infarction. In: *Prostacyclin. Clinical Trials*, edited by J. R. Gryglewski, J. McGiff, and A. Szczeklik. Raven Press, New York.
25. Moncada, S., Gryglewski, R. J., Bunting, S., and Vane, J. R. (1976): A lipid peroxide inhibits the enzyme in blood vessel microsomes that generates from prostaglandin endoperoxides the substance (prostaglandin X) which prevents platelet aggregation. *Prostaglandins*, 12:715–733.
26. Neri Serneri, G. G. (1982): Prostaglandins in patients with ischemic heart disease. In: *Cardiovas-*

cular Pharmacology of the Prostaglandins, edited by A. G. Herman, P. M. Vanhoutte, H. Denolin, and A. Goossens, pp. 361–374. Raven Press, New York.

27. Nizankowski, R., Kròlikowski, W., Bielatowicz, J., Schaller, J., and Szczeklik, A. (1985): Prostacyclin for ischemic ulcers in peripheral arterial disease. A random assignment, placebo-controlled study. In: *Prostacyclin. Clinical Trials*, edited by R. J. Gryglewski, J. McGiff, and A. Szczeklik. Raven Press, New York.

28. Olsson, A. G. (1980): Intravenous prostacyclin for ischaemic ulcers in peripheral artery disease (letter). *Lancet*, 2:1076.

29. Olsson, A. G. (1984): Clinical uses of prostaglandins in cardiovascular disease. In: *Atherosclerosis*, edited by N. E. Miller, pp. 91–104. Raven Press, New York.

30. Pardy, B. J., Hoare, M. C., Eastcott, H. H. G., Campbell, C. M., and Ellis, B. W. (1982): Prostaglandin E_1 in severe Raynaud's phenomenon. *Surgery*, 92:953–965.

31. Pardy, B. J., Lewis, J. D., and Eastcott, H. H. G. (1981): Preliminary experience with prostaglandin E_1 and I_2 in peripheral vascular disease. *Surgery*, 88:826–832.

32. Pickles, H., and O'Grady, J. (1982): Side effects occurring during administration of epoprostenol (prostacyclin, PGI_2) in man. *Br. J. Clin. Pharmacol.*, 14:177–185.

33. Rhodes, R. S., and Heard, S. E. (1983): Detrimental effect of high-dose prostaglandin E_1 in the treatment of ischemic ulcers. *Surgery*, 93:839–842.

34. Rubin, L. J., Groves, B. M., Reeves, J. T., Frosolono, M., Hendel, F., and Cato, A. (1982): Prostacyclin-induced acute pulmonary vasodilatation in primary pulmonary hypertension. *Circulation*, 66:334–338.

35. Sikujara, O., Monden, H., Toyoshima, K., Okamura, J., and Kosaki, G. (1983): Cytoprotective effect of prostaglandin I_2 on ischemia-induced hepatic cell injury. *Transplantation*, 36:238–243.

36. Sinzinger, H., O'Grady, J., Cromwell, M., and Hofer, R. (1983): Epoprostenol (prostacyclin) decreases platelet deposition on vascular prosthetic grafts. *Lancet*, 1:1275–76.

37. Szczeklik, A., and Gryglewski, R. J. (1982): Prostaglandins as therapeutic agents in cardiovascular disease. In: *Cardiovascular Pharmacology of the Prostaglandins*, edited by A. G. Herman, P. M. Vanhoutte, H. Denolin, and A. Goossens, pp. 347–359. Raven Press, New York.

38. Szczeklik, A., Gryglewski, R. J., Musiał, J., Grodzińska, L., Serwońska, M., and Marcinkiewicz, E. (1978): Thromboxane generation and platelet aggregation in survivals of myocardial infarction. *Thromb. Haemostas.*, 40:66–74.

39. Szczeklik, A., Gryglewski, R. J., Nizankowski, R., Musiał, J., Piętoń, R., and Mruk, J. (1978): Circulatory and anti-platelet effects of intravenous prostacyclin in healthy men. *Pharmacol. Res. Commun.*, 10:545–556.

40. Szczeklik, A., Kopeć, M., Sładek, K., Musiał, J., Chmielewska, J., Teisseyre, E., Dudek-Wojciechowska, G., and Palester-Chlebowczyk, M. (1983): Prostacyclin and the fibrinolytic system in ischemic vascular disease. *Thromb. Res.*, 29:655–660.

41. Szczeklik, A., Nizankowski, R., Skawiński, S., Szczeklik, J., Gluszko, P., and Gryglewski, R. J. (1979): Successful therapy of advanced arteriosclerosis obliterans with prostacyclin. *Lancet*, 1:1111–1114.

42. Szczeklik, A., Nizankowski, R., Szczeklik, J., Tabeau, J., and Kròlikowski, W. (1984): Prostacyclin therapy in subgroups of patients with spontaneous angina. In: *Prostacyclin. Clinical Trials*, edited by R. J. Gryglewski, A. Szczeklik, and J. McGiff. Raven Press, New York.

43. Szczeklik, A., Szczeklik, J., and Nizankowski, R. (1981): Prostacyclin, nitroglycerin and effort angina (letter). *Lancet*, 1:1006.

44. Szczeklik, A., Szczeklik, J., Nizakowski, R., and Głuszko, P. (1980): Prostacyclin for acute coronary insufficiency. *Artery*, 8:7–11.

45. Szczeklik, J., Szczeklik, A., and Nizankowski, R. (1980): Prostacyclin for pulmonary hypertension (letter). *Lancet*, 2:1076.

46. Szczeklik, J., Szczeklik, A., and Nizankowski, R. (1980): Haemodynamic changes induced by prostacyclin in man. *Br. Heart J.*, 44:254–258.

47. Uchida, Y., Hanai, T., Hasegawa, K., Kawamura, K., and Oshima, T. (1982): Coronary recanalization induced by intracoronary administration of prostacyclin in patients with acute myocardial infarction. *Circulation (Abstr.)*, 66(part II):1045.

48. Vane, J. R. (1983): Prostaglandins and the cardiovascular system. *Br. Heart J.*, 49:405–409.

49. Watkins, W. D., Peterson, M. B., Crone, R. K., Shandon, D. C., and Levine, L. (1980): Prostacyclin and prostaglandin E_1 for severe idiopathic pulmonary artery hypertension (letter). *Lancet*, 1:1083.

50. Weston, M. J. (1983): Prostacyclin and extracorporeal circulation. *Br. Med. Bull.*, 39:285–288.
51. Whittle, B. J., and Moncada, S. (1983): Pharmacology of prostacyclin and thromboxanes. *Br. Med. Bull.*, 39:232–238.
52. Yui, Y., Nakajima, H., Kawai, C., and Murakami, T. (1982): Prostacyclin therapy in patients with congestive heart failure. *Am. J. Cardiol.*, 50:320–324.
53. Zygulska-Mach, H., Kostka-Trąbka, E., Grodzińska, L., Bieroń, K., Telesz, E., and Gryglewski, R. (1984): Prostacyclin in therapy of central retinal vein occlusion. In: *Prostacyclin. Clinical Trials*, edited by R. J. Gryglewski, A. Szczeklik, and J. McGiff. Raven Press, New York.

Advances in Prostaglandin, Thromboxane, and
Leukotriene Research, Vol. 13, edited by G. G. Neri
Serneri, et al. Raven Press, New York © 1985.

Hemodynamic Changes During Intraarterial Administration of Prostaglandin E₁ in Healthy Subjects

Thomas Brecht and Meltem Eryilmaz-Ayaz

Medical Department, University Hospital, Bonn, Federal Republic of Germany

Prostaglandins have played a continuously increasing role in the field of angiology, particularly in the treatment of arterial occlusive diseases (1,3,4). They have been administered in two different ways for therapeutic purposes. One application was a relatively short-lasting intravenous infusion for 72 to 96 hr, which should lead to healing of trophic lesions, after about 6 to 8 weeks (1). The other application was a long-lasting intraarterial infusion, started by Seki in Japan and continued by Gruss (3) in Europe, who called it the "permanent intraarterial prostaglandin perfusion" (PIPP). Gruss treated patients with inoperable arterial occlusive diseases in stage IV and was successful in avoiding amputation in 47% (1). He inserted an intraarterial catheter into the femoral artery and infused prostaglandin (PG) E_1 in a dosage between 0.1 and 0.2 ng/kg body weight·min using a special infusion pump.

It is not quite clear how to understand the reported therapeutic effects. There is certainly a metabolic effect concerning the platelets and their functions, but in addition a hemodynamic effect should be expected, because PGE_1 is a well-known potent vasodilator, too. Yet only few investigations concerning this problem are known (2). Therefore, we considered it to be of importance to register the hemodynamic effects of intraarterially administered PGE_1 in increasing doses in healthy subjects and to compare these results with the hemodynamic changes during the application of another potent vasodilator with short half-life. For this purpose we used a mixture of nucleotides and nucleosides (NNG), which is a well proven drug in the intraarterial treatment of patients with arteriopathy.

We studied 4 men and 1 woman who had given informed consent. They were physically examined and showed no pathologic findings in laboratory examinations (red and white cell blood count, thrombocytes, electrolytes, transaminases, creatinine, and blood sugar), and they had normal findings in the electrocardiogram and chest X-ray. Two weeks later, these examinations were repeated. In no case were any characteristic changes observed.

For recording the arterial blood pressure, we punctured the brachial artery with a Vigon cannula, and the blood pressure was continuously registered by a Statham strain gauge element P 23 dB. The heart rate was taken from the electrocardiogram. The blood flow volumes of both the lower extremities were analyzed by mercury-in-rubber strain gauges of a venous occlusion plethysmograph (Periquant 2000). The mean values of five single measurements were calculated. The cardiac output was measured with impedance cardiography, using a Minnesota 304 B, also calculated as the average of five single values.

Investigation was started after the subject had rested for 30 min. The values recorded 30, 20, 10, and 0 min before the medication started were defined as 100%. All changings are given in percentages of these values.

For the intraarterial application of the drugs, we punctured one femoral artery with a Vigon cannula and used for the infusion an electrically driven pump. First we infused NNG in routine therapeutic doses, corresponding to 0.6 mg ATP/min during a period of 10 min. After that we gave a 10-min period of infusion of physiological saline. Then we started PGE_1, first in a dosage of 10 ng/min for 10 min, then increasing the dosage stepwise at 5 ng/min up to the last phase, when 37.5 ng/min was administered. This dosage corresponds to an average of 0.5 ng/min·kg for a person of 75 kg body weight.

All subjects tolerated all the dosages very well, without any complaints and without any side effects.

Among the recorded parameters (Fig. 1), the cardiac output showed an increase during the application of NNG, reversible during administration of physiologic saline. After that there were no more impressive changes of the cardiac output, which stayed around the 100% level. A tendency to increase was not of statistic significance.

The functional mean arterial blood pressure of the brachial artery—calculated by the formula of Wezler and Sinn (5)—stayed almost constant and showed no characteristic deviation during the duration of the experiment. Heart rate initially increased slightly for about 10%; later, it became regressive and stayed stable for the duration of the PGE application.

The blood flow volumes of the legs showed a different behavior: during the application of NNG, flow volume of the treated leg increased to almost 400%. This deviation regressed during infusion of physiologic saline. The flow volume of the contralateral extremity remained unchanged. Under the application of PGE_1, initially no characteristic alteration of the flow volume was observed. Starting with 20 ng/min, an increase was seen, remaining a significant trend up to the highest dosage. However, this increase of flow volume never reached the extension of the increase during ATP. Blood flow volume of the untreated extremity stayed unchanged around the 100% level. Interestingly, however, it showed physiological deviations that are much less pronounced, but quite similar to the deviations of the increasing flow volume of the treated leg.

These results suggest that NNG induces a tremendous increase of blood flow volume, abolishing all the regulating mechanisms by a maximum vasodilation. PGE_1 given in the chosen relatively low dosages produces a much less pronounced increase of the flow volume but without removing the regulating mechanisms, only

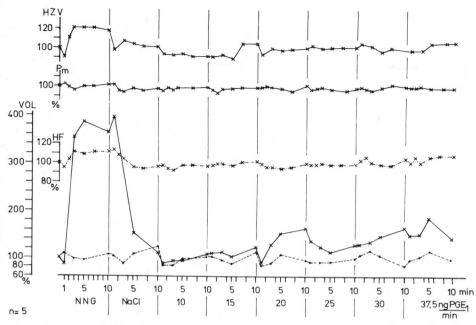

FIG. 1. Percent deviation of cardiac output (HZV), arterial functional mean pressure of the brachial artery (P_m), heart rate (HF), and blood flow volume (VOL) of the treated extremity *(solid line)* and the untreated contralateral extremity *(dashed line).*

lifting them to a slightly higher level. The chosen dosages of PGE_1 as they are used for therapeutic purposes do not change the hemodynamic parameters in an impressive manner. Thus, the increase of blood flow volumes does not change the cardiac parameters. The intraarterial application of ATP produces a marked increase of flow volume by totally reducing the regional vascular resistance, provoking an increase of cardiac output and heart rate without lowering of the systemic arterial blood pressure.

Finally, we conclude that therapeutic effects of PGE_1 in arterial occlusive disease are due more to other sites of action than to hemodynamic effects.

REFERENCES

1. Belch, F. J., McArdle, B., Pollock, J. G., Forbes, C. D., McKay, A., Leibermann, P., Lowe, G. D. O., and Prentice, C. R. M. (1983): Epoprostenol (prostacyclin) and severe arterial disease. *Lancet*, I:315.
2. Fletcher, J. R., and Ramwell, P. W. (1979): Comparison of the cardiovascular effects of prostacyclin with those of prostaglandin E_2 in the rhesus monkey. In: *Prostacyclin*, edited by J. R. Vane and S. Bergström, p. 259. Raven Press, New York.
3. Gruss, J. D., Vargas-Montano, H., Simmenroth, H., Bartels, D., Sakurai, T., and Schaefer, G. (1983): Treatment of the inoperable arterial occlusive disease in stage IV with prostaglandin E_1. XIIIth World Congress of the International Union of Angiology, Abstracts.
4. Sinzinger, H., and Silberbauer, K. (1981): Zum gegenwärtigen stand der prostacyclin-story für die klinik. *VASA*, 10:70.
5. Wezler, K., and Sinn, W. (1963): Das Strömungsgesetz des Blutkreislaufs. Cantor, Aulendorf/ Württemberg.

Advances in Prostaglandin, Thromboxane, and Leukotriene Research, Vol. 13, edited by G. G. Neri Serneri, et al. Raven Press, New York © 1985.

Platelet Responses Observed During and After Infusions of the Prostacyclin Analog ZK 36 374

D. A. Yardumian, I. J. Mackie, H. Bull, and S. J. Machin

Departments of Haematology, Middlesex Hospital and University College Hospital, London, England

The routine clinical use of prostacyclin has been limited by its instability, brevity of action, and unpleasant clinical side effects. Also, some workers (2) have reported a further adverse effect associated with its use: that of rebound platelet hyperactivity following the initial platelet inhibition during and after prolonged infusions, as indicated by platelet release proteins, *ex vivo* aggregability, and platelet count.

A chemically and metabolically more stable analog of prostacyclin, a carbacyclin derivative called ZK 36 374 (Schering A.G.), has recently been developed. This retains the biological properties of native prostacyclin, but has been reported (1) to be more potent as an antiplatelet agent while inducing less vasodilatation and thus fewer adverse clinical side effects.

We wish to report some observations we have made of platelet function during and after infusions of this analog.

VOLUNTEER STUDY

Six healthy male volunteers received a 2-hr infusion of ZK 36 374. An initial baseline blood sample, I, was taken and the infusion commenced through a peripheral venous cannula. The infusion rate was 0.5 ng/kg·min for the first 30 min, increasing to 1.0 ng/kg·min for the second 30 min. A second venous sample, II, was then taken. For the final hour of infusion, the administration rate was increased to 2.0 ng/kg·min; at the end of this time another sample, III, was taken and the infusion was discontinued. Further venous samples were taken at 10, 20, 60, and 120 min after the end of the infusion (samples IV to VII, respectively).

We found no significant changes in platelet count or other blood counts during the infusion or up to 2 hr after its completion. On each of the seven samples from each volunteer, platelet aggregation responses to ADP and collagen were studied. Figure 1 illustrates these in a typical volunteer. The samples taken after 1 and 2 hr of infusion, II and III, show a dose-dependent inhibition of response to both agonists. The 10- and 20-min postinfusion samples show progressive return toward

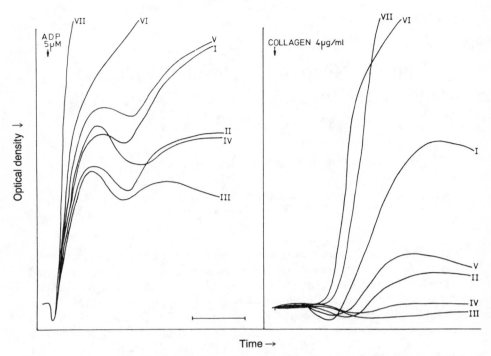

Time →

FIG. 1. Platelet aggregation responses to ADP and collagen, in a typical volunteer. Bar indicates 1 min. Sample numbers I–VII are described in text.

the baseline. However, we observed rebound platelet hyperaggregability in these volunteers after ZK 36 374 infusion, shown here as increased aggregation response in VI and VII as compared to I. The effect was seen in each subject; in 5 subjects it was evident 1 to 2 hr postinfusion (7–46% increase above the baseline response to ADP at 1 μM). In the sixth, the drug's inhibitory action remained until 2 hr after the infusion, but a later (4-hr) sample showed marked rebound hyperaggregability (77%).

PERIPHERAL ARTERIAL DISEASE STUDY

We are also conducting a study of tolerability and efficacy of ZK 36 374 in patients with peripheral arterial disease and stable claudication. These patients attend every 2 weeks for four visits, and receive a 5-hr infusion of placebo or drug at doses of 0.5, 1.0, or 2.0 ng/kg·min, in randomized order so that each patient receives each infusion. A venous sample is taken for tests (including platelet aggregation studies) before the infusion, at the end of the 5 hr, and 1 hr postinfusion on each occasion. We have defined significant hyperaggregability as an increase of response in this postinfusion sample of 50% or more above the preinfusion response.

Of the 14 patients who have to date completed the protocol, we have seen such an effect in 7 following infusion of active drug, and in 1 following placebo.

PLATELET FUNCTION DURING PROLONGED INFUSION

We wish to report the platelet responses occurring in 1 patient who received a prolonged continuous infusion of ZK 36 374. This man, a 64-year-old with systemic sclerosis, was admitted because of acute digital ischaemia with incipient gangrene and intractable pain in three fingers. He first received a 9-day infusion of the drug, as shown in Fig. 2, at a starting rate of 0.5 ng/kg·min, increasing to a final rate of 3.5 ng/kg·min. After a 3-day interval, he then received a daily 5-hr infusion of ZK 36 374 for 5 days. Apart from a headache and generalized flushing at the highest dose (4.5 ng/kg·min), he experienced no adverse effects throughout; in particular, there were no cardiovascular disturbances. The patient derived considerable clinical benefit from the treatment: pain relief was effective within 24 hr of

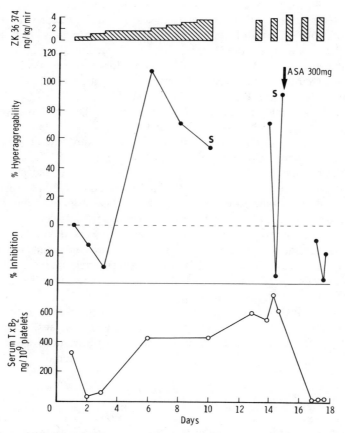

FIG. 2. Platelet responses to infusions of ZK 36 374. **Top:** percent change in maximum aggregation response to ADP at 1 μM, compared to the preinfusion aggregation response. S = spontaneous platelet aggregation. **Bottom:** serum thromboxane B_2 (ng/10^9 platelets).

starting the infusion and remained so until his discharge from hospital 2 weeks after the final infusion.

There were no significant changes in blood count or platelet count throughout. However, there was evidence of decreasing platelet sensitivity to ZK 36 374 from day 3 of treatment. *In vitro* inhibition of platelet aggregation by exogenous ZK 36 374 was studied serially during the infusion. Before the infusion, addition of the drug at 2 ng/ml to platelet-rich plasma prior to the addition of ADP at 5 μM abolished the response (100% inhibition), whereas on day 6 it inhibited the response by only 85% and on day 10 by 38%. *In vitro* platelet sensitivity was restored after the treatment-free 3 days, and did not alter significantly thereafter during the period of interrupted infusions. This falling sensitivity of the platelets to ZK 36 374 was reflected by *ex vivo* aggregation. Initially there was inhibition of response, shown in Fig. 2 for ADP 1 μM, but from day 6 onward the platelets became hyperaggregable, culminating in spontaneous *in vitro* aggregation on the final day of this infusion. Serum thromboxane B_2 levels measured simultaneously were initially reduced, but rose significantly above preinfusion levels as aggregability increased. With platelet sensitivity restored after the interval in treatment, effective inhibition was again seen at the end of each 5-hr infusion. However, a marked postinfusion rebound occurred on day 14, and spontaneous aggregation was again seen in the 1-hr postinfusion sample. Because of the potential clinical risks of such hyperaggregability, the patient received aspirin at 300 mg on day 15. On day 17, 48 hr later, the sample taken 1 hr postinfusion showed only some continued suppression of platelet activity, with no rebound effect. The serum thromboxane B_2 level was very low at this time, following aspirin ingestion.

In conclusion, therefore, we have seen some degree of rebound platelet hyperaggregability after short infusions of ZK 36 374 in both volunteers and patients with arterial disease, with some variability in the time of its occurrence postinfusion. We have seen a similar effect during one prolonged infusion.

The mechanism of this phenomenon has not yet been worked out: it may represent a resetting of the balance in anti- and proaggregatory prostaglandins, resulting from weighing the prostacyclin side of the balance. Alternatively, perhaps there is prolonged occupation of receptor sites by the drug, such that further drug or native prostacyclin is unable to exert an effect.

We wish to stress that similar observations have been made during and after infusions of prostacyclin, so the problem is not unique to this analog, and that the laboratory observations reported have not on any occasion been associated with adverse clinical effects.

REFERENCES

1. Schror, K., Ohlendorf, R., and Darius, H. (1981): Beneficial effects of a new carbacyclin derivative, ZK 36 374 in acute myocardial ischaemia. *J. Pharmacol. Exp. Ther.*, 219:243–249.
2. Sinzinger, H., Horsch, A. K., and Silberbauer, K. (1983): The behaviour of various platelet function tests during long term prostacyclin infusion in patients with peripheral vascular disease. *Thromb. Haemostas,*, 50(4):885–887.

Advances in Prostaglandin, Thromboxane, and
Leukotriene Research, Vol. 13, edited by G.G. Neri
Serneri, et al. Raven Press, New York © 1985.

Control of Human and Animal Platelet Aggregation by a New Prostacyclin Analog

P. Maderna, S. Colli, C. Sirtori, E. Tremoli, and R. Paoletti

Institute of Pharmacology and Pharmacognosy, University of Milan, Milan, Italy

The *in vitro* effects of ZK 36 374, a new chemically stable prostacyclin (PGI_2) analog, on platelet aggregation were studied and compared to those of PGI_2. Significantly lower concentrations of ZK 36 374, versus prostacyclin, were required to inhibit collagen and epinephrine-induced aggregation in human platelet-rich plasma. In contrast, in rat and rabbit platelet rich plasma, PGI_2 was more effective than ZK 36 374 in inhibiting the aggregation elicited by ADP and collagen.

It is concluded that ZK 36 374 is a potent antiaggregatory compound and may be useful in the prevention of cardiovascular disorders.

INTRODUCTION

PGI_2 is the major product of arachidonic acid metabolism via cyclooxygenase in the vessel wall. PGI_2 is both a potent vasodilator and an inhibitor of platelet aggregation *in vitro* (10,16) and *in vivo* (2). PGI_2 inhibits platelet aggregation by interacting with specific receptors (13) and by increasing intracellular cAMP concentrations (7).

Arachidonic acid metabolism in the platelets, via the cyclooxygenase pathway, leads to the formation of thromboxane A_2, a vasoconstrictor and a strong inducer of platelet aggregation (8). Deficiency of PGI_2 formation and/or increase of thromboxane A_2 production may result in pathological states associated to high risk of thrombotic disease. PGI_2 has been recently proposed as a potential therapeutic agent, because of its powerful effect on platelets and on the vascular endothelium, in the treatment of acute and chronic occlusive arterial disease (3,9,15).

A major problem affecting the potential therapeutic value of PGI_2 is the chemical instability of the compound in aqueous solution at physiological pH (11). PGI_2 is rapidly converted to stable but inactive metabolites *in vivo* (14,18). The half-life in blood is, in fact, in the range of a few minutes.

Among the many semisynthetic PGI_2 analogs possessing chemical stability and selectivity against platelet receptors (1,17), the 5-*(E)*-(1*S*,5*S*,6*R*,7*R*)-7-hydroxy-6-*(E)*-(3*S*,4*RS*)-3-hydroxy-4-methyl-oct-1-en-6-yn-yl-bicyclo 3.3.0-octan-3-yliden-pentanoic acid (ZK 36 374) is chemically and metabolically stable and shows a pharmacological profile similar to PGI_2 (5,12).

The aim of this study was to compare *in vitro* the effects of ZK 36 374 and PGI$_2$ on platelet aggregation in humans and experimental animals. The antiaggregatory activity of the two compounds was evaluated by measuring the concentrations required to produce a 50% inhibition of platelet aggregation induced by ADP, collagen, and epinephrine.

MATERIALS AND METHODS

Platelets were collected from healthy human volunteers, who had not taken any drugs known to interfere with platelet function for at least 10 days before the test.

For the animal studies, male Charles River rats (200–250 g) were anesthetized with ether, and blood was collected by cardiac puncture. New Zealand rabbits (3–3.5 kg) were anesthetized (Na thiopenthal at 35 mg/kg) and blood was taken from the carotid artery. Blood was collected in plastic tubes containing 3.8% trisodium citrate (1 volume: 9 volumes blood). Platelet-rich plasma (PRP) was obtained after centrifugation at 150 g for 18 min at room temperature. Platelet-poor plasma (PPP) was prepared by a further centrifugation at 650 g.

Platelet aggregation was performed using the Born turbidimetric technique (Born, 1962) at 37°C in an Elvi aggregometer (Elvi Logos, Milan, Italy). Human platelet studies were carried out at a constant platelet number (3×10^8/ml). Rat and rabbit PRP counts were adjusted to 5×10^8 platelets/ml using autologous PPP. ADP (Sigma Co., St. Louis, Mo.), collagen (Hormon Chemie, Munich), and epinephrine (ISM) were used as aggregating agents.

To obtain comparable aggregation tracings, the concentration of each agent giving the maximal aggregatory response was selected: collagen 1 μg/ml and epinephrine 1.4 μM for human PRP; collagen 4 μg/ml and ADP 4 μM for rat PRP; collagen 4 μg/ml for rabbit PRP.

Synthetic PGI$_2$ sodium salt, a kind gift from Dr. C. Gandolfi, Farmitalia Carlo Erba, Italy, was dissolved in ethanol at 1 mM and stored at $-20°C$.

ZK 36 374 (Schering AG, Berlin) was dissolved in sterile physiological saline at 1.4 mM. Further dilutions were freshly made with Tris-HCl 50 mM (pH 7.4) and kept on crushed ice during the tests.

Different concentrations of PGI$_2$ or ZK 36 374 were incubated with PRP samples for 1 min before the addition of each aggregating agent. The concentration giving 50% inhibition (IC$_{50}$) of aggregation was calculated by plotting the percentage of inhibition of platelet aggregation versus the corresponding concentrations of the inhibitor. The percentage of inhibition was calculated on the basis of the amplitude of the aggregation curve at 3 min after the addition of ADP and collagen and at 5 min after the addition of epinephrine.

Statistical analysis of the results was carried out using Student's *t*-test for paired data.

RESULTS

Effects of ZK 36 374 on Human Platelet Aggregation

ZK 36 374 at concentrations ranging between 0.1 and 1×10^{-8} M dose-dependently inhibited platelet aggregation in human PRP stimulated with collagen at 1 μg/ml and epinephrine at 1.4 μM. The mean concentration of ZK 36 374 required to completely inhibit collagen-induced aggregation was 0.5×10^{-8} M; in the case of PGI_2, a 100% inhibition of platelet aggregation was achieved at 1×10^{-8} M (Fig. 1).

Figure 2 shows the regression curves obtained by plotting PGI_2 and ZK 36 374 concentrations versus percent inhibition of the aggregation.

The mean IC_{50} for both compounds are shown in Table 1. Significantly lower concentrations of ZK 36 374 were required to inhibit 50% of the aggregation induced by fixed concentrations of collagen and epinephrine, in comparison with PGI_2.

Effects of ZK 36 374 on Rat and Rabbit Platelet Aggregation

Higher concentrations of ZK 36 374 were necessary to obtain an inhibition comparable to PGI_2 in rat PRP stimulated by collagen and ADP (Fig. 3). The IC_{50} values for ZK 36 374 were higher than those of PGI_2 (Table 2), suggesting a reduced antiaggregatory potency of ZK 36 374 compared to PGI_2.

Similar results were obtained with rabbit PRP. Again, a relatively higher concentration of ZK 36 374, in comparison to PGI_2, was necessary to completely inhibit the aggregation induced by collagen. The 100% inhibition of platelet aggre-

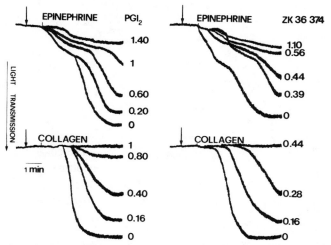

FIG. 1. Effect of ZK 36 374 and PGI_2 ($\times 10^{-8}$ M) on platelet aggregation induced by collagen (1 μg/ml) and epinephrine (1.4 μM). The *arrows* indicate the addition of the inhibitors.

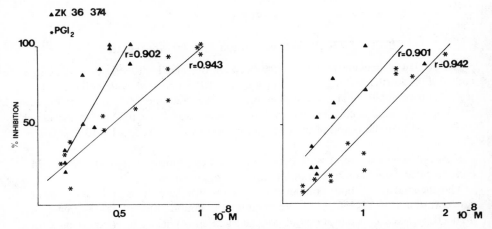

FIG. 2. Dose–response curves obtained by plotting PGI_2 and ZK 36 374 concentrations versus percent inhibition of human PRP aggregation induced by collagen **(left)** and epinephrine **(right)**.

TABLE 1. *Effect of ZK 36 374 and PGI_2 on platelet aggregation in human PRP[a]*

Parameter	Collagen	Epinephrine
PGI_2	$0.49 \pm 0.02 \times 10^{-8}$	$1.06 \pm 0.07 \times 10^{-8}$
ZK 36 374	$0.31 \pm 0.03 \times 10^{-8}$	$0.62 \pm 0.09 \times 10^{-8}$
Significance	$p < 0.01$	$p < 0.02$

[a]The results are IC_{50} expressed as moles/liter, mean $\pm$ SEM, $n = 3$.

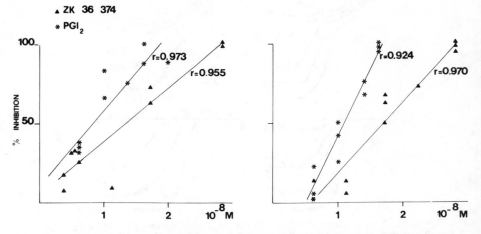

FIG. 3. Dose–response curves obtained by plotting PGI_2 and ZK 36 374 concentrations versus percent inhibition of rat PRP aggregation induced by ADP **(left)** and collagen **(right)**.

TABLE 2. *Effect of ZK 36 374 and PGI₂ on platelet aggregation in rat PRP[a]*

Parameter	ADP	Collagen
PGI$_2$	$0.83 \pm 0.10 \times 10^{-8}$	$1.02 \pm 0.04 \times 10^{-8}$
ZK 36 374	$1.26 \pm 0.22 \times 10^{-8}$	$1.54 \pm 0.14 \times 10^{-8}$
Significance	Not significant	$p < 0.025$

[a]The results are IC$_{50}$ expressed as moles/liter, mean $\pm$ SEM, $n = 3$.

gation was achieved with a 3.36×10^{-8} M ZK 36 374 and with only 2.13×10^{-8} M PGI$_2$ (Fig. 4).

The mean IC$_{50}$ for ZK 36 374 was significantly higher than PGI$_2$, being $1.74 \pm 0.06 \times 10^{-8}$ M and $0.99 \pm 0.13 \times 10^{-8}$ M ($p < 0.01$), respectively.

DISCUSSION

The results of the present study show that ZK 36 374, a chemically stable semisynthetic analog of PGI$_2$, is a potent inhibitor of platelet aggregation elicited by various agents. The inhibitory potency of ZK 36 374 is different in the three studied species. In human PRP, significantly lower concentrations of ZK 36 374, in comparison with PGI$_2$, are required to obtain a 50% inhibition of the aggregation induced by collagen and epinephrine. ZK 36 374 seems to be twice as potent than PGI$_2$, confirming previous results on aggregation induced by ADP in human platelets (4). In contrast, in rat and rabbit PRP, PGI$_2$ is more active than ZK 36 374.

PGI$_2$ at pharmacological doses is a potent platelet antiaggregatory compound and a powerful vasodilator. Its clinical application in diseases associated with increased platelet consumption and/or with atherosclerosis appears to be compli-

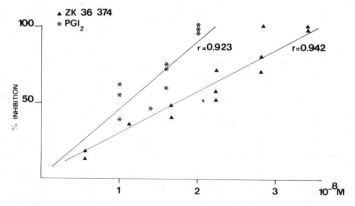

FIG. 4. Dose–response curves obtained by plotting PGI$_2$ and ZK 36 374 concentrations versus percent inhibition of rabbit PRP aggregation induced by collagen.

cated by undesired effects on blood pressure (6). Schrör et al. (12) demonstrated in the cat that the antiplatelet and the blood pressure lowering actions of ZK 36 374 may be dissociated. In addition, ZK 36 374, differently from PGI_2, is chemically and metabolically stable.

In conclusion, this *in vitro* study shows that ZK 36 374 is more potent than PGI_2 in inhibiting human platelet aggregation induced by collagen and epinephrine. It has been hypothesized that the mechanism of action of ZK 36 374 is similar to that of PGI_2. ZK 36 374, in fact, stimulates platelet cAMP formation in a dose-dependent manner, interacting probably with the same receptor site as PGI_2 coupled to adenylate-cyclase enzyme in platelets.

The potent platelet antiaggregatory activity and the relatively lower effects of ZK 36 374 on systemic blood pressure make this compound of particular interest, as compared to PGI_2, for a potential clinical use in the prevention and treatment of thrombotic vascular diseases.

ACKNOWLEDGMENT

Dr. S. Del Mastro (Schering S.p.A., Italy) is gratefully acknowledged for providing ZK 36 374 and for constant encouragement and support to these studies.

REFERENCES

1. Aiken, J. W., and Shebuski, R. J. (1980): Comparison in anaesthetized dogs of the anti-aggregatory and hemodynamic effects of prostacyclin and a chemically stable prostacyclin analog, 6a-Carba-PGI_2. *Prostaglandins*, 19:629.
2. Bayer, B. L., Blass, K. E., and Forster, W. (1979): Antiaggregatory effect of prostacyclin (PGI_2) *in vivo*. *Br. J. Pharmacol.*, 66:10.
3. Belch, J. J. F., McKay, A., McArdle, B., Leiberman, P., Pollock, J. G., Lowe, G. D. O., Forbes, C. D., and Prentice, C. R. M. (1983): Intermittent epoprostenol (prostacyclin) infusion in patients with Raynaud's syndrome. *Lancet*, i:315.
4. Casals-Stenzel, J., Buse, M., and Losert, W. (1983): Comparison of the vasodepressor action of ZK 36374, a stable prostacyclin derivative, PGI_2 and PGE_1 with their effect on platelet aggregation and bleeding time in rats. *Prostaglandins, Leukotrienes Med.*, 10:197.
5. Casals-Stenzel, J., Haberey, M., Loge, P., Losert, W. F., Mannesmann, G., Raduchel, B., Schillinger, E., Skuballa, W., Town, M. H., and Vorbruggen, H. (1980): Pharmacology of a new potent and stable prostacyclin analogue, ZK 36374. *Acta Ther.*, 6(suppl.):37.
6. Fitzgerald, G. A., Friedman, L. A., Miyamori, I., O'Grady, J., and Lewis, P. J. (1979): A double blind placebo controlled crossover study of prostacyclin in man. *Life Sci.*, 25:665.
7. Gorman, R. R., Bunting, S., and Miller, O. V. (1977): Modulation of human platelet adenylate cyclase by prostacyclin (PGX). *Prostaglandins*, 13:377.
8. Hamberg, M., Svensson, J., and Samuelsson, B. (1975): Thromboxanes: A new group of biologically active compounds derived from prostaglandin endoperoxides. *Proc. Natl. Acad. Sci. U.S.A.*, 72:2994.
9. Lewis, P. J., and Dollery, C. T. (1983): Clinical pharmacology and potential of prostacyclin. *Br. Med. Bull.*, 39:281.
10. Moncada, S., Gryglewski, R., Bunting, S., and Vane, J. R. (1976): An enzyme isolated from arteries transforms prostaglandin endoperoxides to an unstable substance that inhibits platelet aggregation. *Nature (Lond.)*, 263:663.
11. Rao, G. H. R., Reddy, K. R., Hagert, K., and White, J. G. (1980): Influence of pH on the prostacyclin (PGI_2) mediated inhibition of platelet function. *Prostaglandins Med.*, 4:263.
12. Schrör, K., Darius, H., Matzky, R., and Ohlendorf, R. (1981): The antiplatelet and cardiovascular actions of a new carbacyclin derivative (ZK 36 374) equipotent to PGI_2 *in vitro*. *Nauyn-Schmiedeberg's Arch. Pharmakol.*, 316:252.

13. Siegl, A. M., Smith, J. B., Silver, M. J., Nicolau, K. C., and Ahern, D. (1979): Selective binding site for ³H prostacyclin on platelets. *J. Clin. Invest.*, 63:215.
14. Sun, F. F., and Taylor, B. M. (1978): Metabolism of prostacyclin in rat. *Biochemistry*, 17:4096.
15. Szczeklik, A., Gryglewski, R. J., Nizankowski, R., Shawinski, S., Gluzko, P., and Korbut, R. (1980): Prostacyclin therapy in peripheral arterial disease. *Thromb. Res.*, 19:191.
16. Whittle, B. J. R., Moncada, S., and Vane, J. R. (1978): Comparison of the effects of prostacyclin (PGI₂), prostaglandin E₁ and D₂ on platelet aggregation in different species. *Prostaglandins*, 16:373.
17. Whittle, B. J. R., Moncada, S., Whiting, F., and Vane, J. R. (1980): Carbacyclin: A potent prostacyclin analogue for the inhibition of platelet aggregation. *Prostaglandins*, 19:605.
18. Wong, P. Y. K., Sun, F. F., and McGiff, J. C. (1978): Metabolism of prostacyclin in blood vessels. *J. Biol. Chem.*, 253:5555.

Advances in Prostaglandin, Thromboxane, and
Leukotriene Research, Vol. 13, edited by G.G. Neri
Serneri, et al. Raven Press, New York © 1985.

Effects of the Prostaglandin H₂/Thromboxane A₂ Antagonist BM 13.177 on Human Platelets

Effects of the Prostaglandin
H_2/Thromboxane A_2 Antagonist BM 13.177
on Human Platelets

*H. Patscheke and **K. Stegmeier

*Institute for Clinical Chemistry, Klinikum Mannheim, University of Heidelberg,
**Department of Medical Research, Boehringer Mannheim,
Heidelberg, Federal Republic of Germany

Thromboxane (TX) A_2 is one of the most potent physiological stimulants of vascular or bronchial smooth muscle contraction and platelet aggregation. It has been claimed that TXA_2 plays a crucial role in certain pathological situations, e.g., myocardial ischemia (1). Therefore, specific antagonists of TXA_2 are of obvious interest both as tools for basic research and as agents with clinical potential. BM 13.177, 4-[2-(benzenesulfonamido)-ethyl]phenoxyacetic acid, is a representative of a new class of antiaggregating and antithrombotic agents. The results presented in this chapter show that this nonprostanoid acts as a selective prostaglandin (PG) endoperoxide/TX antagonist in human platelets.

As the parameter of primary activation, we measured by the turbidimetric method (2) the shape change induced by a series of agonists in acetylsalicylic acid- (ASA-) treated washed platelets or citrated platelet-rich plasma (PRP). Table 1 shows that 10 μM BM 13.177 did not inhibit the shape change induced by ADP, serotonin, collagen, or thrombin in ASA-treated platelets. However, it completely abolished the shape change induced by the stable PGH_2 analogs and TXA_2 mimetics U 46619 and U 44069. These results show that the inhibition by BM 13.177 is selective for

TABLE 1. Effect of BM 13.177 10 μM on the shape change[a]
induced by various agonists

ADP (0.4 μM)	Serotonin (10 μM)	Collagen (10 μg/ml)	Thrombin (0.01 U/ml)	U 46619 (5 nM)	U 44069 (7 nM)
98 ± 2 (5)	96 ± 3 (4)	100 ± 3 (5)	99 ± 2 (4)	4 ± 2 (6)	5 ± 2 (4)

[a]The shape change amplitude was determined with ASA-treated washed platelets and given as the percentage of the control.
Means ± SEM; numbers in parentheses represent number of individuals studied.

the shape change triggered at the PG endoperoxide/TX receptor. As expected from the shape change experiments, BM 13.177 (0.1–100 μM) did not inhibit the ADP-induced primary aggregation but abolished the aggregation induced by U 46619 in ASA-treated PRP. In untreated PRP or untreated washed platelets, BM 13.177 at 10 μM also strongly reduced the aggregating effect of collagen, which is mainly due to PG/TX synthesis. It also blocked the shape change, aggregation, and ^{3}H-serotonin release induced by hydrogen peroxide and arachidonic acid, which essentially require PG/TX synthesis, in the case of hydrogen peroxide (3) from endogenous arachidonic acid. The inhibition by BM 13.177 was also complete when the TX formation was inhibited by the TX synthase inhibitor dazoxiben. It must be emphasized that 20 μM dazoxiben did not inhibit the aggregation by collagen, hydrogen peroxide, or arachidonic acid in the washed platelets, despite blockade of TXB_2 formation. BM 13.177 and dazoxiben exhibited opposite effects: BM 13.177 inhibited aggregation but did not inhibit TXB_2 formation, whereas dazoxiben inhibited TXB_2 formation but did not inhibit aggregation (4,5). Aggregation in the presence of dazoxiben may be due to PG endoperoxides. Additional BM 13.177 even suppressed this aggregation, implying that it also antagonizes the endogenously formed PG endoperoxides.

Figure 1 demonstrates the dose–response curves of the shape change induced by the TXA_2 mimetic U 46619 in the absence of the antagonist and in the presence of 1, 3, and 10 μM BM 13.177. BM 13.177 dose-dependently shifted the curves in parallel to the right without altering the maximal response. This is consistent with a competitive antagonism.

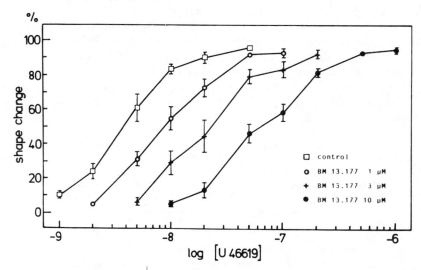

FIG. 1. Inhibitory effect of BM 13.177 on U 46619-induced platelet shape change. Log concentration–response curves for U 46619 alone and in the presence of 1, 3, and 10 μM BM 13.177; means + SEM, $n = 6$.

Comparing the inhibitory effects on platelet function of BM 13.177 and non-steroidal antiinflammatory agents such as ASA or indomethacin, BM 13.177 proved to mimic the inhibitory effects of ASA and indomethacin on stimulation by exogenous or endogenous arachidonic acid, the latter being involved in collagen- or hydrogen peroxide-induced platelet activation. In addition, BM 13.177 suppressed the effects of the stable PGH_2 analog. In further contrast to ASA and indomethacin, BM 13.177 did not alter the arachidonate metabolism. In other words, BM 13.177 is as active an inhibitor of PG/TX-induced platelet activity as ASA or indomethacin but does not share the undesirable effects of these enzyme inhibitors on prostacyclin formation and the redirection of arachidonate metabolism.

ACKNOWLEDGMENT

This study was supported by the Deutsche Forschungsgemeinschaft, Pa 263.

REFERENCES

1. Hirsh, P. D., Hillis, L. D., Campbell, W. B., Firth, B. G., and Willerson, J. T. (1981): Release of prostaglandins and thromboxane into the coronary circulation in patients with ischemic heart disease. *N. Engl. J. Med.*, 304:685–691.
2. Patscheke, H., and Wörner, P. (1978): Platelet activation detected by turbidimetric shape change analysis. Differential influence of cytochalasin B and prostaglandin E_1. *Thromb. Res.*, 12:485–496.
3. Patscheke, H. (1979): Correlation of activation and aggregation of platelets. Discrimination between anti-activating and anti-aggregating agents. *Haemostasis*, 8:65–81.
4. Patscheke, H., and Stegmeier, K. (1984): Investigations on a selective non-prostanoic thromboxane antagonist, BM 13.177, in human platelets. *Thromb. Res.*, 33:277–288.
5. Patscheke, H., and Stegmeier, K. (1984): BM 13.177 is a selective antagonist of prostaglandin H_2 and thromboxane A_2 in human platelets. *IRCS Med. Sci.*, 12:9–10.

Advances in Prostaglandin, Thromboxane, and
Leukotriene Research, Vol. 13, edited by G. G. Neri
Serneri, et al. Raven Press, New York © 1985.

Effects of Selective Thromboxane Synthetase Inhibitor OKY-046 on Plasma Prostaglandins in Patients with Coronary Artery Disease During Exercise

M. Shikano, K. Ogawa, T. Ito, L. S. Chen, Y. Ito, M. Imaizumi, T. Uno, S. Tsutsumi, and T. Satake

Second Department of Internal Medicine, Nagoya University School of Medicine, Nagoya, Japan

Platelet activation in coronary vessels occurring during stress has been implicated as a mechanism of inbalance between myocardial blood supply and demand. The actions of thromboxane (TX) A_2 are balanced by release of prostacyclin (PGI_2). If the TXA_2–PGI_2 equilibrium is altered during stress, it may provide a mechanism of abnormal platelet–vessel wall interaction and development of myocardial ischemia in certain patients (2,3). This study was designed to examine this prostaglandin equilibrium and the effects of selective thromboxane synthetase inhibitor OKY-046 in patients with coronary artery disease (CAD) during exercise stress.

METHODS

The study subjects included 15 normal volunteers and 25 patients with CAD. Ten of 25 patients with CAD had exercise-induced angina pectoris by the treadmill test. In these 10 patients we administered OKY-046 (600 mg/day) for 2 weeks and repeated the treadmill test. All patients had refrained from intake of platelet-active drugs. The exercise was terminated if the patients reported submaximal symptomatic limit, if the electrocardiogram (EKG) showed at least 0.2mV ST-segment depression, or if the patients reported chest pain.

Blood was collected for prostaglandins and platelet aggregation before exercise and at peak exercise. TXB_2 and 6-keto-$PGF_{1\alpha}$ were measured in duplicate by radioimmunoassay as stable metabolites of TXA_2 and PGI_2, respectively, according to Caldwell et al. (1). Results were expressed as mean ± standard error. Student's t-test was used for statistical analysis.

RESULTS

Plasma prostaglandin and platelet aggregation responses to exercise stress test are shown in Table 1. At rest, plasma TXB_2 levels and platelet aggregation (to ADP

TABLE 1. *Prostaglandin and platelet aggregation responses to exercise*

Subjects	TXB$_2$ (pg/ml)		6-Keto-PGF$_{1\alpha}$ (pg/ml)		Platelet aggregation (%)	
	Rest	Exercise	Rest	Exercise	Rest	Exercise
Normal subjects	221 ± 19	218 ± 20	198 ± 20	[d]343 ± 46	37 ± 8	37 ± 7
CAD without chest pain	[b]358 ± 33	406 ± 68	[a]135 ± 28	176 ± 32	[a]57 ± 6	59 ± 7
CAD with chest pain	[b]338 ± 36	[c]410 ± 58	[b]125 ± 16	135 ± 17	[a]48 ± 7	[c]62 ± 6

[a]$p < 0.05$ compared with normal subjects.
[b]$p < 0.01$ compared with normal subjects.
[c]$p < 0.05$ compared with rest values.
[d]$p < 0.01$ compared with rest values.

TABLE 2. *Effect of OKY-046*

Parameter	Control	OKY-046[a]
Exercise duration (min)	7.5 ± 0.8	[b]8.6 ± 1.0
Double product (beats · mm Hg/min)	18,200 ± 1,750	[a]20,000 ± 1,510
Peak TXB$_2$ (pg/ml)	451 ± 55	[b]177 ± 38
Peak 6-keto-PGF$_{1\alpha}$ (pg/ml)	129 ± 14	153 ± 22
Peak platelet aggregation (%)	68 ± 6	[a]50 ± 4

[a]$p < 0.05$ compared with control.
[b]$p < 0.01$ compared with control.

at 1 μM) in normal subjects were significantly less than in CAD patients. Plasma 6-keto-PGF$_{1\alpha}$ levels in normal subjects were higher than in CAD patients. By treadmill exercise stress, only CAD patients with exercise-induced chest pain showed significantly increased plasma TXB$_2$ levels and platelet aggregation. Normal subjects showed significantly increased plasma 6-keto-PGF$_{1\alpha}$ levels from exercise.

Effects of OKY-046 in CAD patients with exercise-induced chest pain are shown in Table 2. Compared with the control, OKY-046 increased the duration of treadmill exercise time and the peak double product significantly. Plasma TXB$_2$ levels and platelet aggregation were significantly lower than those of control both at rest and during exercise.

DISCUSSION AND SUMMARY

An alteration in TXA$_2$–PGI$_2$ equilibrium became apparent during exercise stress. With exercise, CAD patients with exercise-induced chest pain exhibited greater generation of TXA_2 and lower production of PGI_2. Furthermore, the selective thromboxane synthetase inhibitor decreased plasma TXB_2 levels and platelet aggregation and improved exercise tolerance. The alteration in TXA_2–PGI_2 equilibrium described here may be a contributory mechanism in exercise-induced myocardial ischemia in certain CAD patients, and the selective thromboxane synthetase inhibitor may be useful to improve their exercise tolerance.

REFERENCES

1. Caldwell, B. V., Burstein, S., Brock, W. A., and Sperott, L. (1971): Radioimmunoassay of the F prostaglandins. *J. Clin. Endocrinol. Metab.*, 33:171–175.
2. Meta, J., Metha, P., and Horalek, C. (1983): The significance of platelet vessel wall prostaglandin equilibrium during exercise-induced stress. *Am. J. Cardiol.*, 105:895–900.
3. Sobel, M., Salzman, E. W., Davies, G. C., Handin, R. I., Sweeny, I., Ploetz, J., and Kurland, G. (1981): Circulating platelet products in unstable angina pectoris. *Circulation*, 63:300–306.

Advances in Prostaglandin, Thromboxane, and
Leukotriene Research, Vol. 13, edited by G.G. Neri
Serneri, et al. Raven Press, New York © 1985.

Closing Remarks

John C. McGiff

A good symposium provides a few answers and raises many questions but may hesitate to take a hard look into the future. However, in this volume we have seen the shape of the future, and very likely with few distortions. Professor Neri Serneri and his colleagues have striven to offer a balanced view of this field, consolidating some areas and offering several points of departure for exciting future developments. We are all grateful to them for providing an exceptional collection of material.

We have been reminded once again by several authors that the definition of the pathophysiological abnormality must precede the elaboration of the therapeutic strategy if the treatment is to accomplish the greatest benefit. Thus, it is important to define vascular disease in terms of either a deficiency state, such as one resulting from reduced formation of vasodilator–antiaggregatory substances, or a state of overproduction of proaggregatory–vasoconstrictor substances. Perhaps it is simplistic to conceive of vascular disease as resulting from an imbalance of two autacoids: that is, if the thromboxane/prostacyclin ratio (TXA_2/PGI_2) exceeds 1, then thrombosis (and worse) occurs. Yet this paradigm, however inattentive to so much else, has served as a spur to the development of drugs that reduce thromboxane formation or antagonize its effects, as well as drugs that promote PGI_2 formation. As the casuist would put it: better a fecund misconception than a barren truth.

We have been reminded, and rightly so, that there are several pathways affecting platelet aggregation, and that under *in vivo* conditions it is very difficult to estimate the importance of thromboxane generation to platelet aggregation relative to other factors as ADP release, thrombin activation, or production of platelet-activating factor (PAF-acether), as these can dominate events leading to platelet aggregation. We have also been made aware that what occurs in the platelet aggregometer *ex vivo* may not reflect accurately the proaggregatory forces unleashed in the circulation with the generation of thrombin or the release of collagen.

Persuasive reasons have been advanced to use drugs that inhibit platelet cyclooxygenase in order to forestall heart attacks and strokes. All of us are familiar with the aspirin controversy: very low versus low versus moderate doses of aspirin, given daily or every second or third day. It is uncertain whether all of the benefits to be derived from aspirin accrue from inhibition of cyclooxygenase and prevention of thromboxane generation *in vivo*. As we know little about the lipoxygenase pathway in platelets, at least in terms of its functional implications, and as aspirin has multiple effects on several systems affecting platelet function, it seems "the better part of valor" to sidestep this burning issue and to be mindful that in several years it will probably make no difference. Thus, we can expect the arrival in the clinic of thromboxane antagonists, i.e., drugs that affect the response of the thromboxane receptor. Unfortunately, thus far, thromboxane-synthase inhibitors have not achieved their predicted high therapeutic usefulness.

Other approaches to the problem of containing the circulatory effects of thromboxane depend on promotion of prostacyclin formation and/or release. Indeed, in this area as in many others of this remarkable field, it pays to stay awake, as unexpected therapeutic benefits in seemingly unrelated areas may intervene. Thus, nafazatrom, which was introduced to prevent thromboembolism by increasing prostacyclin formation, has proved effective as an antimetastatic agent, preventing the dissemination of animal tumors. This observation has resulted in extensive clinical trials to determine the usefulness of nafazatrom in the management of tumors in man.

The conceptual framework that we have erected should not retard the acceptance of novel observations or new ideas, as our knowledge is incomplete, if not sparse. We were all puzzled by the reports of long-term benefits in patients with peripheral vascular disease conferred by infusing PGI_2 intraarterially. We all know that PGI_2 has a brief biological half-life and were unaware of any biological properties of PGI_2 that would cause benefit of several weeks or months duration in subjects having peripheral vascular disease. This study has been repeated and now enjoys all the statistical advantages of a double-blind study, although we still do not understand the prolonged therapeutic effects of infused PGI_2. One can predict that the confusion will be resolved when we bring to light unexpected effects of PGI_2, e.g., on fibrinolysis and blood clotting, as well as effects mediated through active stable metabolites of PGI_2 such as 6-keto-PGE_1. It is worth repeating that open-mindedness, particularly in a rapidly evolving field, is the wisest and sometimes the most difficult course.

Many of the recent developments in this field, particularly those achieved through studies based on the biochemical pharmacology of arachidonic acid metabolism, have provided new insights into the mechanism of action of old drugs. Aspirin, nitroglycerin, dipyridamole, sulfinpyrazone, and many other cardiovascular drugs have primary and secondary effects on prostaglandin and thromboxane formation that influence their cardiovascular actions and side effects. Furosemide and other "loop" diuretics, as well as hydralazine and β-receptor blocking agents, have been shown to interact with prostaglandin-dependent mechanisms that contribute to, modify, or mediate the drugs' effects.

Among the most important recent developments have been those issuing from studies that reexamined the pathogenesis of diseases in terms of activation and subsequent infiltration of white blood cells. The damage resulting from ischemia of the kidney, the heart, and other organs may be limited or contained by denying polymorphonuclear leukocytes and monocytes access to the ischemic area. Invasion of white blood cells occurs earlier than was thought and is responsible for the local formation of leukotrienes and lipid hydroperoxides, as well as generation of free radicals. These products of white blood cells reduce myocardial contractility, diminish blood flow, and extend the zone of injury. The interaction of these products of injury also plays a decisive role in adult respiratory distress syndrome and other forms of lung injury. The evolution of autoimmune diseases may also yield to those therapeutic interventions aimed at decreasing white-blood-cell invasiveness.

One can see from this random survey of the topics of this volume that we are approaching the ideal state in which diseases will be defined in terms of biochemical mechanisms and chemical mediators of tissue injury and repair, and that in so doing, we are placing therapy on a more rational and less empirical footing. This volume has provided an unsurpassed opportunity to review the major advances of the past several years and to use them as a sort of "launching pad" for future developments.

Subject Index

Subject Index[1]

---

[1]British and American spelling are used in text. For consistency this index uses American spelling only.

383